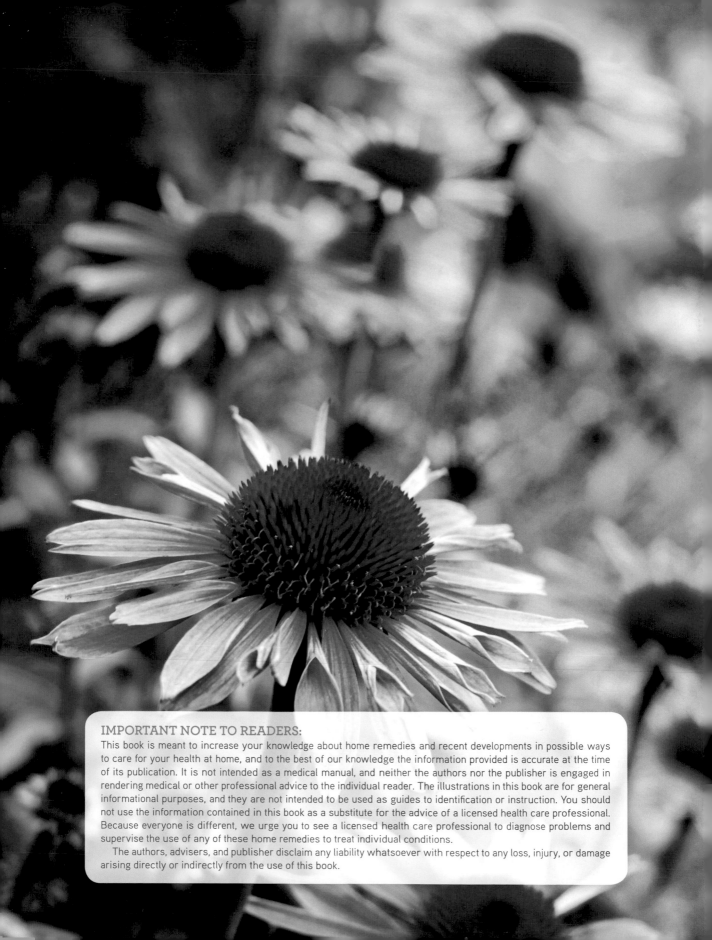

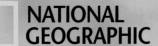
NATIONAL
GEOGRAPHIC

COMPLETE GUIDE TO

natural
home
remedies

1,025 Easy Ways
to Live Longer, Feel Better,
and Enrich Your Life

Foreword by Joe and Terry Graedon
of The People's Pharmacy

NATIONAL GEOGRAPHIC
WASHINGTON, D.C.

CONTENTS

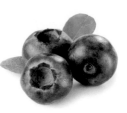

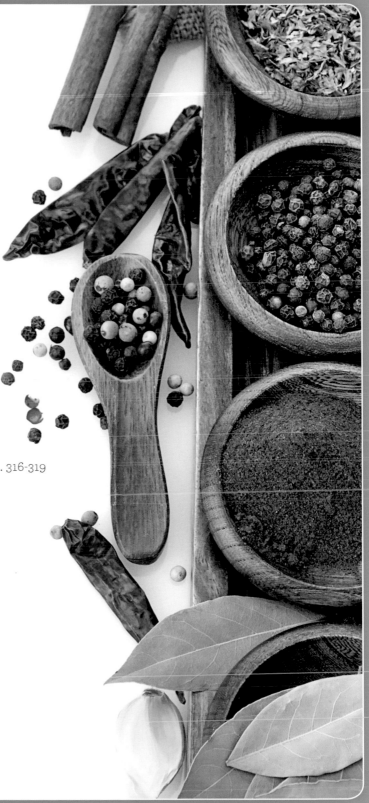

Foreword

Before the development of scientific medicine, healers had to rely on common sense, compassion, and experience. For eons, people experimented with the plants in their natural environments. Sometimes they got sick from toxic ingredients, but they learned from their mistakes. Often, native peoples were able to harness the healing power of Mother Nature's bounty. For example, Quechua Indians in the Andes

discovered that the bark of the cinchona tree could alleviate fever. They taught the Spanish. Quinine, derived from cinchona tree bark, is still a useful treatment for malaria.

Being attentive to the healing power of plants has led to the discovery of many powerful drugs, from the heart medicine digoxin, derived from foxglove, to the anticancer compound Taxol, developed from the bark of the Pacific yew tree. Research often builds on accidental discoveries. Penicillin is our most famous example, but some modern drugs such as Viagra also owe their existence to serendipity and careful observation, along with randomized, double-blind, placebo-controlled trials to help reduce bias, suggestibility, and chance.

Trial & Error

Many people assume that when the Food and Drug Administration (FDA) approves a medication based on such scientific studies, the drug is highly effective. That's not always true. All a drug company has to demonstrate is that its product is statistically better than an inactive sugar pill. In many cases, that means it's only a bit more effective than nothing at all.

There are relatively few placebo-controlled studies to determine the effectiveness of home remedies. But observation and millennia of human experience cannot be discounted. If a spoonful of yellow mustard eases your nighttime leg cramps promptly, you probably don't care that the FDA has never blessed this treatment. On the other hand, not every treatment works for all of us. That is just as true for natural approaches as it is for drugs. Doctors have dozens of blood pressure medicines to choose from; ordinary people, too, have discovered many natural approaches to ease joint pain. If one doesn't work, another might.

It is worthwhile to learn something about the healing traditions in which botanical knowledge has stood the test of time. Using food as medicine stretches back to the father of medicine, Hippocrates, some 2,400 years ago. The details have been refined, but it's still a good idea to use techniques that bolster the body's natural ability to heal itself.

Taking Control of Your Health

Grandmothers in northern climates like Scandinavia figured out that cod liver oil was good for their families' health, especially in the winter. They did not know why. But common sense and observation told them to persist. We now know that cod liver oil is rich in vitamin D, which can help bolster immunity against infections like colds and flu. In Scandinavia's dark winters, people don't get the sun exposure to make vitamin D naturally. Blood levels drop, and cod liver oil is a good way to supplement this critical nutrient.

Today many people are eager to try natural healing methods and home remedies. The high cost of conventional drug treatments, both financially and physically, is often daunting. Serious side effects often appear long after a medication has been on the market, exposing people to potentially damaging consequences. For example, the diabetes drug Avandia (rosiglitazone) ended up causing some of the very problems it should have prevented—heart attacks and other cardiovascular complications. This was discovered after millions had taken it for years. The drug is now restricted in the United States and banned in many other countries.

Home remedies, herbs, and healing foods are less likely to cause serious side effects. Lowering blood pressure with beet juice has been shown in scientific experiments to be about as effective as medications, without the adverse reactions. Walnuts can lower bad low-density lipoprotein (LDL) cholesterol and help lower the risk for heart attacks. But natural remedies are not safe for everyone. People may develop allergic reactions to almost anything. Some herbs, spices, and foods may interact with medications. St. John's wort, for example, can make many medicines less effective, including oral contraceptives. Grapefruit, on the other hand, may raise blood levels of certain cholesterol-lowering drugs so that side effects could become more troublesome. Knowing the benefits and risks of all your healing strategies is essential.

Long ago, advice on living well would have come from grandmothers or other trusted elders. In today's mobile society, it has become more difficult to tap the wisdom of the ages. So a book that captures the experience of generations as well as the essence of modern knowledge and common sense can be very useful. National Geographic's *Complete Guide to Natural Home Remedies* offers a wonderful range of healing traditions for common ailments. You'll find yourself referring to it again and again.

Joe & Terry Graedon
of The People's Pharmacy

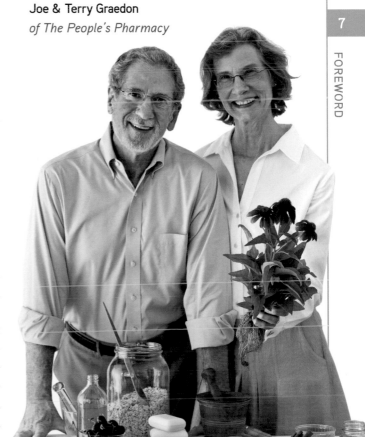

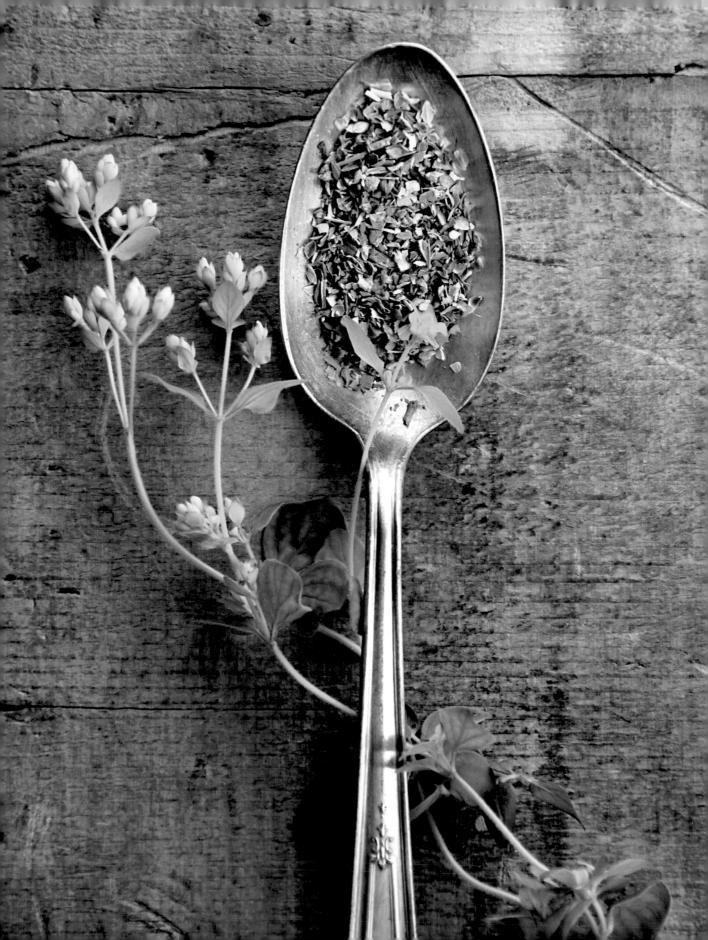

Board of Advisers

Linda B. White, M.D.

Home Remedies on Hand A frequent lecturer and contributor to books and magazines on the subject of herbal remedies and other facets of integrative medicine, Linda B. White teaches at the Metropolitan State College of Denver in Colorado. She has authored or contributed to six books, including *The Herbal Drugstore* (Rodale, 2000) and *Kids, Herbs, and Health* (Interweave Press, 1998). She writes regularly for *The Herb Companion, Mother Earth News, Alternative Therapies,* and the website AllHerb.com.

Steven Foster

Herbs for Healing The author of 17 books including three Peterson field guides—*Medicinal Plants and Herbs: Eastern North America* (2nd ed., 2000 with Jim Duke), *Venomous Animals and Poisonous Plants of North America* (1994, with the late Roger Caras), and *Medicinal Plants and Herbs: Western North America* (with Christopher Hobbs)—he is also co-author of National Geographic's top-selling *Desk Reference to Nature's Medicine* (2006, named "Best of Reference" by the New York Public Library) and *Guide to Medicinal Herbs* (2010), which also featured photos from his noted archive of photography of medicinal plants from around the world.

Barton Seaver

Foods for Health Author of the currently popular *For Cod and Country,* Seaver graduated with honors from the Culinary Institute of America and first worked at a small family restaurant in southern Spain. His influence as executive chef of Hook, a sustainable-seafood restaurant in Washington, D.C., brought the restaurant onto *Bon Appetit*'s top 10 eco-friendly restaurant list. *Esquire* named Seaver Chef of the Year in 2009. He serves on the board of D.C. Central Kitchen, an organization fighting hunger through job training and life skills, and is a National Geographic Fellow, participating in Mission Blue, an international initiative to increase awareness and action to save the ocean.

Annie B. Bond

Clean, Safe, & Beautiful The best-selling author of five books, many e-books, and thousands of articles, Bond has been called "the foremost expert on green living" by *Body & Soul* magazine. Her books include *Better Basics for the Home* (Three Rivers Press, 1999), *Home Enlightenment* (Rodale, 2008), *Clean & Green* (Ceres Press, 1990), and *True Food* (National Geographic, 2010). Her e-books include *Homemade Detox Baths, Natural Skin Care Baths, Clean Green for Pennies, Natural Flu Protection,* and more. She is the founder and CEO of GreenChiCafe.com.

Tieraona Low Dog, M.D.

Healing Traditions A faculty member at Andrew Weil's Center for Integrative Medicine at the University of Arizona and an internationally known speaker on health topics ranging from the responsible use of dietary supplements to integrative approaches to women's health, Low Dog also maintains a clinical practice in integrative medicine. She has served on the White House Commission of Complementary and Alternative Medicine and the National Institutes of Health Advisory Council for Complementary and Alternative Medicine. She delivers more than 50 public lectures annually and has appeared on E!, ABC's *20/20*, CNN, and *The People's Pharmacy.*

Dan Buettner

A Healthy Lifestyle Dan Buettner is the founder and chief executive officer of Blue Zones and author of the *New York Times* best-seller *The Blue Zones: Lessons for Living Longer from the People Who've Lived the Longest* (National Geographic, 2008). An internationally recognized explorer, educator, public speaker, and co-producer of an Emmy Award–winning travel documentary, Buettner has appeared as a longevity expert on *The Oprah Winfrey Show, Good Morning America,* the *Today* show, ABC's *World News,* CBS's *The Early Show,* and CNN. National Geographic published his book *Thrive: Finding Happiness the Blue Zones Way,* in 2010.

About This Book

With health care costs rising, doubts about drug safety swirling, and many seeking ways to live a more natural life, a book from the National Geographic Society on safe and practical home remedies seems, well, a natural. Following our mission to care about the health of the planet, we have sought the best ideas from around the world and, with the help of our writers and advisers, put them to the test of current science.

The result is a book that may define "home remedies" a bit more broadly than some would expect. It may take some explanation, but think of this as a full array of possibilities from which you can choose your favorites. Mix and match, learn something new, fine-tune your understanding of practices already part of your health routine.

A New Definition of Home Remedy

Chapter 1 follows the traditional definition, including teas and poultices that our grandparents may have used, along with other handy aids that you already have on hand, from lemons to vinegar, from glue to duct tape. Chapters 2 and 3 feature medicinal herbs and the foods best known to promote health; Chapter 4 carries the same principles over to the realms of beauty and housekeeping.

But the stretch comes—literally—in Chapter 5, as we cast our eyes to the ancient traditions of wellness and healing from which we can all learn. And, finally, Chapter 6 wraps everything up into the most important message of all, namely that your lifestyle choices shape your health.

Our team of authors, editors, and advisers has orchestrated a combination of ways in which you can read and learn from this book. As those in the fields of natural healing show us, a healthy body is an integrated combination of complex parts. We hope that this book manifests the same wholeness.

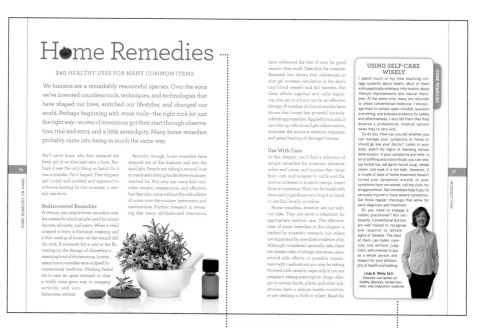

...CHAPTER INTRODUCTION
Each chapter begins with an overview of this realm of natural healing.

...ADVISER INTRODUCTION
Meet each adviser through the message shared at the beginning of a chapter.

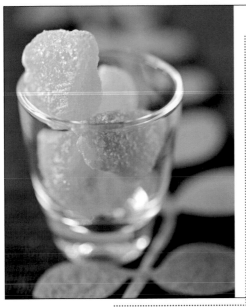

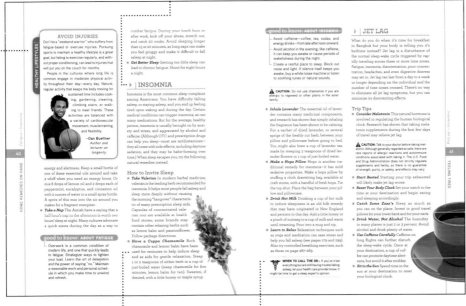

...SECTION INTRODUCTION
Each chapter covers
many topics, arranged
alphabetically.

...GOOD TO KNOW
Helpful suggestions, cautions,
and rules of thumb related to
the current topic.

...CAUTION
These messages
convey important
exceptions and medi-
cal contraindications.

...ADVISER CROSS-REFS
Every adviser shares ideas in
every chapter, showing how
healthful lifestyles intersect.

...LOOK FOR SUBTOPICS
Every topic is subdivided, so
you can find ailments and the
remedies you need quickly.

...SIMPLE SOLUTIONS
Browse these points
or read them one after
another. Lots of good ideas.

...CALL THE DOCTOR
Sometimes home remedies aren't enough.
These warnings advise when an illness
warrants professional attention.

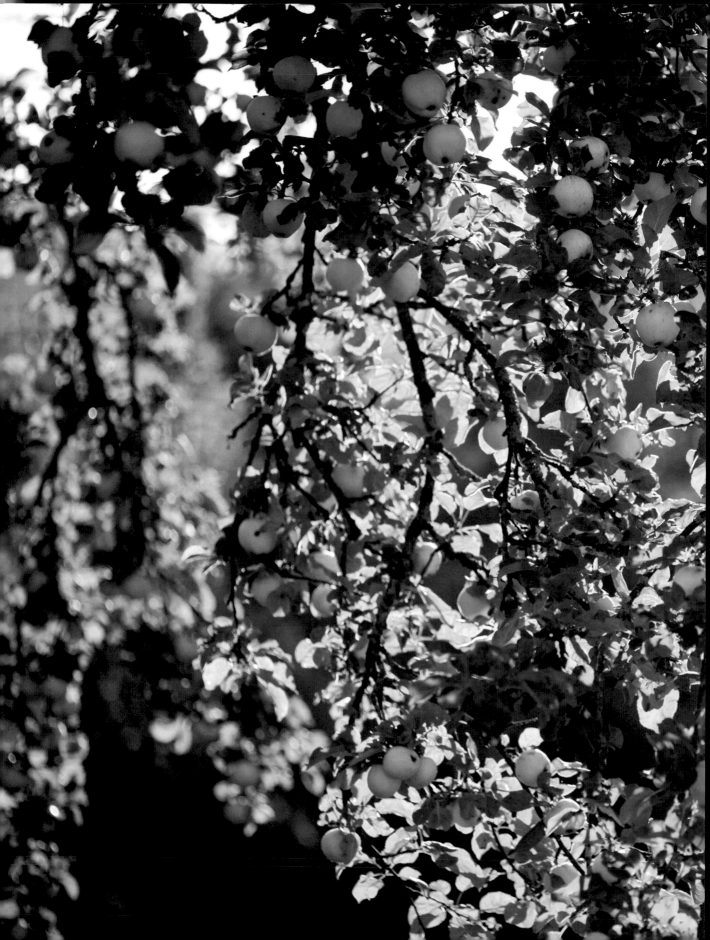

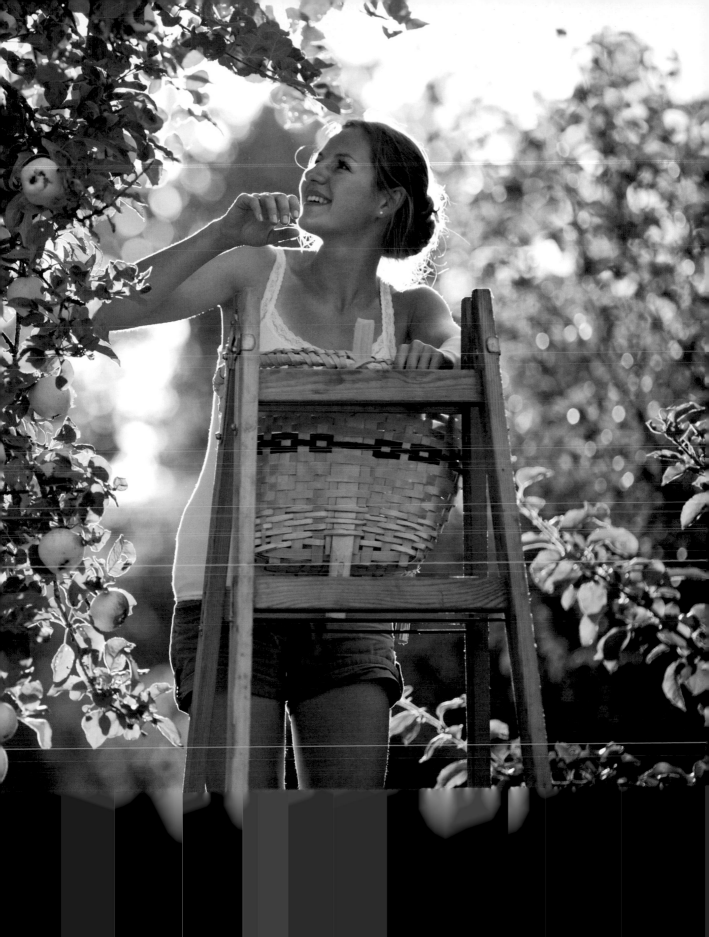

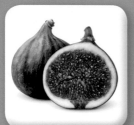 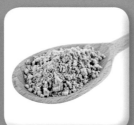 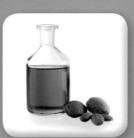 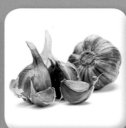 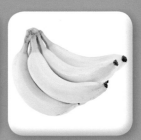

CHAPTER ONE

home remed

ies on hand

H me Remedies

240 HEALTHY USES FOR MANY COMMON ITEMS

We humans are a remarkably resourceful species. Over the eons we've invented countless tools, techniques, and technologies that have shaped our lives, enriched our lifestyles, and changed our world. Perhaps beginning with stone tools—the right rock hit just the right way—scores of inventions got their start through observation, trial and error, and a little serendipity. Many home remedies probably came into being in much the same way.

We'll never know who first smeared the fresh gel of an aloe leaf onto a burn. Perhaps it was the only thing on hand. Or it was a mistake. Yet it helped. That slippery gel cooled and soothed and appeared to enhance healing. In that moment, a remedy was born.

Rediscovered Remedies

A century ago, simple home remedies were the means by which people cared for minor injuries, ailments, and pains. When a child scraped a knee, a thorough washing and a thin coating of honey on the wound did the trick. If someone felt a cold or the flu coming on, the therapy of choice was a steaming bowl of chicken soup. In time, many home remedies were eclipsed by conventional medicine. Drinking herbal tea to ease an upset stomach or clear a stuffy nose gave way to popping antacids and anti-histamines instead.

Recently, though, home remedies have stepped out of the shadows and into the spotlight. People are taking a second look at treatments their grandmothers routinely reached for. Not only are many folk remedies simple, inexpensive, and effective, but they also come without the side effects of some over-the-counter treatments and medications. Further, research is revealing that many old-fashioned treatments

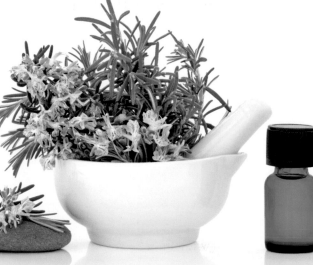

have withstood the test of time for good reason—they work. Take aloe, for instance. Research has shown that substances in aloe gel increase circulation in the skin's tiny blood vessels and kill bacteria. Put these effects together and voila! Applying aloe gel to a burn can be an effective therapy. A number of clinical studies have shown that honey has powerful bacteria-inhibiting properties. Applied to wounds, it can clear up infections, fight inflammation, stimulate the immune system's response, and speed healing of damaged tissues.

Use With Care

In this chapter, you'll find a selection of simple remedies for common ailments, aches and pains, and injuries that range from cuts and scrapes to colds and flu, motion sickness to muscle cramps, insect bites to insomnia. Most can be made with items and ingredients you've got on hand, or can find locally or online.

Home remedies, however, are not without risks. They are never a substitute for appropriate medical care. The effectiveness of some remedies in this chapter is backed by scientific research, but others are supported by anecdotal evidence only. There are always risks of allergic reactions, side effects, or possible interactions with medications you may be taking. Proceed with caution, especially if you are pregnant, taking prescription drugs, allergic to certain foods, plants, and other substances, or are treating a child or infant. Read the warnings and cautionary notes. When in doubt, call your doctor without delay.

USING SELF-CARE WISELY

I spend much of my time teaching college students about health. Most of them enthusiastically embrace information about lifestyle improvements and natural therapies. At the same time, many are reluctant to utilize conventional medicine. I encourage them to remain open-minded, question everything, and evaluate evidence for safety and effectiveness. I also tell them that they deserve a professional, medical opinion when they're very sick.

So do you. How can you tell whether you can manage your symptoms at home or should go see your doctor? Listen to your body; watch for signs of mending versus deterioration. If your symptoms are mild—a bit of sniffling and a sore throat, you can rest, sip herbal tea, eat garlic-laced soup, inhale steam, and soak in a hot bath. However, if a couple of days of home treatment haven't turned your symptoms around, or your symptoms have worsened, call the clinic for an appointment. Get immediate help if you're seriously injured or have severe symptoms. Get those regular checkups that allow for early diagnosis and treatment.

Do you need to engage a holistic practitioner? Not necessarily. Conventional doctors are well trained to recognize and respond to telltale signs of disease. The best of them can listen carefully and without judgment, with interest in you as a whole person and respect for your philosophy of health and healing.

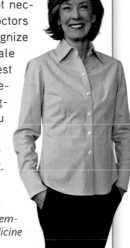

Linda B. White, M.D.
Educator and author on healthy lifestyles, herbal remedies, and integrative medicine

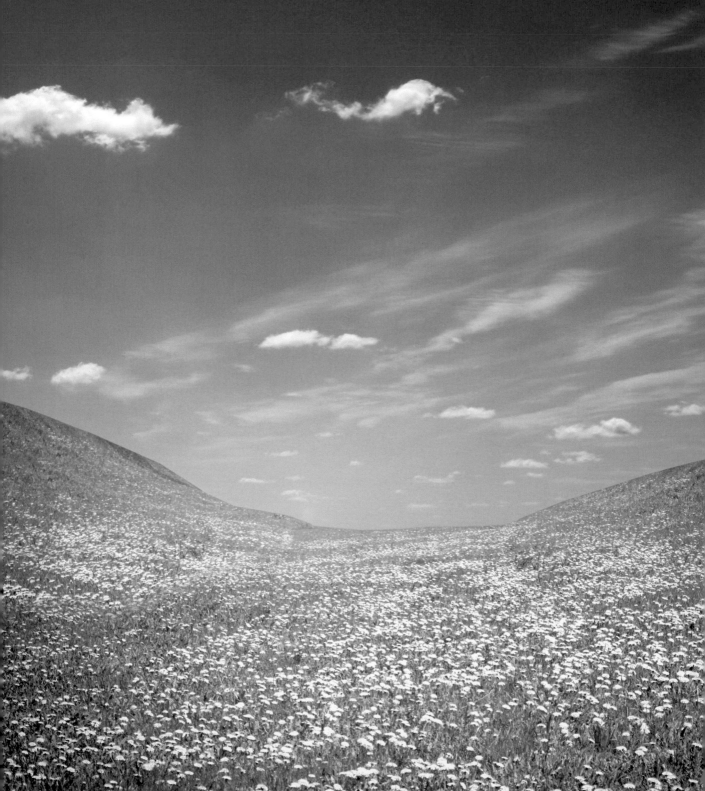

Breathing Difficulties

15 WAYS TO TAKE A DEEPER BREATH

At rest, a healthy adult takes between 8 and 16 breaths per minute. Most of the time, you're hardly aware of your breathing. It's a largely unconscious reflex controlled by the nervous system, much like blinking or the beating of the heart. But you notice immediately when breathing becomes even the slightest bit difficult, or when something interferes with that rhythmic and usually effortless intake and release of air. Serious breathing problems, including those associated with asthma, severe allergic reactions, injuries, or something caught in the airways, always require immediate medical attention. But minor breathing difficulties such as the annoying stuffy nose that often accompanies a cold usually can be relieved by taking simple steps at home.

▶ | CONGESTION

When tissues and blood vessels lining the nasal passages become inflamed and swollen, it's difficult—and sometimes nearly impossible—to breathe through your nose. Doctors call this stuffy, plugged-up condition "nasal congestion." Colds and flu can bring it on. So can common allergens such as pet dander, pollen, and mold, as well as airborne irritants like dust and smoke. Most acute cases of nasal congestion eventually clear up on their own, but try the following tips and techniques to make breathing a little easier.

Breathe Easier

- ***Try a Nasal Wash*** Nasal lavage is a time-honored technique for flushing out nasal passages with a saltwater solution. A nasal wash helps rinse away mucus, germs, and allergens that contribute to congestion. Here's how: Stir ½ teaspoon noniodized salt into 1 cup warm water (use distilled water only) until completely dissolved. Alternatively, use a store-bought nasal saline solution. Two of the most common tools for getting the salt water into your nose are a small bulb syringe or a neti pot. If using a syringe, draw up some of the solution into the bulb. While leaning over a sink, place the tip of the syringe in one nostril and gently squeeze the bulb, causing the solution to fill the nostril, run through the sinuses, and flow out the other nostril. Blow your nose gently to get all the water out. Then flush the other nostril in the same way. If using a neti pot, tip your head forward and slightly sideways and then pour the solution into the uppermost nostril; repeat on the other side. Thoroughly clean and air-dry the bulb syringe or neti pot after each use. Discard any unused salt solution.

- ***Use Steam Therapy*** Inhaling steam is an old-fashioned remedy for helping clear congestion. Carefully pour 4 cups just-boiled water into a large,

---

good to know: ABOUT CONGESTION

- Avoid alcohol, which can make congestion worse.
- Dehydration can also aggravate congestion. Drink plenty of water, herbal teas, and clear broth to stay hydrated.
- Avoid lying flat. Keeping your head slightly elevated when lying down can promote mucus drainage.

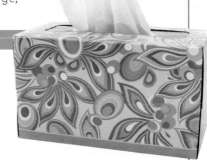

heatproof bowl. Place a towel over your head and shoulders and lean over the bowl, keeping your face at least 12 inches above the water's surface. If the temperature feels comfortable, inhale deeply. Continue inhaling the steam for about 10 minutes. To boost the congestion-clearing power of the steam, add 1 or 2 drops of eucalyptus essential oil to the hot water in the bowl before you begin.

⚠ **CAUTION:** People with asthma or other reactive airway diseases, or who are allergic to eucalyptus, should not breathe eucalyptus fumes. Not appropriate for children under the age of three.

■ *Go Warm and Cold* Place a warm, wet washcloth across the bridge of your nose. Hold it against your face for about a minute. Then switch to a cold, wet washcloth and hold for about the same length of time. Repeat several times.

■ *Have a Cup of Herbal Tea* A steamy cup of an aromatic herbal tea, such as peppermint (see pages 107–109) or ginger (see pages 95–97) can help clear a stuffy nose. To brew peppermint tea, place 1 heaping teaspoon of dried peppermint in a cup, fill with just-boiled water, cover, and steep ten minutes. Strain and add honey or maple syrup to sweeten, if desired. To brew ginger tea, steep 1 teaspoon freshly grated ginger root in a cup of just-boiled water for ten minutes. Sweeten as needed, or add a squeeze of fresh lemon juice.

⚕ **WHEN TO CALL THE DR.:** If nasal congestion lasts for more than a week to ten days, see your doctor. You may have something more serious than a simple stuffy nose, such as a sinus infection. • Also see your doctor if congestion is accompanied by a high fever, if you have asthma or emphysema, if you are taking immune-suppressing medications, or if nasal discharge contains blood.

▶| SNORING

Snoring is the rough, rattling, sometimes thunderous sound that occurs when a person's breathing is partially obstructed while sleeping. This can happen when muscles in the roof of the mouth, tongue, and throat relax. As air flows past, these relaxed tissues vibrate, which creates the irritating noises. Habitual snoring, especially if marked by episodes of breath holding, can be a sign of a serious condition (see the following When To Call the Dr. section). Infrequent light snoring, such as that caused by temporary nasal congestion, is less serious. The following remedies may help.

Snuff Out Snoring

■ *Raise Your Head* Try a different pillow, one that lifts your head while keeping your neck relatively straight. This may alleviate minor blocking of your airways caused by sagging muscles in your mouth and throat.

■ *Try Your Side* When you sleep on your back, your tongue and soft palate (the soft area on the roof of your mouth) may move down as they relax to contact the back of your throat. Sleeping on your side helps prevent this. If you've been a back sleeper most of your life, however, changing position isn't easy. Try the tennis ball trick: Sew a pouch on the back of a T-shirt or pajama top and tuck a tennis ball inside. Whenever you start to roll onto your back, the bulge of the tennis ball may help keep you on your side.

■ *Tape Your Nose* Those nasal strips football players wear do actually help to spread the nostrils and increase airflow through the nose. Available at most drugstores, they are worth a try.

■ *Control Allergens* If allergies are causing congestion, they can make snoring much worse. Wash sheets frequently in

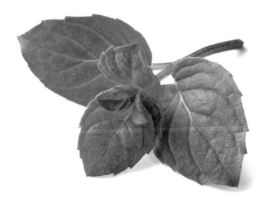

hot water, and zip up your pillow in an allergen-blocking case. Vacuum and dust your bedroom at least once a week. And keep your pets off the bed.

WHEN TO CALL THE DR.: When airflow is restricted enough to cause interruptions in breathing, a serious condition known as sleep apnea may develop in which a snorer stops or nearly stops breathing repeatedly throughout the night. The more restricted the airway, the greater the negative impacts on health. Sleep apnea and very loud snoring warrant a visit to the doctor.

good to know: ABOUT SNORING

- Avoid drinking alcohol at least two hours before bedtime. Alcohol can cause excessive relaxation of muscles, including those in the throat, which can aggravate snoring.
- If you smoke, quit. Smoking greatly aggravates snoring.
- Being overweight is a common cause of snoring. Make weight loss a healthy goal.

▶ | HICCUPS

The annoying and often embarrassing hics of hiccups are caused by involuntary contractions of the diaphragm, the large sheet of muscles underlying your lungs. The contractions lead to abrupt, uncontrollable intakes of air. Spicy foods, overeating, swallowing air, drinking carbonated beverages or too much alcohol, sudden excitement, and emotional stress can bring on a case of hiccups. Hiccups usually resolve within a few minutes or hours. But these time-tested remedies can help bring them under control.

Nix the Hics

- *Hold Your Breath* Take a deep breath and hold it as long as you can. Swallow when you feel a hic coming. Alternatively, take a deep breath and hold it for ten seconds. Without exhaling, take another breath and hold for five seconds more. Without exhaling, take a third small breath and hold for an additional five seconds. Holding your breath causes a buildup of carbon dioxide in your lungs, which can help restore normal breathing.
- *Gargle* Try gargling with water. This essentially forces you to hold your breath.
- *Increase the Carbon Dioxide* Cup your hands around your nose and mouth and keep rebreathing your exhaled breath. You can get the same effect by breathing into a paper bag. Both these remedies lead to a buildup of carbon dioxide in your lungs.
- *Sip or Suck* Take quick sips from a glass of water, or suck on a slice of lemon, a dill pickle, or an ice cube.
- *Try Sugar* Swallow a teaspoon of white sugar. The challenge of getting the dry crystals down your throat is distracting and can interrupt breathing and the hiccup response.
- *Compress the Chest* Lean forward or lie down and pull your knees up to your chest. Compressing your chest in this way may help calm a diaphragm that is in spasms.
- *Do What Granny Says* A number of simple cures for the hiccups have been passed down through the generations. Drink a glass of water from the opposite side of the glass. Breathe into a paper bag for half a minute. Pull on your earlobes. Some claim that having someone sneak up on you and yell "Boo!" will scare the hiccups out of you. Not a one of these can be proved, but they won't hurt either.

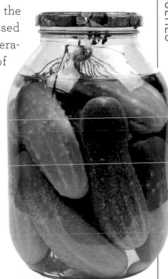

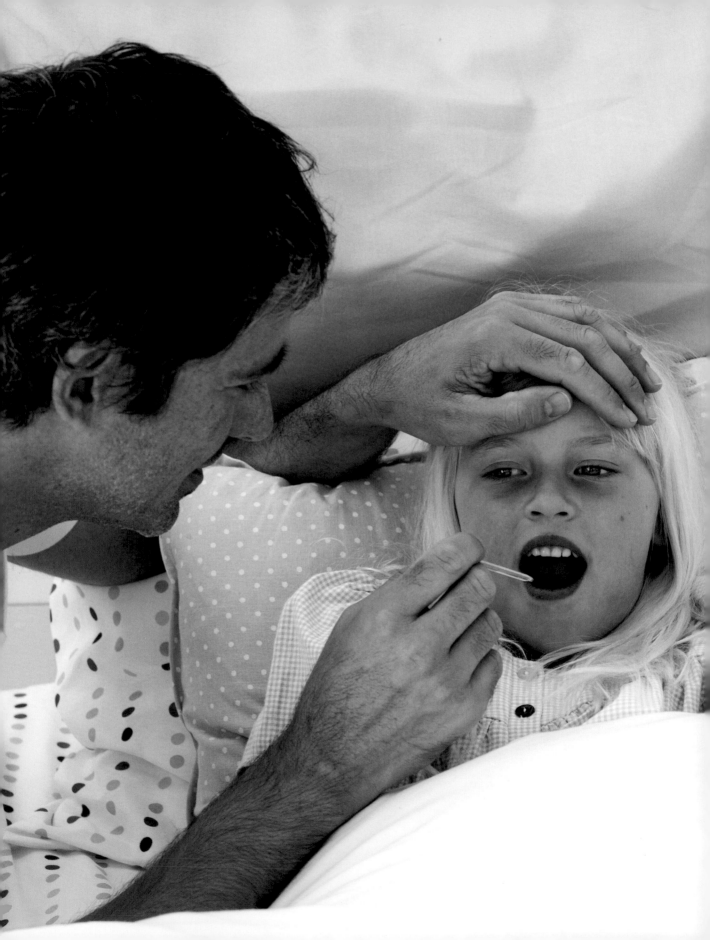

Chest & Throat Ailments

20 AIDS TO EASE COLD & FLU ILLS

Runny nose, scratchy throat, sneezing, coughing, and watery eyes. Sound familiar? These are all classic symptoms of colds and flu, two common ailments caused by viruses. Unfortunately, there is no cure for either one. Part of the reason is that viruses have a knack for mutating quickly, which is why new strains of colds and flu make the rounds every year. Antibiotics are no help—they have no effect on viruses. Over-the-counter cold and flu medicines suppress some symptoms but often have undesirable side effects. Home remedies can be a healthier, safer alternative.

▶ | COLDS & FLU

Though they share some symptoms, colds and flu are caused by different types of viruses. So how can you tell which illness you've got? An old rule of thumb states that if your symptoms tend to be from the neck up, you've probably got a cold. With the flu, you may also have a runny nose and sore throat, but on top of that, expect body aches, fever, and fatigue. Colds tend to last longer, but the flu generally causes more discomfort.

Upper Respiratory Rescue

- **Hydrate** "Drink plenty of fluids" is the mantra. Water is best, but clear broth, green and herbal teas, and diluted juices are also good choices.
- **Try Chicken Soup** It's a time-honored treatment backed up with modern research. Chicken soup—especially recipes rich in garlic and onions—does indeed provide more than comfort. Some ingredients fight inflammation or thin mucous secretions to help relieve congestion.

- **Rinse the Sinuses** Nasal irrigation can help relieve congestion caused by colds and flu (see page 19). Even just spritzing your nasal passages with saline nasal drops several times a day can make a difference.
- **Suck on Zinc** Clinical trials have shown that sucking lozenges that contain zinc (in the form of zinc gluconate or zinc acetate) may help shorten the duration of a cold by several days. Follow package directions. Be aware that zinc lozenges can leave a bad taste in your mouth or make some people nauseated.
- **Go Herbal** Andrographis and echinacea are two herbs that top the list of cold and flu treatments. Research supports *Andrographis paniculata*'s effectiveness in relieving the symptoms of colds, flu, and some other

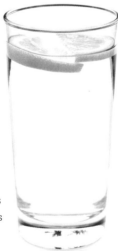

---

good to know: ABOUT COLDS & FLU

- When you have a cold or flu, avoid alcohol and caffeinated drinks. Both tend to promote water loss.
- Avoid zinc-based nasal sprays and gels. Research has shown these products can harm your sense of smell; the damage can be permanent.

upper respiratory conditions. Preparations of the dried herb are available in some health food stores and online. Follow package directions. Echinacea has been a popular herbal treatment for respiratory ailments for centuries (see pages 87–88). Echinacea tinctures (also available at health food stores) tend to be more effective than teas for treating the symptoms of colds and flu. Follow package directions.

⚠ **CAUTION:** Because echinacea acts on the immune system, anyone with an autoimmune condition should exercise caution using this herb. Echinacea may also inhibit production of certain liver enzymes, so check with your doctor before using the herb while also taking medications, including birth control pills. People who are allergic to ragweed and other plants in the Asteraceae (daisy) family should avoid echinacea.

■ *Reach for Elderberry* A number of recent studies have shown that extracts of elderberries (*Sambucus nigra*) have virus-inhibiting properties. Elderberry syrup (marketed as Sambucol) has been shown to be effective for treating colds and flu in some people. You might also try lozenges that combine elder extracts and zinc. Follow package directions.

☤ **WHEN TO CALL THE DR.:** See your health care provider if you have a fever between 100°F to 101°F that persists for more than three days or a fever of any duration above 103°F. • See your doctor if you develop a cough that produces bloody, brownish, or greenish phlegm. • If you have any difficulty breathing or have severe lung, chest, or throat pain, see your doctor immediately. • Also see your health care provider if sinus congestion continues for more than ten days, especially if accompanied by a green or brown discharge.

▶ | COUGH

Coughing is the body's way of trying to keep the airways clear of mucus and other substances. People suffering from colds and flu often develop "productive" coughs that help get rid of mucus from the back of the throat or the bronchial tubes. A nonproductive or "dry" cough is a dry, hacking—often tickling—cough that usually doesn't bring up anything. Dry coughs can

sometimes develop after you've recovered from a cold, and they may linger for several weeks.

Slough Off a Cough

■ *Reach for Horehound* If you have a productive cough, try old-fashioned horehound drops. The bittersweet herb has expectorant properties.

■ *Suck Slippery Elm* For centuries, Native Americans used slippery elm (see pages 119–121) to treat coughs and other respiratory ailments. Slippery elm contains mucilage, a substance that, when mixed with water, becomes a slick gel. Slippery elm lozenges can soothe irritated throats and dry coughs.

■ *Sip Syrup* Here's a home remedy that has withstood the test of time: Mix 2 tablespoons of freshly squeezed lemon juice with 1 tablespoon honey. Heat gently until warm. Take 1 teaspoon every hour, as needed.

■ *Swig Ginger Tea* Ginger (see pages 95–97) has been shown to have anti-inflammatory, antibacterial, and antiviral properties. Ginger tea can soothe throats made raw by coughing. Add about a tablespoon of freshly grated, peeled ginger to a cup and fill with just-boiled water. Steep for ten minutes, strain, and sweeten if desired. Alternatively, try thyme tea (see recipe opposite).

■ *Rub On a Rub* Chest rubs can help loosen congestion. Mix 5 drops of eucalyptus essential oil with 2 teaspoons of almond oil. Rub some of this mixture on your chest and cover with a hot water bottle or heating pad wrapped in flannel or a soft thin towel. Leave on 20 minutes. Repeat once or twice a day.

▶ | SORE THROAT

A sore throat often goes hand in hand with a cold or the flu. The feeling is unmistakable—a painful, raw scratchiness that intensifies when you swallow. Sore throats usually resolve on their own in a few days. But there's no need to suffer while you wait. Try the following remedies to ease throat discomfort.

WHEN TO CALL THE DR.: If you have severe sore throat pain, especially if it's accompanied by swollen lymph nodes in the neck region, headache, fever, or upset stomach, see your health care provider.

Thwart a Sore Throat

- **Reach for the Salt Cure** Gargling with salt water is a simple and effective sore throat remedy. Stir a teaspoon of salt into a cup of warm water until the salt is completely dissolved. Take a mouthful, gargle, and spit. Repeat hourly.
- **Sip or Gargle With Thyme** Thyme tea (see recipe) is also a time-tested sore throat remedy. Sip hot thyme tea to soothe a sore throat or transform it into an effective gargle by adding a teaspoon of salt to a cup of cooled tea. Stir until the salt is dissolved and gargle with small mouthfuls. Spit; don't swallow.
- **Sip Sweet and Sour** Another old remedy calls for mixing equal amounts of honey and apple cider vinegar (try 2 teaspoons of each) in a cup of hot water. Take frequent small sips of this mixture to ease sore throat pain.
- **Pop a Lozenge** Zinc lozenges can soothe a sore throat as well as help shorten the duration of a cold (see page 23).

⚠ **CAUTION:** Do not use zinc lozenges to treat a cold or a sore throat for more than seven days.

THYME TEA
Thyme has a long history of use in Europe as an herbal treatment for coughs.

Place 2 teaspoons fresh thyme leaves, or 1 teaspoon dried thyme leaf, in a cup. Cover with just-boiled water and let steep for ten minutes. Strain, and sweeten with honey, stevia, or maple syrup, if desired.

▶ | # LARYNGITIS

Laryngitis is an inflammation of the larynx, or voice box. Straining your voice from loud talking or shouting can bring it on. It can also develop as a result of irritation or infection during a cold or a bout of the flu. Although persistent hoarseness can be a sign of a more serious medical condition, temporary (acute) laryngitis typically clears up in a few days. If you're stricken with temporary silence, the following simple remedies may help.

Talk Back
- **Breathe Moist Air** Inhale steam by pouring just-boiled water into a large bowl, draping a towel over your head and shoulders, and leaning over the water (keep your face at least 12 inches from the water's surface).

⚠ **CAUTION:** Not appropriate for children under age three.

- **Keep Your Throat Moist** Take steps to stay hydrated. Sucking on soothing lozenges, chewing gum, and sipping warm water can help too.
- **Drink Tea** A variety of herbal teas can soothe a stressed throat. Try making a cup of tea from the herb mullein. Place 2 teaspoons of dried mullein leaves in just-boiled water. Steep, strain, and sweeten, if desired. Drink a cup one to three times daily.
- **Spoon in Honey and Cayenne** Mix together a teaspoon of lemon juice, a teaspoon of honey, and a pinch of cayenne pepper in the bowl of a large spoon. Put the spoon in your mouth and slowly suck off the mixture, letting it coat your throat. Repeat two or three times a day.

WHEN TO CALL THE DR.: See your health care provider if your voice disappears suddenly, for no apparent reason.
• If a case of laryngitis persists for more than a week, it may be a sign of something more serious. Seek medical advice.

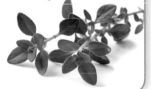

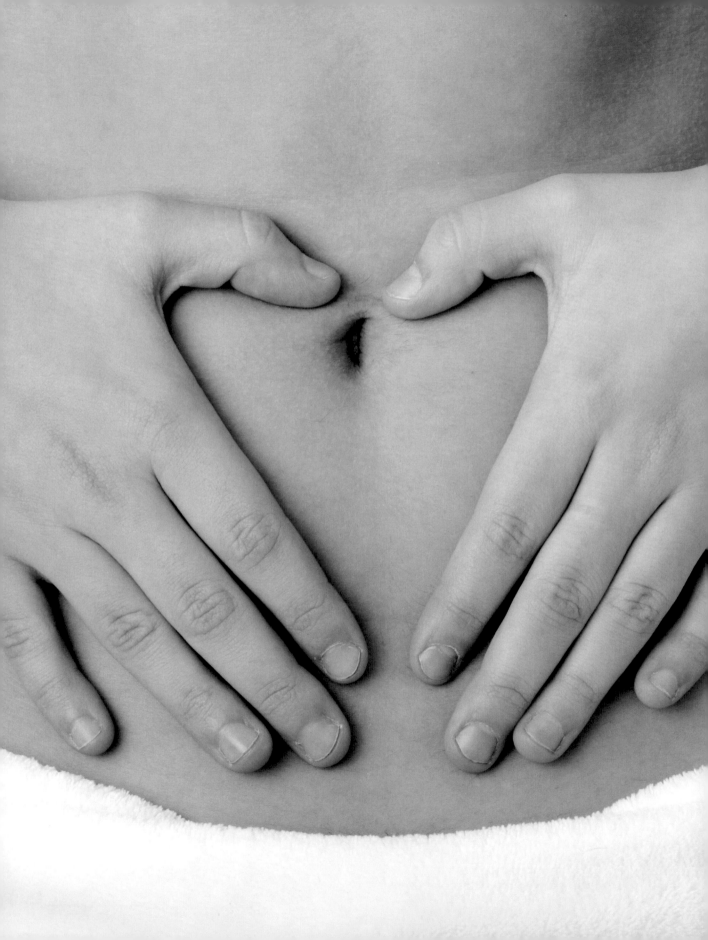

Digestive Upsets

16 STOMACH SETTLERS

An upset stomach. A bout of belly-churning diarrhea. Painful bloat from constipation. An uncontrollable attack of gas. Sound familiar? Don't worry; you're not alone. It's probably safe to say that everyone has had some form of digestive disorder at one time or another. These upsets are among the most common of all health complaints. Persistent, long-lasting digestive problems can be warning signs of a serious underlying condition. But occasional upsets tend to be triggered or at least aggravated by what—and how—we eat and drink. Viruses, bacteria, stress, smoking, and pregnancy can be contributing factors, too. The good news is that tried-and-true remedies can tame unsettled tummies and deliver relief.

▶ | INDIGESTION

When your last meal seems to be sitting uncomfortably in your stomach, roiling around enough to make you queasy, or even threatening to come back up, you've probably got a classic case of indigestion. Eating too much or too fast can bring it on, even in people who claim they have cast-iron stomachs. Certain foods are also known indigestion makers. Many home remedies for indigestion rely on time-tested herbs to help relieve spasms and bloating. Some promote normal digestion, helping move food out of the stomach and into the intestines so you can be comfortable again.

Tame the Tummy
- **Choose Chamomile** A tea made from the herb chamomile (see page 84) has been used to relieve indigestion for centuries. Chamomile exerts healing and protective effects on the digestive tract lining. It also relieves cramping, expels gas, and stimulates normal digestion. Chamomile tea is easy to make

and very safe. Add a heaping teaspoon of the dried herb to a cup, pour in just-boiled water, and steep for five minutes. Strain and add a little honey to sweeten, if desired.

⚠ **CAUTION:** Chamomile is generally considered to be very safe, although rare allergic reactions have been reported in people who are allergic to ragweed, asters, chrysanthemums, and other plants in the Asteraceae family.

- **Chew Seeds** Many Indian restaurants have a dish of fennel seeds available as a digestive aid for departing diners. Fennel (see page 91) is a carminative, an herb that aids digestion and alleviates cramping and gas. Try chewing a teaspoon of fennel seed to soothe an upset stomach, particularly one triggered by eating spicy foods.
- **Try Peppermint** Studies have shown that peppermint tea has a relaxing effect on gastrointestinal tissues and can relieve pain too. Steep 1 heaping teaspoon of dried peppermint leaf in a cup of boiling

good to know: ABOUT INDIGESTION
- Avoid eating large meals or eating any meal fast. Small meals, eaten slowly, are less likely to cause indigestion.
- Don't eat just before going to bed. Give yourself at least three hours to digest your dinner before you turn in.

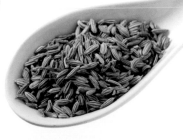

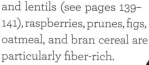

water, strain, and sip. Research has also shown that small doses of peppermint oil may help relieve indigestion, as well as the symptoms of irritable bowel syndrome (see pages 107–108). Peppermint oil may cause heartburn; if so, try coated capsules, available in health food stores.

- **Chew Ginger** Ginger (see page 95) has been used for thousands of years to settle unsettled stomachs. Studies have shown that ginger calms intestinal spasms and can significantly reduce nausea. Try slowly chewing a few pieces of candied ginger when indigestion strikes. Ginger is available in health food stores and many supermarkets.
- **Sip Soda** Although drinking carbonated beverages may sometimes cause indigestion, slowly sipping a small amount of club soda or real ginger ale may help alleviate the discomfort.

▶ | CONSTIPATION

Constipation may be nearly as common as indigestion. It's the reason behind roughly 2.5 million doctor visits each year. Although what constitutes "regularity" varies widely from person to person, you're constipated from a medical perspective if you haven't had a bowel movement for more than three or four days. Typically, constipation is the result of too little fiber, not enough water, and too little exercise, although stress and certain medications can also play a role.

Restore Regularity
- **Add Fiber** If constipation is a problem, try gradually increasing the amount of fiber in your diet. Expand your daily menu to include more whole grains (see page 187), fruits, and vegetables. Foods such as beans and lentils (see pages 139–141), raspberries, prunes, figs, oatmeal, and bran cereal are particularly fiber-rich.
- **Hydrate** Make sure you are drinking at least eight eight-ounce glasses of water a day. Keep an eye on your coffee or tea intake, though. Both are diuretics that can promote water loss.
- **Drink Hot Lemonade** Warm drinks can stimulate the digestive tract, especially first thing in the day. Even before you have your morning coffee, try drinking a hot "lemon-aid" made by adding a tablespoon or two of freshly squeezed lemon juice to a cup of hot water. Sweeten with a little honey, if desired.
- **Get Going** Physical activity can help stimulate the digestive tract to move things along. It also reduces stress, which can contribute to constipation (as well as indigestion). Walking (see pages 340–342) is one of the simplest and best exercises. Try including a 20- to 30-minute walk as part of your daily activities.

▶ | DIARRHEA

Diarrhea often strikes without warning and can send you running to the bathroom many times a day. Viruses can cause it. So can food poisoning, antibiotics, and foreign strains of the bacterium *E. coli* picked up while traveling. Fortunately, most cases of common diarrhea usually clear up in a few days. Simple remedies—and staying hydrated—can help you cope until the crisis has passed.

Ditch Diarrhea
- **Keep Hydrated** Diarrhea can be very dehydrating. Fight dehydration by sipping your way through eight glasses of water every day. Herbal teas and diluted vegetable and fruit juices are also good choices.

---

good to know: ABOUT CONSTIPATION

– Avoid stimulant laxatives. They are effective but can also be habit-forming.

– Never strain. Straining can cause hemorrhoids and anal fissures, small but extremely painful tears in the tissues around the anal opening.

good to know: ABOUT DIARRHEA

- Avoid drinking full-strength fruit juices, as they can make diarrhea worse.
- Avoid artificial sweeteners like xylitol and sorbitol, which can also aggravate diarrhea.

- **Drink Blackberry Tea** Blackberry tea is an old folk remedy for diarrhea. Traditionally, though, the tea was made from blackberry roots, which may not be easy to find. An alternative is tea made from blackberry leaf. Steep 2 teaspoons of dried blackberry leaf in a cup of just-boiled water for ten minutes. Drink up to three cups a day.
- **Keep It Light** Avoid eating solid food for 12 to 24 hours. Then eat small amounts of simple foods such as applesauce, bananas, yogurt, white rice, soda crackers, and toast.
- **Try Probiotics** Antibiotics can kill off large numbers of "good" bacteria that normally inhabit your intestines. You may be able to replenish these helpful microbes—and speed recovery from diarrhea—by eating yogurt, kefir, and other probiotic foods (see page 179) that contain live bacterial cultures, including strains

of *Lactobacillus*. Helpful bacteria are also available in pill form at natural food stores.

 WHEN TO CALL THE DR.: See your health care provider if diarrhea persists for more than five to seven days. • Also check with your health care professional if you are experiencing extremely severe abdominal cramps or have blood or mucus in your stool, or if onset of diarrhea followed a trip to a foreign country or an outdoor excursion during which you drank water from a lake or stream.

▶ | GAS

Most intestinal gas is produced in the colon, where undigested food, such as plant fibers, ferments with the help of billions of bacteria. Excessive gas can form if you eat too fast or too much, swallow air, consume lots of fatty or gas-producing foods such as beans and raw vegetables, or are unable to digest lactose, a natural sugar found in milk and other dairy products. Gas can also result from constipation, and when the normal balance of bacteria in your intestines is disrupted by taking antibiotics and certain other medications.

Fight Flatulence

- **Slow Down** Gulping food encourages overeating and the swallowing of air, both of which can contribute to gas formation.
- **Go Easy With Fiber** Some high-fiber foods tend to produce intestinal gas. Among the worst offenders are beans, lentils, cabbage, onions, broccoli, cauliflower, bananas, raisins, prunes, whole wheat bread, and bran cereal. If gas is an issue, try cutting back on these foods.
- **Experiment With Herbs** A number of herbs, including fennel (see page 91), peppermint (see page 106), and lemon balm (see page 103), can also help relieve intestinal gas. A handful of fennel seeds or a cup of lemon balm tea can be a very effective flatulence fighter!

THE IMPORTANCE OF FOOD SAFETY

Don't risk digestive upsets (or worse!) by employing unsafe methods in the kitchen. Wash your hands thoroughly and often—before cooking and after touching raw meat, seafood, or eggs. Make sure to sanitize any cutting boards that have had raw meat on them before reusing them. And beware of the "danger zone": Between 40°F and 140°F, foods are at a prime temperature for bacterial growth. Prevent problems by keeping cold foods cold and hot foods hot. If leftovers in your fridge don't smell right to you, follow your instincts. When in doubt, throw it out!

–Barton Seaver
Chef and sustainable food expert

good to know: ABOUT GAS

- Avoid carbonated beverages.
- Don't drink through a straw; you'll swallow air, which can lead to gas formation.

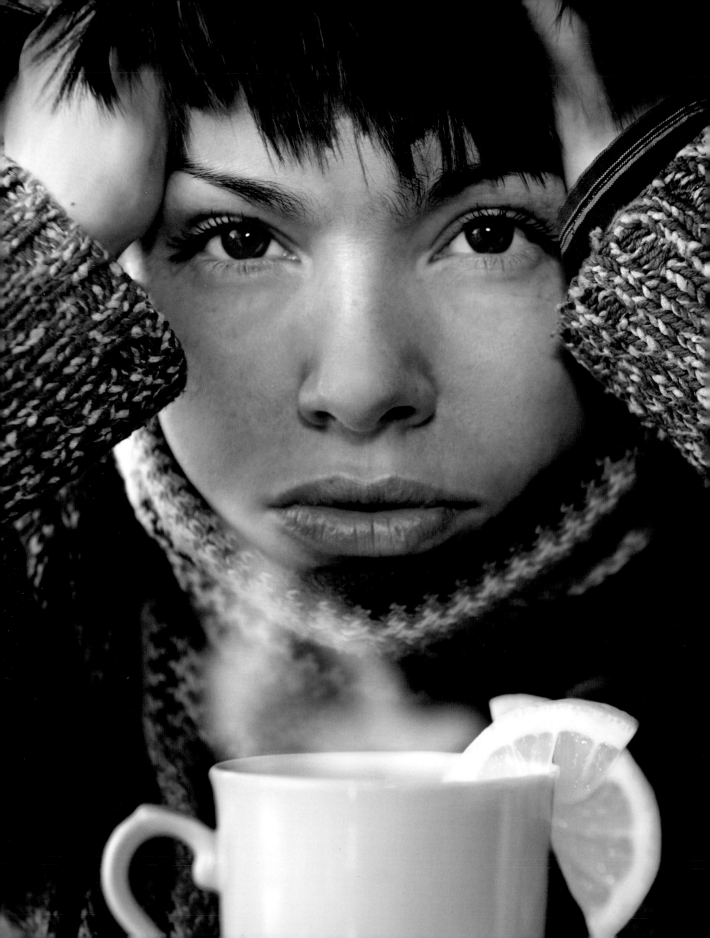

Everyday Aches

14 SOOTHING SOLUTIONS FOR PAIN

Begin with the alarm not going off. Add a frantic commute. Sprinkle liberally throughout the day with deadlines and meetings. Top with screaming children and a stack of bills. If this sounds like a recipe, it is: for a headache. Headaches often come on quite suddenly. So can other painful conditions, such as earaches or toothaches. When something hurts, our first instinct is often to reach for over-the-counter (OTC) painkillers. Although these handy pills do effectively kill pain, they may not always be the best choices for the job. Aspirin, acetaminophen, and naproxen, the most common OTC options, all have potentially serious side effects. The alternative? Natural remedies may often quell pain as well, or even better, than these medicine cabinet staples.

▶ | HEADACHE

Headaches come in different sizes and intensities, but there are two common types. Tension headaches typically begin as a constant dull ache at the back of the head or in the forehead. At their worst, they spread into a sensation that your head is being squeezed in a vise. Tension headaches can be brought on by stress, anxiety, eyestrain, or lack of sleep. Migraine headaches are often characterized by a throbbing, stabbing, or aching pain in one part of the head that may be coupled with nausea, vomiting, and sensitivity to light and sound. The triggers for migraines may include foods, hormones, stress—even a change in the weather. If you have chronic headaches or excruciating pain, see your doctor immediately. But for the typical headache after a hard day, try the following approaches.

Head Off a Headache

- **Grab an Ice Pack** When your head is pounding, using an ice pack may bring relatively speedy relief. You can use a frozen gel pack, a bag of frozen peas or corn, or a do-it-yourself pack made by placing a few ice cubes with a little water in a zip-top bag. Cover your ice pack with a paper towel or a thin dish towel and apply it to the part of your head that hurts for ten minutes every hour.
- **Combine Heat and Cold** If ice doesn't ease the pain of a headache, try heat. Heat can help relax tight muscles, which can contribute to tension headaches. Try putting a warm, moist compress on the back of your head and neck, or wherever the pain seems to be concentrated. Repeat as needed.
- **Apply Acupressure** Several acupressure points (see page 257), when activated, can

---

TENSION TAMER

When you are feeling stressed out or overwhelmed, you can use the power of essential oils to lift your spirits and ease tension. The oil from the rind of sweet orange helps promote feelings of cheerfulness and warmth, while its cousin bergamot orange is said to ease irritability and sadness. Vetiver oil is known as the "oil of tranquillity" because it relaxes and grounds us. You can find these oils at most health food shops. The following is a recipe to tame your tension:

5 drops bergamot
5 drops sweet orange
3 drops vetiver

Fill a four-ounce spray bottle with water and add essential oils. Mist in the room or on bedding when you need some serenity.

—Tieraona Low Dog, M.D.
Author and integrative medicine expert

HEALING TRADITIONS

ease headache pain. Here's one to try: With the thumb and index finger of one hand, grip the meaty webbing between the thumb and index finger of the other hand. Apply firm, squeezing pressure for several seconds, release gently, and then squeeze again. Repeat this massaging action for about a minute, and then switch hands.

- **Use Essential Oils** Massaging your temples with a diluted aromatic essential oil may bring headache relief. Mix a drop of either peppermint or lavender oil with a teaspoon of a neutral carrier oil, such as sweet almond oil. Wet your fingertips with this mix and rub your temples gently using small circular motions. Be careful not to get the oil in your eyes.
- **Try a Scalp Massage** Use your fingertips to massage the skin all over the head and neck, but focus mostly on the sides of the head above and around the ears. Ideally, ask someone to do this for you, so you can more completely relax.

....

WHEN TO CALL THE DR.: See your health care provider if you have frequent, recurring headaches, or if you have headaches accompanied by numbness, blurred vision, dizziness, or memory loss. • Seek medical help quickly if you develop a severe headache following a head injury or after exercising.

....

▶ | EARACHE

Earaches caused by infections of the middle ear (otitis media) are one of the most common ailments of childhood, especially in children younger than three. But this type of earache can strike adults too. The problem often begins following a cold or a bout of sinusitis. Bacteria or viruses migrate into the middle ear via the Eustachian tube—the tubular structure that connects the middle ear to the back of the throat—where they cause inflammation and swelling.

Swelling may block the Eustachian tube, trapping accumulating fluids and microbes and causing a painful throbbing along with a feeling of fullness. Consult your health care provider to rule out medical problems such as a perforated eardrum, then consider home remedies to ease the discomfort.

Ease an Earache

- **Try Heat** Make a warm compress by soaking a hand towel in hot water (not hot enough to burn skin); wring out the excess. Fold the towel in thirds the long way and position it under your chin, wrapping the ends up alongside the jaw line and continuing up to your ears. Hold in place. When the compress cools, rewarm the towel in hot water, and repeat. Do this two or three times a day.
- **Ease Pain With Oil** Pierce a garlic oil capsule (available at health food stores). Squeeze a few drops of the garlic oil onto a small cotton ball and place the oil-dampened portion gently inside your ear (leave enough sticking out to make it easy to remove); leave in for several hours. Recent studies have shown that warm olive oil, applied in the same manner, can also relieve earache pain.

....

⚠ CAUTION: Avoid applying oil to ears shortly before seeing your health care provider, as the presence of the oil may interfere with an ear examination.

....

- **Massage à la Qigong** Qigong (pronounced chee gung) is an ancient Chinese form of

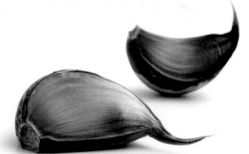

....

good to know: ABOUT EARACHE

- When you have a cold, blow your nose gently. Hard blowing can force bacteria back into your middle ear from your sinuses or throat and cause an ear infection.
- During the night, keep your head elevated with pillows to encourage drainage from the ear canal.

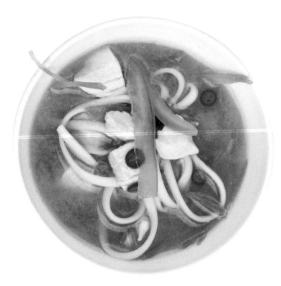

healing movement therapy (see page 283). To encourage circulation and drainage of fluid trapped in the ear canal, try a qigong-inspired massage. Place your middle and index fingers on either side of your ear (middle finger in front, index finger behind). Starting near the earlobe, press firmly while moving your fingers (maintained in a V shape) upward alongside the ear. Release the pressure when you reach the top of the ear. Return to the starting position and repeat about two dozen times. Repeat twice a day.

■ *Drink and Gargle* Make sure you're drinking lots of fluids. The act of swallowing tends to stimulate the muscles surrounding the Eustachian tube to contract, which may help trapped fluid to drain. Gargling with warm water can have a similar effect.

WHEN TO CALL THE DR.: If your ear pain persists after two days of approved home care, seek medical help. • If your ear becomes extremely painful, discharges blood or green or yellow pus, or if you have a fever of 100°F or higher, see your doctor immediately. • Earaches in children need to be treated quickly and appropriately, and diagnosis can sometimes be difficult. If your child is younger than six months, call your doctor before using any home remedy for earache. Take your child to the doctor immediately if the child has a fever that exceeds 103°F, if pain or redness develops along the bone behind the ear, if small amounts of mucus or blood are visible in the ear canal, on clothes, or on bed linens, or if the child in any other way looks or acts very sick, has a stiff neck, cannot touch chin to breastbone, or has extreme irritability or lethargy.

▶ | TOOTHACHE

Toothache can be caused by untreated tooth decay or gum disease, a broken or cracked tooth, a missing cap, or a lost filling. Professional care is required as soon as possible, either from your dentist or a medical doctor. But if toothache strikes late at night or over a weekend and you can't get an appointment until Monday morning, these simple steps can help ease the pain temporarily.

Contain the Pain

■ *Use Salt and Cloves* Add ¼ teaspoon salt and 3 drops of pure clove essential oil to about 6 ounces of warm water in a glass. Stir until the salt dissolves. Swish small mouthfuls of this mixture around the painful tooth. Spit; don't swallow. Repeat as needed.

⚠ **CAUTION:** Rare allergic reactions to clove oil have been documented in a few people. This clove oil–containing mouth rinse is very dilute, but use it for no more than three days. If you experience any sign of irritation on your gums or the lining of your mouth, stop using it immediately.

■ *Apply a Spicy Paste* Mix about a teaspoon of powdered ginger and a teaspoon cayenne pepper in a small dish. Add enough water to make a paste. Scoop up some of the paste onto a cotton swab and hold it on the tooth for several minutes. Be careful not to get this mixture on your gums, your tongue, or the lining of your mouth, as it could cause irritation.

■ *Mix a Peppermint Mouthwash* Make a cup of peppermint tea. Swish small mouthfuls of the liquid gently around the affected tooth.

■ *Ice It* Place an ice pack on your cheek (with a paper towel or thin, soft cloth in between to protect your skin) over the painful tooth. Apply for five minutes every hour.

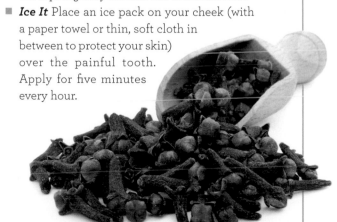

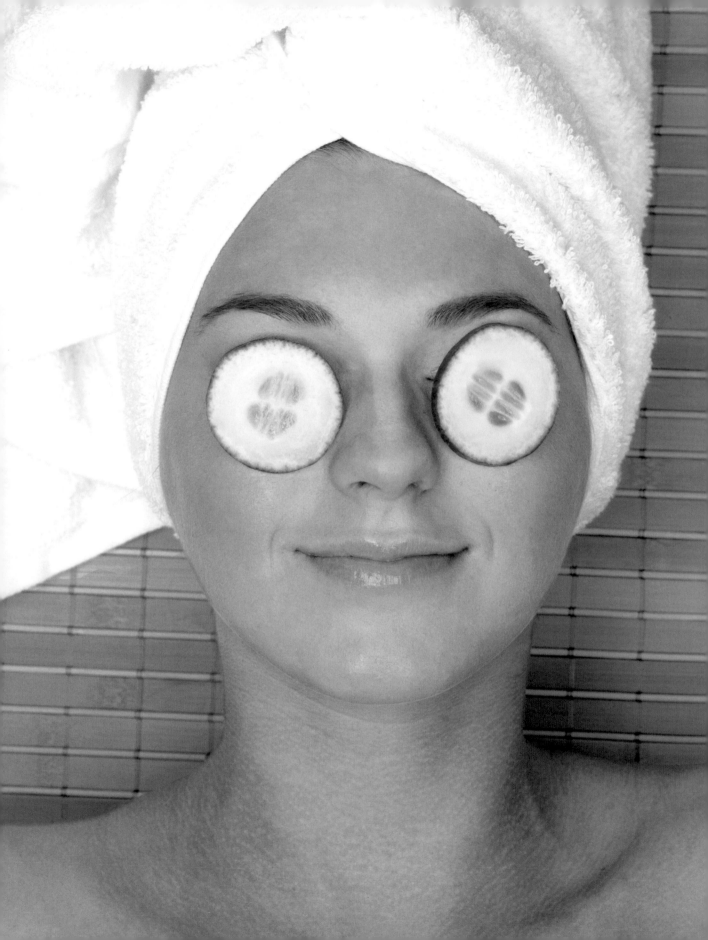

Eye Troubles

17 EYE-EASING IDEAS

Eyes can reveal much about our health, environment, and levels of stress. Are they moist, clear, and bright? Or tired and rimmed in red? Dust, allergens, and pollutants can irritate and inflame delicate eye tissues. Eyes fixed on a computer screen all day or a television screen at night almost guarantee a good case of eyestrain. Bacteria and viruses can cause eye infections. And, if you've ever collided with a door—or someone's fist—you know that eyes can be easily injured. See your doctor immediately about a serious eye problem or injury. But when your eyes simply need a little tender loving care, here are some remedies to try.

▶ | DRY, IRRITATED EYES

Whether you live in the city or the country, daily life can be downright dirty. Dust, smog, sand, tobacco smoke, vehicle exhaust, and pollen—it's all out there, swirling around. Invariably, some of it ends up in your eyes. Even the smallest particle of dirt or dust can feel like the proverbial mote when it's trapped beneath an eyelid. Allergens can trigger reactions that leave eyes tearing and flaming red. Dry air and wind can whisk away moisture, and unfortunately, so does aging.

Protect Your Peepers

For removing particles:

- **Lift Your Lids** Here's what to do if you get a bit of dirt or sand in your eye. First, don't rub—rubbing might drag whatever's in your eye across the cornea (the eyeball's clear covering) and scratch it. Instead, gently grip the lashes on your eyelid and lift it slightly away from the eyeball. Then look up, down, and around. With luck, tears washing across the surface of the eyeball may flush the particle down and out into the corner of your eye.

- **Flush It** Tears alone will sometime flush out an irritating particle, but if not, use a glass or plastic eye wash cup, available from any drugstore. Fill the cup with lukewarm water or sterile saline solution, hold it firmly enough against the eye socket to create a seal, and then open your eye and blink with it "underwater" several times. Refill the cup and repeat until the irritation is gone.

For soothing dryness and irritation:

- **Cool the Eyes** One simple way to sooth irritated eyes is to apply a cool, moist compress. Soak a washcloth in cold water, wring it out, and lay it over closed eyes for at least ten minutes. Repeat as often as needed.

- **Calm Your Eyes** Use a tea bag to create a mini-compress. Black, green, or herbal tea will work. Wet two bags in cold water, squeeze out, chill in the refrigerator a few minutes, and then place one over each closed eye.

good to know: ABOUT DRY, IRRITATED EYES

- Wear swim goggles when you swim in chlorinated pools.
- Wear protective goggles when using machinery, mowing the lawn, or using a leaf blower.
- Avoid eye drops designed to eliminate redness. They contain chemicals that cause blood vessels to constrict and may sap moisture from your eyes. A better option might be artificial tears, available at most pharmacies.

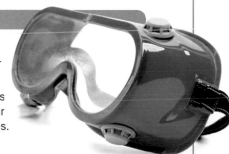

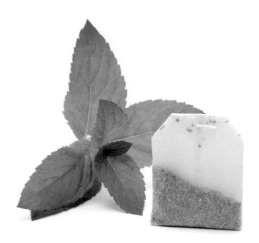

■ *Soothe With Cucumber* Here's an old folk remedy for soothing dry or irritated eyes: Slice off a half dozen ⅛-inch-thick slices of chilled cucumber. Place a slice over each closed eye; keep the rest in the fridge. As the slices warm up, replace with fresh cool ones.

WHEN TO CALL THE DR.: If you are unable to flush a particle out of your eye, or you think there's a foreign object embedded in the eye's surface, seek immediate medical care. • See your health care provider if there is no improvement in red, inflamed eyes after several days, or they begin to produce matter or pus; you could have an infection.

▶ EYESTRAIN

Six small muscles control the movement of our eyes. And like all muscles, from biceps to hamstrings, eye muscles become fatigued when they're overused and don't get a chance to relax. Hours of staring at a computer screen, peering through a microscope, driving cross-country, or poring over books will do just that. Symptoms of eyestrain include burning, watery, or itchy eyes, and possibly blurred vision and headaches. Fortunately, tired eye muscles usually recover once they get a break and a bit of rest.

Go Easy on the Eyes

■ *Blink* Blinking is the body's way of cleansing the eye's surface and keeping it moist. But often when we're concentrating or staring at a fixed point for long periods of time, we tend not to blink. Try to consciously blink more often to keep eyes moist and help reduce strain. For example, blink every time you reach the end of a sentence, or hit "enter" on the keyboard.

■ *Refocus* If you sit at a computer screen or do other close work, look away from the screen every 20 minutes and focus on something in the distance. Look up, down, and from side to side. Set a timer to help you remember.

■ *Close Your Eyes* Simply closing your eyes can help eye muscles relax. Find ways to shut your eyes for several minutes every hour. Try it while talking on the phone.

■ *Relax* For a restful break, rub your hands briskly together to create friction and heat. Quickly cup your warm hands over your eyes, lean back, and relax. Do this every hour.

good to know: ABOUT EYESTRAIN

— Get a regular eye exam. Not only will you find out if you need glasses or a prescription upgrade (which may be why your eyes are strained), but an eye doctor may spot signs of serious health problems, such as diabetes, while checking your eyes.

— Increase contrast on your computer screen, and use a bigger font.

— Wear sunglasses in bright light, both in summer and winter.

■ *Cool, Then Warm* Alternate cool and warm compresses. Wet a washcloth with cool water and lay over your eyes for a few minutes. Then wet the cloth with warm water and repeat.

■ *DIY Massage* Using the tips of your index, middle, and ring fingers, press gently on the orbital bones above your eyes for five seconds, and then on the bones below for five seconds. Repeat this routine several times. Caution: Press only on the bones, not the eye itself.

▶ STIES

A stye (also spelled sty) is an infection at the edge of the eyelid that's caused

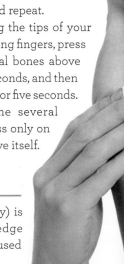

when an oil gland or eyelash follicle becomes clogged with dirt or oil, and then invaded by bacteria. Sties often look like small boils or pimples and can be extremely painful. Most run their course along familiar lines: They fill with pus that gradually comes to a head, after which they rupture and heal. It's possible to speed this process with uncomplicated therapies.

Stymie Sties

- **Warm It Up** Gentle heat may help bring a stye to a head more quickly. Try applying a moist compress for five to ten minutes several times a day. Just wet a washcloth in warm water, wring it out, and hold it over the stye. Launder the cloth in hot water after each use to reduce the chance of spreading infection.

- **Boil an Egg** Wet compresses tend to cool quickly. For something with more staying power, boil an egg in a pot of water until hard-boiled (about four minutes). Remove, dry, and wrap the egg in a piece of clean, soft, dry cloth. Hold this wrapped, warm "compress" against the outside of the affected eyelid.
- **Just Add Calendula** This herb has antiseptic properties and can help soothe irritated tissues. Up the clout of a wet compress by using calendula tea instead of water. Add 2 cups just-boiled water to 2 teaspoons of dried calendula blossoms and let steep for 20 minutes. Cool and strain. Wet a washcloth with the tea, and apply as a compress.

 WHEN TO CALL THE DR.: Most sties heal in a few days. If a stye persists, see your doctor.

▶ | BLACK EYES

A black eye is essentially a bruise around the eye. A hard blow damages tissues and breaks tiny capillaries. Blood and other fluids then collect in the space around the eye, resulting in swelling and a very dark blue discoloration. As the bruise heals, the pooled blood is slowly reabsorbed, usually producing a kaleidoscope of colors.

WHEN TO CALL THE DR.: Seek medical help immediately after any eye injury because it's difficult to judge the true extent of the damage. • Most black eyes resolve on their own in a week or two. However, if the eye becomes increasingly swollen and inflamed, or if you experience headaches, blurred vision, or any other vision problem, see your doctor right away.

See to It

- **Ice First** Apply a cloth-wrapped ice pack (a gel pack or a bag of frozen vegetables) for 10 to 15 minutes every hour you're awake for the first 2 days. This will ease swelling and help constrict blood vessels, reducing the pooling of blood. After 48 hours, apply warm, moist compresses to increase circulation and speed healing.
- **Try a Tea Bag** A soaked tea bag is another home remedy for bruising. Substances in tea are astringent and also anti-inflammatory. Saturate a tea bag of black or green tea, squeeze out the excess water, and hold gently to the bruised areas. Repeat several times a day.
- **Dab on Arnica Gel** Arnica has been used for centuries to treat injuries. Dab a little arnica gel on the bruised skin around a black eye several times a day.

⚠ **CAUTION:** Be careful not to get any of the arnica gel in your eyes.

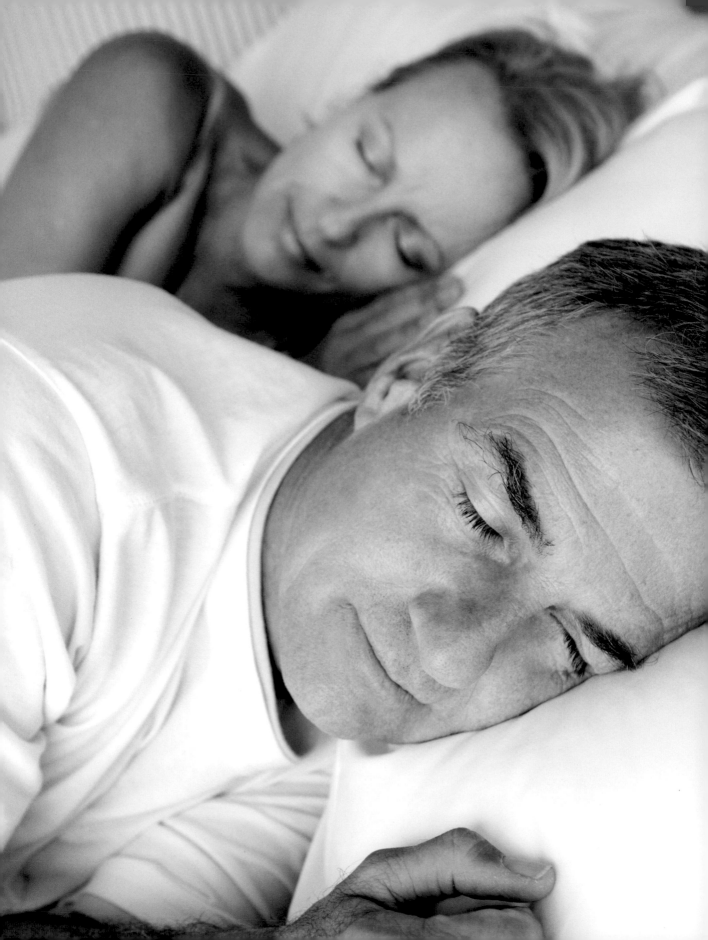

Feeling Tired

20 WAYS TO WAKE UP RESTED

You claw your way out of the covers in response to the beeping alarm, but you're just as tired now as you were when you went to bed. Sound familiar? Every day, more than two million Americans complain of being weary, worn-out, and done in. A lingering feeling of tiredness can be a symptom of an undiagnosed medical condition, so start by getting a thorough medical checkup. If you're otherwise healthy, bouts of fatigue usually stem from having too much to do and too little time to do it, coupled with energy-stealing habits. Periods of insomnia, when sleep won't come no matter what you do, can also lead to feeling chronically exhausted. So can long-distance travel, which leaves your jet-lagged body unsure of what time zone it's in.

▶ | FATIGUE

Call it exhaustion. Lethargy. Sluggishness. Lassitude. Fatigue by any name is the feeling that you simply don't have the energy, and maybe not even the interest, to do what you need to do. Fatigue strikes everyone at some point or another. The usual prescription is to get more rest and exercise. Eat a balanced diet. Squeeze in a little R&R. If you've done all those things and you're still dragging—and there's nothing medically wrong—strategies for de-stressing and re-energizing may help.

War on Weariness

- **Eat Breakfast** Fatigue can be a side effect of skipping meals, especially breakfast. Start your day with a little low-fat yogurt or some scrambled eggs. Or try an almond-rich Ayurvedic smoothie traditionally used to battle fatigue (see recipe at left).

- **Go for Mini-Meals** Having three small meals and two snacks helps keep blood sugar and energy levels stable all day long. These meals and snacks should contain a mix of complex carbohydrates, protein, and a small amount of fat.

- **Exercise to Energize** Although it may seem counterintuitive, exercising gives you energy. Just taking a brisk walk every day for 20 to 30 minutes may be enough to release stress and add bounce to your step. With a little creativity and planning, you can find many easy ways to work exercise into your day (see pages 339–343) to help banish fatigue.

- **Try Morning Yoga** At first glance, yoga may seem like something people do to relax, but it can be invigorating and energizing. Try starting your day with a few simple yoga postures (see pages 301–303).

- **Perk Up** Some aromas can calm you down; others perk you up. Eucalyptus, clove, cinnamon, lemon, and peppermint are some natural scents used in aromatherapy (see pages 260–261) to reduce drowsiness and increase

---

RECIPE FOR HEALTH

ALMOND ENERGY BOOSTER

Almonds are high in protein, healthy fats, and soluble fiber (see pages 167–168). They have also been shown to help prevent a post-meal spike in blood sugar that can lead to an energy crash later on.

Put 10 almonds in a small bowl. Cover with water and let them soak overnight to soften. In the morning, peel off the papery brown skins. Combine the almonds, a cup of hot skim or soy milk, a teaspoon of maple syrup or palm sugar, and a pinch each of powdered cardamom, cinnamon, and ginger in a food processor or blender. Process until smooth.

AVOID INJURIES

Don't be a "weekend warrior" who suffers from fatigue-based or overuse injuries. Pursuing sports to maintain a healthy lifestyle is a great goal, but failing to exercise regularly, and without proper conditioning, can lead to injuries that will put you on the couch for months.

People in the cultures where long life is common engage in moderate physical activity throughout their day—every day. Natural, regular activity that keeps the body moving for sustained time includes cooking, gardening, cleaning, climbing stairs, or walking to meet friends. These activities are balanced with a variety of cardiovascular movement, muscle training, and flexibility.

–Dan Buettner
Author and lecturer on longevity

energy and alertness. Keep a small bottle of one of these essential oils around and take a whiff when you need an energy boost. Or mix 8 drops of lemon oil and 2 drops each of peppermint, eucalyptus, and cinnamon oil with 8 ounces of water in a small spray bottle. A spritz of this mix into the air around you makes for a fragrant energizer.

■ *Take a Nap* The Amish have a saying that a half hour's nap in the afternoon is worth two hours' sleep at night. Many cultures advocate a quick siesta during the day as a way to

good to know: ABOUT FATIGUE

Overwork is a common condition of modern life, and one that quickly leads to fatigue. Strategize ways to lighten your load. Learn the art of delegation and the power of saying "no." Maintain a reasonable work and personal schedule in which you make time to unwind and refresh.

combat fatigue. During your lunch hour or after work, kick off your shoes, stretch out, and catch 20 winks. Avoid sleeping longer than 15 or 20 minutes, as long naps can make you feel groggy and make it difficult to fall asleep at night.

■ *Get Better Sleep* Getting too little sleep can lead to chronic fatigue. Shoot for eight hours a night.

▶ | INSOMNIA

Insomnia is the most common sleep complaint among Americans. You have difficulty falling asleep, or staying asleep, and you end up feeling tired upon waking and during the day. Certain medical conditions can trigger insomnia, as can many medications. But for the average, healthy person, insomnia is usually brought on by anxiety and stress, and aggravated by alcohol and caffeine. (Although OTC and prescription drugs can help you sleep—most are antihistamines—they all come with side effects, including daytime sedation, and they may be habit-forming over time.) When sleep escapes you, try the following natural remedies instead.

How to Invite Sleep

■ *Take Valerian* In modern herbal medicine, valerian is the leading herb recommended for insomnia. It helps most people fall asleep and sleep more deeply without causing the morning "hangover" characteristic of many prescription sleep aids. Capsules of concentrated valerian root are available at health food stores; some brands may contain other relaxing herbs such as lemon balm and passionflower. Follow package directions.

■ *Have a Cuppa Chamomile* Both chamomile and lemon balm (see pages 103-105) have been used for centuries to help induce sleep and as aids for gentle relaxation. Steep 1 or 2 teaspoons of either herb in a cup of just-boiled water (steep chamomile for five minutes, lemon balm for ten). Sweeten, if desired, with a little honey or maple syrup.

- Avoid caffeine—coffee, tea, sodas, and energy drinks—from late afternoon onward.
- Avoid alcohol in the evening; like caffeine, it can keep you awake or cause periods of wakefulness during the night.
- Create a restful place to sleep. Block out noise and light. If silence itself keeps you awake, buy a white noise machine or listen to soothing tunes or natural sounds.

⚠ **CAUTION:** Do not use chamomile if you are allergic to ragweed or other plants in the aster family.

■ *Inhale Lavender* The essential oil of lavender contains many medicinal components, and research has shown that simply inhaling the fragrance can be calming. Put a sachet of dried lavender, or several sprigs of the freshly cut herb, between your pillow and pillowcase before going to bed. You might also brew a cup of lavender tea, made by steeping 2 teaspoons of dried lavender flowers in 1 cup of just-boiled water.

■ *Make a Hops Pillow* Hops is another traditional remedy for insomnia—it has mild sedative properties. Make a hops pillow by stuffing a cloth drawstring bag, available at craft stores, with a handful of fresh hops. Tie the top shut. Place the bag between your pillow and pillowcase.

■ *Drink Hot Milk* Drinking a cup of hot milk to induce sleepiness is an old folk remedy that may have originated in New England and persists to this day. Add a little honey or a pinch of nutmeg to a cup of milk and warm until steaming. Pour into a mug and sip.

■ *Learn to Relax* Relaxation techniques such as yoga and meditation can ease stress and help you fall asleep (see pages 299 and 279). Also try controlled breathing exercises, such as those on pages 267–269.

⚕ **WHEN TO CALL THE DR.:** If you've tried everything but are still having trouble falling asleep, let your health care provider know. It might be time to get a sleep expert's opinion.

▶ JET LAG

What do you do when it's time for breakfast in Bangkok but your body is telling you it's bedtime instead? Jet lag is a disturbance of the normal sleep-wake cycle triggered by rapidly traveling across three or more time zones. Fatigue, insomnia, disorientation, poor concentration, headaches, and even digestive distress may set in. Jet lag can last from a day to a week or longer depending on the individual and the number of time zones crossed. There's no way to eliminate all jet lag symptoms, but you can minimize its disorienting effects.

Trip Tips

■ *Consider Melatonin* This natural hormone is involved in regulating the human biological clock. Research has shown that taking melatonin supplements during the first few days of travel may relieve jet lag.

⚠ **CAUTION:** Talk to your doctor before taking melatonin. Although generally regarded as safe, there are rare reports of allergic reactions and autoimmune conditions associated with taking it. The U.S. Food and Drug Administration does not strictly regulate supplements and herbs, so there is no guarantee of strength, purity, or safety, and effects may vary.

■ *Start Rested* Starting your trip exhausted will likely make jet lag worse.

■ *Reset Your Body Clock* Set your watch to the time at your destination and begin eating and sleeping accordingly.

■ *Catch Some Zzzz's* Sleep as much as you can on the plane. Invest in good travel pillows for your lower back and for your neck.

■ *Drink Water, Not Alcohol* The humidity in many planes is just 2 or 3 percent. Avoid alcohol and drink plenty of water.

■ *Use Caffeine Carefully* Caffeine on long flights can further disturb the sleep-wake cycle. Once at your destination, a cup of coffee can promote daytime alertness, but avoid it after midday.

■ *Sit in the Sun* Spend time in the sun at your destination to reset your biological clock.

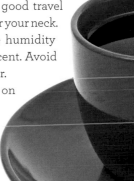

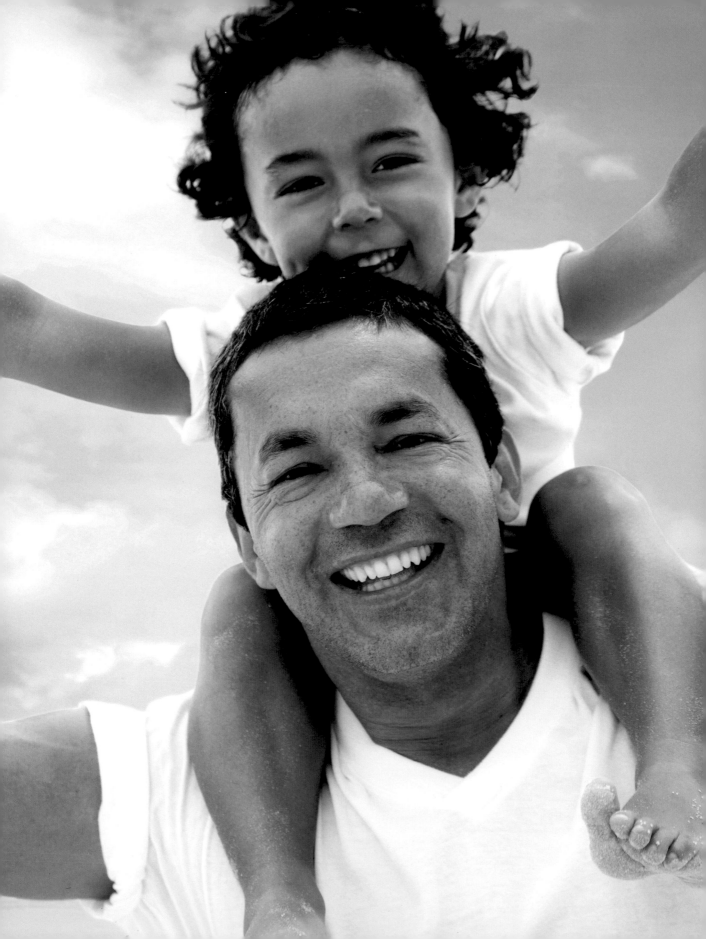

Mouth Problems

18 CLUES FOR CLEANER MOUTHS

The mouth is many things: It is the source of smiles and frowns; the home to teeth and tongue and taste buds; the organ that shapes our speech and laughter, savors and chews our food, and acts as the gateway to our digestive tract. The eyes may be the windows to the soul, but the mouth in many ways is a window to our overall health. Health problems, from dehydration to stress to an immune-system challenge, can manifest themselves in and around the mouth. Bad breath, cold sores, canker sores, and even chapped lips are things we often think of as minor irritations. Yet they can also be warning signs that something else is amiss.

▶ BAD BREATH

Sometimes bad breath is simply the aftereffect of a recent meal. A garlicky Alfredo, raw onions on a salad, or a slice of stinky cheese can leave us with breath vile enough to make other people flee face-to-face conversations. But bad breath can also be a sign that bacteria—our mouths teem with them—have somehow obtained the upper hand. Brushing up on dental hygiene is an obvious first step. Then try the following simple steps and remedies. If these self-care techniques don't solve the problem, make an appointment with your dentist to rule out gum disease, an abscessed tooth, sinus infection, or some other condition.

Banish Bad Breath

- **Chew Spices** Skip sugary breath mints; sugar acts as food for odor-causing bacteria. Instead, take a tip from the ancients—refresh your breath with aromatic spices that are as close as your spice rack. Try chewing or sucking on a small piece of cinnamon bark, a peeled cardamom pod, or a few fennel or anise seeds.
- **Try Parsley** The little green herb that often garnishes restaurant plates is both nutritious and a natural breath cleanser. Chew a sprig or two of fresh parsley to help improve breath quickly.
- **Drink More Water** Dehydration can be a cause of bad breath. Up your water intake to at least eight eight-ounce glasses of water each day. Green tea and juice can also be helpful, but be careful with coffee and other caffeinated beverages. These can tend to act as diuretics, causing water loss. Coffee itself can also be a source of bad breath.
- **Use a Natural Mouthwash** The brightly colored mouthwashes that line drugstore shelves may contain ingredients that are far from healthful (see page 229). Peppermint tea makes an effective and natural mouthwash. Steep a heaping tablespoon of dried peppermint leaf in a cup of just-boiled water for 15 minutes. Cool and strain. Swish and gargle with a mouthful of the cooled tea; spit. Repeat several times a day. Use as needed to freshen your breath.
- **Change Your Toothbrush** Toothbrushes harbor bacteria, which can multiply astronomically in a very short time. Let your toothbrush thoroughly dry between brushings. Replace it every two or three months.
- **Scrape Your Tongue** The surface of the tongue harbors millions of bacteria. Scraping

good to know: ABOUT BAD BREATH

- Carry a toothbrush and brush after every meal to fend off bad breath.
- Smoking causes unpleasant mouth odor. Breaking the habit will help.

your tongue to remove some of them can help keep breath fresher. Tongue scrapers are available at most drugs stores; follow package directions and use at least once a day. When finished, rinse your mouth thoroughly.

▶ COLD SORES

Cold sores are caused by an insidious virus known as herpes simplex type 1. It lurks in most of us, lying dormant along nerves, waiting for the immune system to drop its guard. Stress, illness, too much sun, and changing hormones are common triggers for an attack. The virus heads toward the mouth region, where it typically invades cells in or near the lips. Within hours, it causes small blisters that erupt into ugly, painful sores. Shortly before the blisters appear, though, there is often a telltale tingling or itching sensation at the skin's surface. That's your call to action. Although these natural remedies can't cure or prevent cold sores from developing, they can lessen their severity and speed healing.

Conquer Cold Sores

- **Try the Tea Bag Trick** Saturate a black tea bag with cold water. Squeeze to remove excess and then hold the damp bag over the site where you feel the cold sore coming on. Apply for ten minutes every hour.
- **Use a Mini-Pack** Place an ice cube in a zip-top bag or wrap in a piece of damp paper towel. Hold the wrapped cube against the site for up to two minutes (keep the cube moving slightly to avoid any one spot from getting too cold). Repeat hourly.
- **Go for Lemon Balm** Research has shown that lemon balm, an aromatic herb with a strong lemony fragrance, contains compounds that

can inhibit the herpes virus, and so shorten the duration and severity of an outbreak. Apply lemon balm ointment (available at health food stores) to the site where a cold sore feels like it's developing; follow package directions.
- **Apply a Compress** Dip a cotton swab or cotton ball in cold milk, and hold on the site for five seconds. Resaturate the cotton and repeat this procedure for several minutes, then rinse. Do this four to five times a day.

WHEN TO CALL THE DR.: Get medical advice if you are plagued by frequent cold sores. Prescription antiviral medications can help. • Head to your health care provider if a cold sore fills with pus, which could indicate a bacterial infection.

CRANKY OVER CANKER SORES?
Goldenseal's bright yellow root has long been used as a traditional remedy for canker sores. The best product form available at a natural food store is a goldenseal tincture, with the root's active components extracted in alcohol. Put up to ½ teaspoonful of goldenseal tincture in a shot glass and fill the glass about half full of warm water. Swish the mixture around in the area of the canker sore for a minute or two, and then spit it out. Don't swallow it! You will be tempted to rinse your mouth out because of the bitter taste, but refrain from doing so. Let the goldenseal's medicinal compounds go to work. This remedy is not recommended for children because of its taste.

–Steven Foster
Herbalist and lecturer

good to know: ABOUT COLD SORES

- Avoid picking at a cold sore at any stage. Leave it alone to heal. Wash your hands after applying anything to a sore to avoid spreading to other parts of your face or your eyes.
- Herpes virus is highly contagious and passes from one person to another through skin-to-skin contact. If you have a cold sore, take special care to avoid touching others, particularly infants, anyone with eczema, or people with suppressed immune systems.
- If sun exposure triggers your cold sores, apply a sun block liberally to your lips before going outside.

CANKER SORES

Canker sores are usually small but painful eroded areas in the lining of the mouth caused by food allergies, eating acidic foods, overly aggressive tooth brushing, ill-fitting dentures or braces, or an accidental cheek bite. Sodium lauryl sulfate, a common ingredient in toothpastes and mouthwashes, may also be a factor. A variety of home remedies can help relieve the painful symptoms.

WHEN TO CALL THE DR.: Consult your health care provider if your canker sores are large, seem to be spreading, or last longer than two to three weeks. • Tell your doctor if you develop a high fever as canker sores appear.

Soothe a Sore

- ***Swish With Myrrh*** This fragrant plant resin is a traditional remedy for mouth and gums. Buy tincture of myrrh at most health food stores. Put several drops in a glass, add about 4 ounces of warm water, and then sip, swish, and spit two to three times a day. Do not swallow.
- ***Rinse With Salt Water*** Simply dissolve a teaspoon of salt in a small glass of warm water. Use this solution to rinse the area of the canker sore several times a day.
- ***Gargle With Flowers*** Calendula (see page 79) has been used since antiquity for a wide variety of skin and mouth irritations. Steep 1 or 2 teaspoons of dried calendula flowers in a cup of just-boiled water for ten minutes. Cool and use as a mouth rinse.

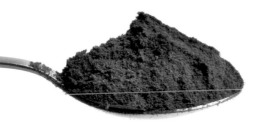

- ***Try Cayenne*** This pungent spice contains capsaicin, a chemical that can temporarily desensitize nerve endings in skin. Place a tiny pinch of cayenne on a canker sore to ease the pain. Or look for cayenne pepper lozenges at a health food store.

HOMEMADE PEPPERMINT LIP BALM

2 ounces almond kernel oil
¼ ounce beeswax
1 teaspoon vegetable glycerin
1 to 2 drops peppermint essential oil

Place the almond kernel oil and beeswax in the top of a double boiler over medium heat. Warm, stirring gently, until the beeswax melts completely. Remove from heat and stir in glycerin and essential oil. Beat with a whisk or electric mixer until the mixture takes on a creamy consistency. Store up to six months in a glass jar with a screw-top lid.

CAUTION: Discontinue the use of cayenne if this makes your canker sore seem to worsen.

CHAPPED LIPS

Unlike the rest of our skin, lips lack glands that produce protective, moisture-trapping oils. Lip skin is also thin and delicate. So it's no surprise that lips can easily dry out to become parched, cracked, and sore. Exposure to sun and wind are common offenders. So are certain ingredients in toothpastes, lipsticks, and medications.

Tips for Lips

- ***Try Natural Balms*** Coat your lips with a thin layer of almond, sesame, or almond kernel oil. Or pierce a capsule of vitamin E, squeeze out a bit, and apply.
- ***Slather On Lanolin*** Natural waxes work well as lip balms, and tend to last longer than oils. Try lanolin, derived from wool, or beeswax. Many health food stores carry natural lip balms made of these waxes with few or no other ingredients.
- ***Hydrate and Humidify*** Lips chap because they are losing moisture. Drink more water and other fluids to keep your body well hydrated. If your environment is cold and dry, run a humidifier to add warm moisture to the air.

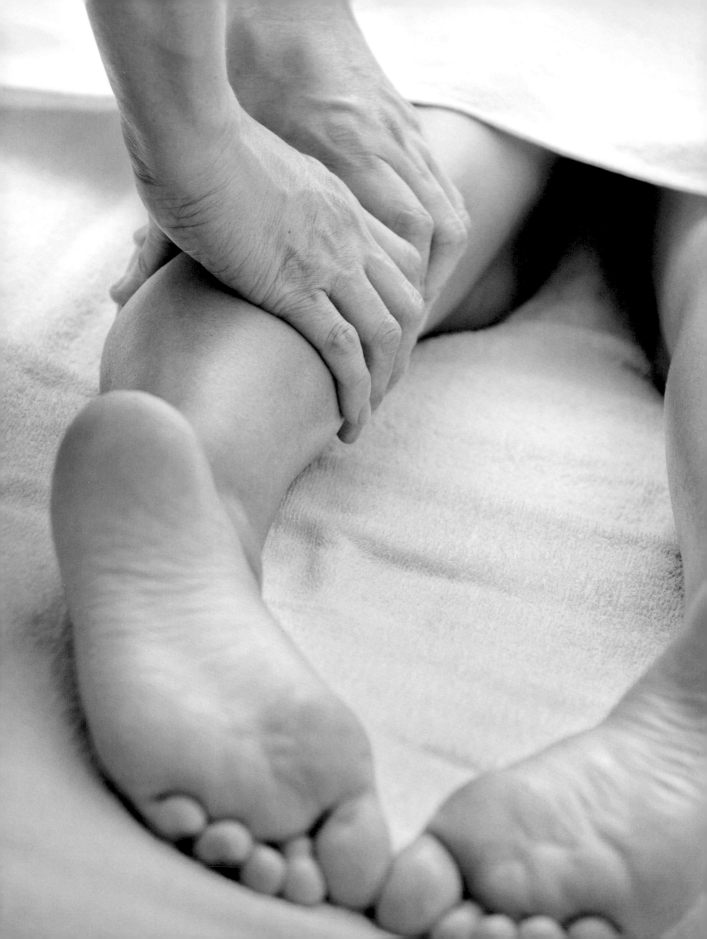

Muscle Cramps & Spasms

17 WAYS TO DECREASE CRAMPING

The runner in the lead seems sure to win. Then suddenly, her stride shortens. She clutches her calf and limps to the sidelines. It's obvious what has just happened: a classic muscle cramp. A cramp can last anywhere from a few seconds to several hours, and the pain can be breathtakingly severe. Muscles cramp for a variety of reasons: overuse, dehydration, an irritated nerve, certain medications, or a position held too long. Muscles can also cramp as a result of an imbalance in the key minerals that play a role in normal muscle contraction. Though painful and annoying, muscle cramps are rarely serious enough to require medical care. Simple steps can help ease the pain and prevent a recurrence.

▶ | CHARLEY HORSE

A charley horse is the colloquial term for a muscle cramp, especially one in the calf or in the front or back of the thigh. These muscle spasms usually strike during some type of exercise, but they can also happen when we're asleep. Nocturnal charley horses, or nighttime leg cramps, are quite common and are not typically a sign of disease. Fortunately, most are short-lived and simple measures can bring them under control.

Rein In That Charley Horse

- **Drink Plenty of Fluids** Doctors think dehydration may be a trigger for muscle cramps in some people. Avoid dehydration by drinking plenty of water, especially before, during, and after exercising. If nighttime cramps are a problem, try drinking a glass of water before bedtime, and keep one on the nightstand, too.
- **Act Fast** At the first sign of cramping, stop whatever you are doing and begin stretching and massaging the affected muscle. Putting your weight on a cramping leg may help stop the spasm.
- **Apply Heat and Cold** As a rule of thumb, apply heat—warm towels, a hot water bottle or heating pad—initially to help a cramped

muscle relax. Once the spasm begins to ease, apply a cold pack or cold compress to relieve pain.

- **Slip Into a Warm Bath** There's nothing quite as soothing as a warm bath to help relax muscles. Add ½ cup Epsom salts to the bath water for a therapeutic soak.
- **Take Time to Stretch** You can lessen the chance of muscle cramping by stretching regularly. Before engaging in any type of exercise, limber up. To help prevent nocturnal muscle cramps (which usually occur in the legs), perform this easy stretching routine before bed: Face a wall and place your palms against the wall at shoulder level. Step backward with one leg, extending it as far behind you as is comfortable. Keep the other knee slightly bent. Keeping the heel of the extended leg on the floor, lean forward until you feel a pulling sensation in the extended leg. Hold for ten seconds, and then relax and repeat three more times. Switch legs and repeat the same stretch on that side.

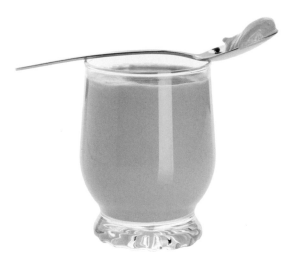

■ *Sip Something Sour* An old folk remedy for nighttime leg cramps is to drink a small amount of pickle juice at the first sign of a spasm. Swallowing a teaspoon of prepared mustard (also high in vinegar and salt) works for some people too.

 WHEN TO CALL THE DR.: See your health care provider if you have a cramp that doesn't ease after a few days, or if you get muscle cramps in the same place on a regular basis.

▶ | SIDE STITCHES

It feels like a sharp, intense pain in your right side, just under the lower edge of the rib cage. With each breath the pain becomes more intense. Side stitches, sometimes called side aches, are the result of sudden, spontaneous cramping of muscles in the diaphragm. The diaphragm is the large, flat sheet of muscle between your lungs and your abdominal organs that plays a critical role in helping to draw air in and out of your lungs. No one is really sure what causes side stitches. But almost everyone who engages in vigorous exercise, especially running, will probably experience one at some point.

Sideline a Side Ache
■ *Breathe From Your Belly* A possible cause of side stitches is shallow breathing. When you exercise, focus on breathing deeply by slowly expanding the belly, as well as the chest area, as you breathe in.
■ *Don't Run Through It* If a side stitch strikes, don't continue running or exercising. Working "through" the pain can intensify the muscle cramping. Stop and breathe deeply, and wait for the cramping to ease.
■ *Push and Blow* To alleviate a side stitch, try pushing your fingers deeply into your belly just below your ribs where the cramping seems to be most severe. At the same time, purse your lips and blow out as hard as you can. The combination may help interfere with the muscle contractions causing the pain.

▶ | MENSTRUAL CRAMPS

Most women experience menstrual cramps at one time or another. The cramping is a result of powerful contractions of the muscles in the uterus during the monthly cycle. Hormone-like substances called prostaglandins, known to cause inflammation and pain, are largely responsible for triggering the uterine contractions that lead to menstrual cramps. While mild menstrual cramps are normal, predictable, and temporary, they can be debilitating, and simple home remedies can offer welcome relief.

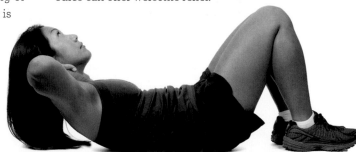

good to know: ABOUT SIDE STITCHES
└ Avoid eating for at least an hour before running or engaging in any type of vigorous exercise.
└ Never try to run or move through pain of any type of muscle cramp in the arms, legs, or torso. Stop whatever you're doing to give the muscle a chance to recover.

Hamper the Cramps

- **Take a Tea Break** Raspberry leaf tea, available at grocery or health food stores, contains fragrine, a substance that can help ease cramping in some women. Brew a cup and sip it as you try to relax—ideally while soaking in the tub. Alternatively, try ginger tea, made with fresh gingerroot. Ginger contains a substance that inhibits the production of prostaglandins. Grate a teaspoon of fresh, peeled gingerroot into a cup, add just-boiled water, steep, strain, and sweeten to taste.

- **Try Exercise** Research has shown that moderate exercise can ease menstrual cramps in many women. Go for a brisk walk, swim, or take a bike ride.

- **Try a Little Pressure** Using an acupressure point on your leg may help relieve menstrual cramps. Place your finger on the bony point of the inner ankle of one of your legs. The acupressure point in question is approximately four finger widths above that point, on the inside surface of the leg. When you've located it, apply gradually intensifying pressure to the spot with your thumb or forefinger. Hold for three minutes, then release. Repeat several times on each leg.

⚠ **CAUTION:** Do not do this acupressure exercise if you are pregnant or experiencing heavy menstrual flow.

- **Go for a Soak** A warm bath can do wonders for menstrual cramps. The heat from the water helps relax cramped muscles in the uterus as well as the lower back.

- **Hug a Hot Water Bottle** If a bath is not an option, fill a hot water bottle with very warm water, wrap in a soft thin towel, and place it on your abdomen or against your lower back.

▶ | RESTLESS LEGS

Restless legs syndrome (RLS) is a nervous system disorder that triggers an irresistible urge to move the legs (and sometimes arms) to relieve uncomfortable sensations—muscle cramping, itchiness, and creepy-crawly feelings—in the legs. Up to 10 percent of Americans suffer from this strange affliction; it seems to occur most often in middle-aged and older adults. Doctors aren't sure what causes the odd sensations of restless leg syndrome, although they suspect that genes play a role because the condition of RLS tends to be seen in families. Research also suggests that how the brain uses iron may be a possible contributing factor.

Calm the Crazy Legs

- **Try Immediate Massage** As soon as you are awakened by RLS sensations in your legs, grab your calf muscles firmly (the meaty part at the back of the calf) and pull them gently outward. Squeeze the muscle mass gently several times, and then release. Repeat this massaging action for at least five minutes.

- **Experiment With Heat and Cold** Try bathing legs in warm water, and then apply ice packs. Alternate these temperature extremes every few minutes.

- **Shed Stress** Worry and stress appear to make RLS worse in most people who have it, although the reason for this is unclear. Try relaxation techniques such as meditation and yoga (see pages 279 and 299) to relieve stress and improve sleep.

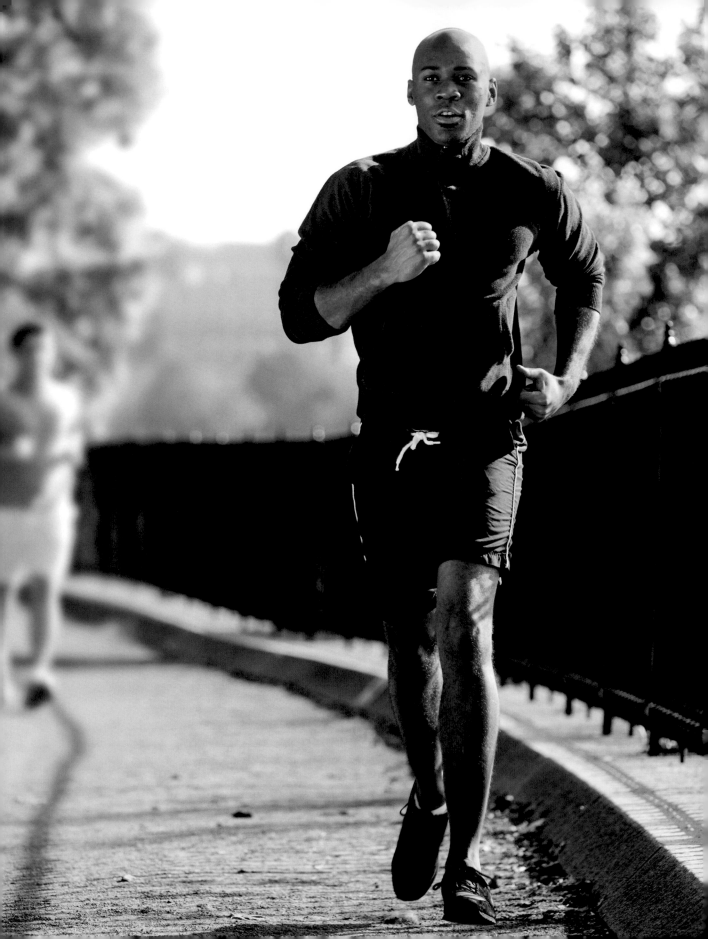

Painful Joints

17 METHODS TO EASE THE MOVES

Joints are places where bones meet. They are the body's bending, rotating, and pivoting points, enabling you to move in infinitely marvelous ways—until something goes wrong. When a joint is swollen, painful, inflamed, and not working the way it should, you're quickly reminded that, for all their versatility and apparent strength, joints are not indestructible. Like every other part of your body, they need care and tending. Joint problems can strike in a moment or develop slowly over time. Bursitis, tendinitis, sprains, and arthritis are among the most common. Home remedies are appropriate for treating minor joint complaints. Anything more serious should be examined first by your health care provider.

▶ | INFLAMED JOINTS

Your new exercise routine is going well—so well, in fact, that it feels like it's time to up the challenge. Rather than progressing gradually, though, you add an extra 20 pounds on the barbell instead of 10. You run another five miles instead of one. You move further into a yoga posture than ever before. In other words, you overdo. And what happens? A joint complains, often in the form of painful bursitis or tendinitis. Bursitis is inflammation of the tiny fluid-filled pads called bursae that cushion the structures making up a joint. Tendinitis is inflammation of the tendons—the thick fibrous cords that attach

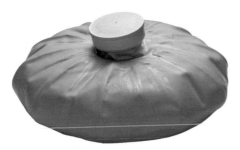

muscles to bones—around a joint. If you're experiencing either of these joint conditions, try the following remedies—in conjunction with medical care and your doctor's approval—to relieve the pain and speed healing.

Points for (Painful) Joints

- **Apply Ice, Then Heat** Chill down a complaining joint with an ice pack, applied for 10 to 20 minutes every four hours. Keep icing for three days, or until the joint no longer feels warm or appears swollen. At that point, start alternating cold with heat (warm compresses, a hot water bottle, or a heating pad). End with a cold application during cold/heat alternations.
- **Go for Ginger** This herb has been shown to have anti-inflammatory properties. Make a ginger compress by chopping 2 tablespoons of fresh, peeled ginger. Combine with 3 cups just-boiled water and let steep for 20 minutes. Strain. Soak a washcloth in the warm liquid, wring it out, and place over the sore

---

good to know: ABOUT BURSITIS & TENDINITIS

When bursitis or tendinitis strikes, take a long break from the activity that caused it. If you start again before the joint is completely healed (or overdo again), you'll simply reinjure it. However, it's also important to continue gently moving the joint through its range of motion to avoid a "frozen" joint, a condition in which scar tissue causes pain and reduced mobility.

Always stretch properly before and after exercise.

joint for five minutes. Repeat three or four times a day.

- **Rub on Arnica** Salve made from the herb arnica is used extensively in Europe to help reduce swelling and inflammation in injuries. You can find arnica gel or salve at most health food stores. Follow package directions.

> ⚠ **CAUTION:** Always remember: Arnica is for external use only.

- **Try Turmeric** This yellow "curry spice" contains curcumin, a substance found to help reduce inflammation and joint pain and stiffness. Turmeric is available in capsules, as is a standardized extract of curcumin (it's often combined with bromelain, a natural enzyme from pineapple that has also been shown to possess anti-inflammatory properties). Alternatively, add a teaspoon of turmeric powder to warm milk and drink once or twice daily.

- **Soothe With Hot Stuff** Capsaicin is the substance that gives hot peppers their heat. Distilled and made into an ointment, it can help ease pain when applied to the skin overlying a sore joint. Follow package directions.

> ⚠ **CAUTION:** Wash hands well after each application and avoid contact with eyes and other sensitive mucous membranes.

- **Massage With Oils** Try mixing several drops of lavender, thyme, or eucalyptus essential oil with a teaspoon of sweet almond oil. Gently massage some of this mixture into the joint several times a day.

▶ | SPRAINS

Sprains don't just happen on ski trips. All it takes is an awkward, unbalanced step off a curb and you can end up with an ankle that is swollen, painful, bruised, and difficult to move. A sprain is an injury to a joint that has been severely stressed, so much so that the ligaments holding the bones together have been overstretched or torn. Always have an injured joint examined by a doctor to make sure it's a sprain, not a fracture.

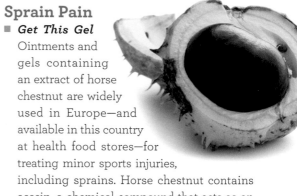

Sprain Pain
- **Get This Gel** Ointments and gels containing an extract of horse chestnut are widely used in Europe—and available in this country at health food stores—for treating minor sports injuries, including sprains. Horse chestnut contains aescin, a chemical compound that acts as an anti-inflammatory to help reduce swelling. Follow package directions.

- **Think RICE** To treat a doctor-confirmed minor sprain, first REST; if possible, immobilize the injured area. ICE the injury as soon as possible with an ice pack or a bag of frozen peas or corn for 10 to 15 minutes every two hours. (Place a thin towel between the ice pack and bare skin.) COMPRESS the joint with dressings or elastic bandages to provide support and control swelling, but not so tight as to interfere with circulation. Finally, ELEVATE the sprain in relation to the rest of your body, if possible. After 48 hours, cautiously use the injured joint.

> ⚠ **CAUTION:** Get your doctor's advice if swelling and pain do not subside.

- **Choose the Ayurvedic Way** In between icing, try this ancient Hindu treatment: a salt compress to help reduce swelling. Mix together one part ordinary table salt and two parts powdered turmeric. Add just enough water or aloe vera gel to make a paste. Apply the paste to the sprain for 20 to 30 minutes. Cover with a piece of cloth to protect clothing and furniture from turmeric stains. Do this once or twice a day.

- **Arm With Arnica** Another herb to try is arnica, which has been used topically to help heal sprains and other joint injuries for hundreds of years. It's available as a gel from some grocery and most health food stores.

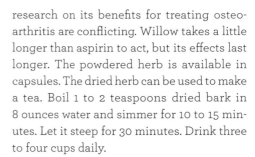

WHEN TO CALL THE DR.: Call your doctor if the pain and swelling don't diminish after 48 hours, if you have numbness in or around any part of the injured joint, or if you notice redness or red streaks spreading out from it.

▶ | OSTEOARTHRITIS

Both common forms of arthritis—osteoarthritis and rheumatoid arthritis—are characterized by moderate to severe pain in the joints. Osteoarthritis occurs when the cartilage that cushions the ends of bones begins to deteriorate, so bone rubs directly on bone. This type of arthritis is age-related, and is usually the result of normal joint wear and tear. Rheumatoid arthritis is an autoimmune disease in which dysfunctional antibodies attack joint linings. Millions of arthritis sufferers typically reach for over-the-counter nonsteroidal anti-inflammatory drugs (NSAIDs). Although these drugs can ease pain in the short term, they come with serious side effects. Natural remedies are a viable alternative.

Fight Fire in the Joints

- **Try a Glucosamine Supplement** Glucosamine sulfate, derived from the shells of shrimp, lobsters, and crabs, can help the body make and repair cartilage. Several studies suggest that glucosamine supplements can help joint pain and mobility.
- **Experiment With Willow** The medicinal use of willow bark dates back thousands of years. Some studies have shown that willow bark preparations are as effective as aspirin in relieving pain and inflammation. However

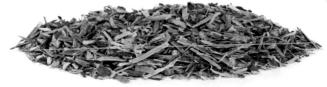

research on its benefits for treating osteoarthritis are conflicting. Willow takes a little longer than aspirin to act, but its effects last longer. The powdered herb is available in capsules. The dried herb can be used to make a tea. Boil 1 to 2 teaspoons dried bark in 8 ounces water and simmer for 10 to 15 minutes. Let it steep for 30 minutes. Drink three to four cups daily.

- **Treat It With Capsaicin** Gels and creams containing capsaicin can temporarily reduce arthritis pain in some people. Apply externally to painful joints, following package directions.
- **Add Omega-3s** Evidence continues to mount that omega-3 fatty acids in the body help fight inflammation and so may help control pain. Increase the omega-3s in your diet by eating more nuts, especially walnuts, fish, and flaxseed (see pages 169 and 159).
- **Try Massage** Massaging the skin with aromatic oils can be very soothing. Mix 3 drops rosemary essential oil and 3 drops chamomile essential oil into ¼ cup sweet almond or sesame oil. Apply liberally to skin and gently massage.
- **Zap It With Ginger** As a remedy for arthritis pain, ginger has a long history. Studies show ginger may block the formation of inflammation-causing chemicals. Make a refreshing tea by placing 3 to 4 slices peeled fresh ginger in 1 cup boiling water. Steep for ten minutes and strain. Sweeten with honey, if desired. Or incorporate ½ teaspoon powdered ginger or up to 6 teaspoons fresh ginger into your day's diet.
- **Eat Cherries** Eating cherries to ease arthritis pain is an old folk remedy supported by modern research: Studies show that cherries contain compounds that inhibit enzymes that cause inflammation.

good to know: ABOUT OSTEOARTHRITIS

- Always check with your health care provider before beginning any type of exercise program, including yoga or qigong.
- A diet low in saturated fats (see page 331) may reduce the body's production of prostaglandins, hormone-like substances known to contribute to inflammation.

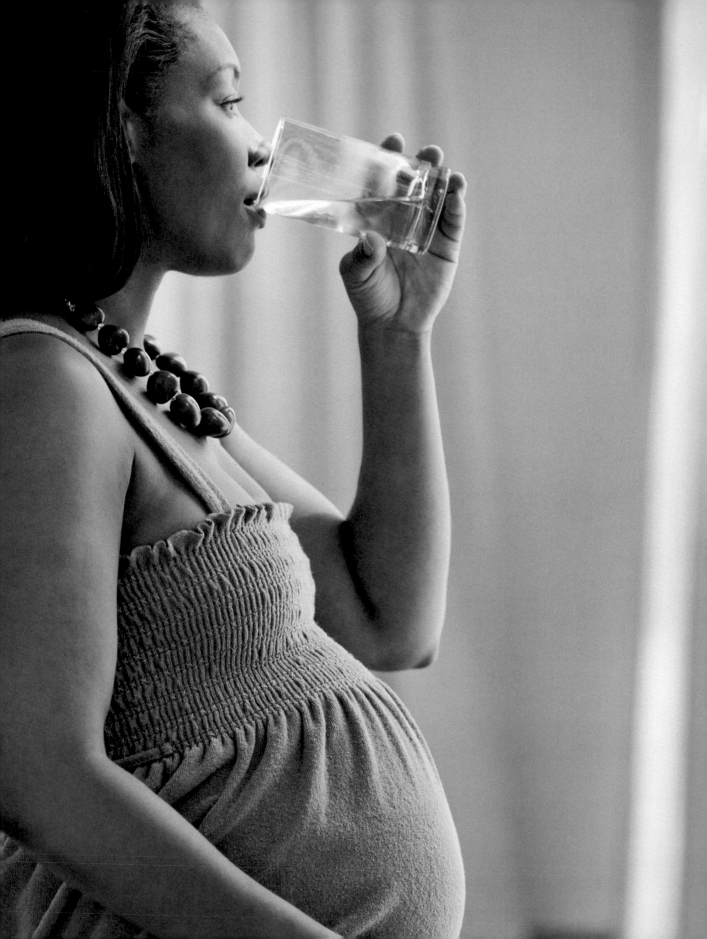

Queasiness

20 STEPS TO SETTLING YOUR STOMACH

The world is full of things that can make your stomach heave: a meal wolfed down in haste, stuffy rooms, the smell of fryer grease at a fast food restaurant, roller coasters and Tilt-A-Whirls, fishing off the back of a boat. You've probably experienced that awful twisting, turning feeling in the pit of the stomach, when you're poised on the edge of nausea, or worse. Muscle contractions are at the core of this queasiness. Normally, the stomach walls contract gently and rhythmically, about three times a minute, to help digest food in the stomach and keep it moving through the digestive tract. When contractions come faster than that, the stomach starts to flutter and that horrible feeling ensues. Natural remedies can help.

▶ | MOTION SICKNESS

The Greek physician Hippocrates penned what appears to be the first description of motion sickness more than 2,000 years ago. Ancient Greece was a country of seafarers who were no doubt intimately familiar with the "motion of the ocean." In fact, the word *nausea* originates from *naos*, the Greek word for ship. But you don't have to be at sea to have a queasy and rebellious stomach. Motion sickness can strike whether you're traveling by car, train, airplane, or elevator—even camel! The queasiness is triggered when there's a discrepancy between the messages the eye and balance organs in the inner ear send to the brain. Sooner or later, you will begin to experience the feelings of motion sickness. The thing to do is stay calm and try some of the following suggestions.

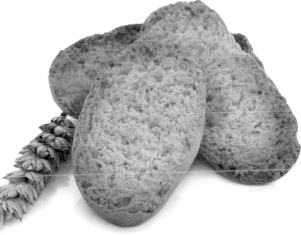

Trials of the Traveler

- **Stay Focused** If possible, keep your eyes on the horizon and keep your head stationary. The middle of a boat and the front seat of a car exhibit the least motion; move there if you can.
- **Eat Something** Hunger can make motion sickness worse. Eat a light meal before taking a trip, and then, during the ride, nibble on crackers or a piece of bread. Avoid heavy, greasy foods.
- **Reach for Ginger** Many people find ginger combats queasiness, and several studies support its effectiveness. Try eating small amounts of candied ginger to avoid or treat nausea. For most purposes, take a gram of ginger daily, in divided doses (for example, 250 mg four times a day). To prevent motion sickness, it is best to begin treatment one to two days before a trip; continue taking it for the duration of travel.
- **Keep Hydrated** Dehydration can also aggravate motion sickness. Drink water, in small sips. Sometimes sipping carbonated beverages, such as club soda or real ginger ale, can also help. So can sucking on ice chips.

- **Flee Strong Odors** Distance yourself from diesel fumes, lavatories, galleys where food is being cooked, and tobacco smoke.
- **Keep Cool** Open a window or go out on deck. Open the overhead vents above your seat on the plane. Hold an ice cube to your wrists.
- **Try Acupressure** Place your right thumb on the center of the inside of your left forearm, about three finger widths above the wrist crease. Apply firm pressure for a minute, while breathing deeply. Alternate arms. Repeat as needed.

▶ | MORNING SICKNESS

Doctors are still somewhat mystified by morning sickness. The exact cause of these bouts of nausea, and sometimes vomiting, remains unknown. Possible culprits are changing hormones, fluctuating blood sugar levels, stress, and fatigue. Morning sickness is also a bit of a misnomer, as it can strike anytime of the day or night. It typically begins during the first month of pregnancy and continues for several months, and sometimes throughout a pregnancy. However, the good news is that natural remedies can go a long way toward counteracting the queasiness.

Mothers' Malaise

- **Eat Small Meals** To reduce nausea, eat something every few hours, but not a lot. Start with crackers or dry toast when you first get up in the morning. Eat small meals, concentrating

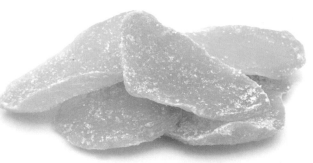

on foods that are high in protein and complex carbohydrates. Keep healthy nibbles, such as crackers or nuts, on your bedside table for those times when you wake up at night.
- **Keep Hydrated** Keeping well hydrated may help keep nausea at bay. Try to drink eight eight-ounce glasses of water a day. Set a timer to remind yourself to drink, drink a glass of water every time you go to the bathroom, or drink one with and between every meal.
- **Go for Ginger** Ginger tea is a time-tested remedy for morning sickness. Put a few slices of fresh, peeled ginger in a cup, pour in just-boiled water, and let steep for ten minutes. Strain, sweeten with a little honey or stevia, and sip slowly. Also try nibbling on ginger candy or sipping real ginger soda.

⚠ **CAUTION:** Pregnant women should limit their intake of ginger to no more than a gram/day.

- **Try Herbal Teas** Several other herbal teas may be helpful for morning sickness. Peppermint, chamomile, and lemon balm are particularly good for relieving nausea. Red raspberry leaf is another herb herbalists often recommend for pregnancy problems, including morning sickness.
- **Slip On a Wristband** Acupressure wristbands, available at drug, health food, travel, and boating stores, put pressure on a point known to ease nausea.
- **Sniff a Little Citrus** Inhaling the fragrance from a freshly cut lemon, grapefruit, or orange can help ease morning sickness in some people. Try adding a piece of fresh citrus peel to a cup of hot herbal tea so you can sniff as you sip.

good to know: ABOUT MORNING SICKNESS

- Keep a positive attitude. Morning sickness usually stops after the first three or four months.
- Avoid foods that are high in fat and salt. Anything fried seems to intensify nausea in most pregnant women.

▶ | NAUSEA & VOMITING

OK, so what started out as a little queasiness just isn't going away. You've nibbled crackers and sipped some ginger tea. But your mouth has gone dry, you're perspiring, and suddenly you're pretty sure you're about to lose whatever is roiling around in your stomach. What do you do? Doctors agree that if something inside your stomach wants to get out, go ahead and let it. But don't try to make yourself throw up. Let whatever is going to happen happen naturally. With luck, vomiting will leave you feeling better. After the initial storm has passed, try the following tips to soothe your stomach and your soul.

That Sickening Feeling

- **Lie Still** Moving around can aggravate the balance centers in your inner ear and continue to generate feelings of nausea. Lie down with your upper body slightly elevated (put an extra pillow under your head and torso). Or if lying down doesn't feel good, relax into a comfortable chair in which you can lean back and rest your head.

- **Chill Out** Place a cool washcloth over your forehead or against the back of your neck. Concentrate on the coolness as you breathe slowly and smoothly.

- **Try Heat Near Your Stomach** Sometimes vomiting can leave the stomach area feeling painfully cramped and tight. To relax those muscles, try putting a hot water bottle against the left side of your body, beside, but not on, your stomach (the weight of the bottle pressing on your stomach could make you feel nauseated again).

- **Freshen Your Mouth** The vile taste that vomiting leaves in your mouth can keep the cycle of nausea going. To neutralize it, try rinsing your mouth with a solution of 1 teaspoon baking soda and ¾ teaspoon salt mixed into 4 cups of water. Swish and spit. Alternatively, brush your teeth or suck on a piece of hard candy.

- **Replace Fluids** As soon as you feel a little better, begin replacing some of the fluids (and salts) that vomiting causes you to lose. Start slowly by sipping cool, plain water. If this goes down well, sip a little Gatorade, or make a homemade version. Add 1 teaspoon of salt and 8 teaspoons of sugar to a quart of water. Stir until the crystals are completely dissolved. Sip small amounts at a time.

- **Divert Yourself** Just thinking about being sick again can make it happen. Get your mind off the way you feel by watching television or a DVD. As you get caught up in a program or movie, you'll think less about your stomach.

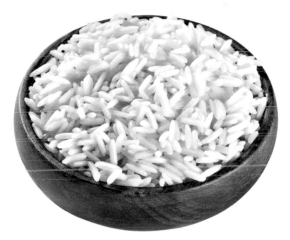

- **Start With Carbs** As you start to improve, it may help to put a little bland food in your stomach. Toast, crackers, and boiled white rice are good choices, as are gelatin dessert and clear soup.

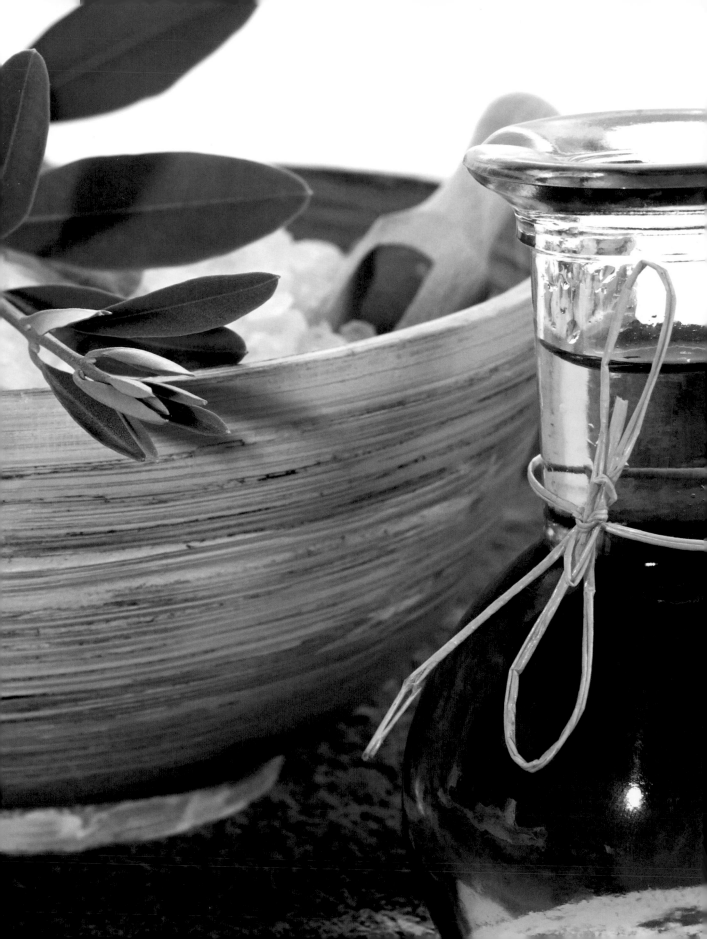

Sensitive Skin

20 WAYS TO SOOTHE AND SOFTEN

Skin is a bit like a barometer—it's exquisitely responsive to conditions in and around you. When you're too warm, skin flushes. When you're too cold, it blanches, and may even turn blue. And when something is irritating either inside or out, skin lets you know in no uncertain terms. It can become red and itchy, inflamed and sore. Tiny bumps and blisters can pop up. The more sensitive your skin is, the more dramatic the reaction. Fortunately, there are ways to soothe sensitive skin and help keep its overreactions under control.

▶ | ECZEMA

Eczema is a general term for several types of itchy skin rash. The condition is sometimes called the "itch that rashes" because the itch often precedes any sign of redness. Atopic dermatitis is the most common form. It's due to an overactive immune system response (similar to an allergic reaction) to certain foods or something in a person's environment, resulting in itchy, inflamed, sometimes crusty patches on the skin. Atopic dermatitis can run in families, and people who have it often have hay fever or asthma too. Contact dermatitis is eczema caused by direct contact with irritating substances such as detergents, fragrance, or chemicals. Doctors often prescribe steroid creams to treat eczema, but natural remedies can help calm and cool its flaming itch as well.

 WHEN TO CALL THE DR.: See your health care provider if eczema becomes very widespread, if nothing relieves the itching, or if any patches begin to show signs of infection.

Rout the Rash

- **Be a Detective** Eczema flare-ups can be triggered by food, pollen, dust mites, animal dander, wool, soaps, dyes, fragrances, sudden changes in temperature—the list is almost endless. Keep a record of whatever seems to make your eczema worse. Then try eliminating suspects one by one, from your diet or your environment.
- **Cool Off With Milk** Heat tends to make most eczema worse, so cooling the skin may help ease the discomfort. Some people find that cooling skin with cold milk can be more effective than cold water. Pour a cup of milk

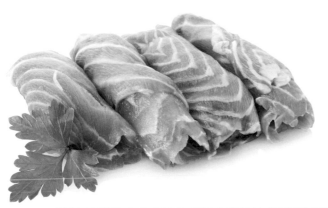

---

good to know: ABOUT ECZEMA

- Keep your body out of water whenever possible. Take short, lukewarm showers, don't over-wash your hands, and skip doing dishes by hand.
- If your environment is dry, run a humidifier to help moisten the air.
- The temptation to scratch can be overwhelming during an eczema flare-up. Keep your fingernails short. If you scratch in your sleep, wear thin cotton gloves to bed.

into a bowl and add a few ice cubes. Saturate a washcloth, wring out any excess, and use as a compress on affected areas several times daily.

■ **Apply Avocado** Rich in oil and vitamins, avocado is an old remedy for soothing skin irritations. Mash a few slices of ripe avocado and apply it directly to affected areas. Leave on for 20 minutes, and then rinse clean. Eating avocado is also a good way to get essential fatty acids into your diet (see pages 172–173).

■ **Reach for Chamomile** People have used the herb chamomile for many centuries to soothe both internal and external irritations (see page 83). Brew a cup of strong chamomile tea by pouring just-boiled water over a tablespoon dried chamomile in a cup. Steep five minutes, strain, and let cool to room temperature. Saturate a cotton ball and apply liberally to the affected area. Repeat several times a day.

⚠ **CAUTION:** People allergic to ragweed, chrysanthemums, and other plants in the Asteraceae family may have adverse reactions to chamomile.

■ **Take an Oatmeal Bath** Finely ground, or colloidal, oatmeal has natural skin-soothing properties. Add a packet or two of commercially available colloidal oatmeal (such as Aveeno) to a tepid bath and submerge your skin for up to ten minutes.

■ **Try Olive Oil** It creates a seal on skin to prevent moisture loss. Gently massage a little olive oil into affected areas. Sweet almond oil is a good alternative if olive oil seems too greasy.

■ **Go for Truly Clean Laundry** Chemicals and fragrances in laundry soaps and softeners may aggravate eczema in some people. Use laundry products that are free of dyes and fragrances or make you own (see page 248). Run clothes through the rinse cycle several times to eliminate any soap residue.

▶ | PSORIASIS

Psoriasis is a condition in which skin cells proliferate and accumulate at an abnormally fast rate, causing raised, red, itchy, sometimes painful patches topped with silver, flaky scales of dead skin. These irritated patches can form anywhere, including on the scalp. Often passed down in families, psoriasis can appear suddenly or slowly, and flare-ups are often triggered by stress, illness, injuries, sunburn, dry air, and medications.

Psoothe, Psun, & Psoak

■ **Sit in the Sun** Sunlight is often the best remedy. Expose affected areas to direct sunlight for 15 minutes a day. Protect healthy skin with a skin-safe sunscreen (see page 224).

■ **Go With Aloe** An extract cream of aloe vera has been shown to help reduce itching, scaling, and other symptoms of psoriasis.

■ **Soothe With Salts** For itch relief and to help exfoliate dead skin cells, add a handful of Epsom salts to tepid water and soak the affected area for 20 minutes.

■ **Try Massage** Take a cool to tepid bath and then gently massage areas with olive, sweet almond, or jojoba oil.

■ **Oil Your Scalp** For psoriasis on the scalp, warm a tablespoon of olive oil before bed and massage down into roots of hair. Don a shower cap to protect bed linens overnight. In the morning, wash your hair to remove the oil. Repeat nightly, then once or twice a week as needed.

good to know: ABOUT PSORIASIS

- Avoid hot water, which can make psoriasis worse.
- Don't rub or pick at flaky skin.

▶ | HIVES

The seafood crepe was delicious. But now your arms are covered with little bumps that itch like crazy and turn white at the slightest touch. You've got urticaria—aka "hives"—an outbreak of bumps or welts with raised edges (doctors call them wheals). Hives are caused when white blood cells release the chemical histamine into the skin in response to an allergen. Hives are usually harmless, and often disappear within minutes or hours after the allergic reaction has run its course. Doctors usually recommend over-the-counter antihistamines, but try a more natural approach.

Drive Away Hives

- **Be Cool** Cold shrinks blood vessels and may help block further release of histamine. Take a cool shower or a tepid bath with colloidal oatmeal (see the section on eczema) or make a soothing, cooling compress by adding 10 drops of lavender essential oil to a basin of cold water, saturate a washcloth, wring it out, and apply for 20 minutes.
- **Reach for Nettle** Leaves of stinging nettle contain quercetin, a substance shown to inhibit the release of histamines. Herbalists often recommend nettle as an alternative to antihistamines. Dried nettle capsules are available at health food stores.

> ⚠ **CAUTION:** Consult your doctor before using nettle if you are taking medicines for diabetes, high blood pressure, anxiety, or insomnia.

- **Try Astringents** Astringents tend to shrink or constrict tissues, including small blood vessels in skin. This can decrease blood flow to an area and thus histamine release. Old-fashioned calamine lotion is an astringent that can help with hives. Witch hazel can also help (be sure to use real extract). Saturate a cotton ball with witch hazel and apply several times a day.
- **Make a Paste** To ease the itching, mix a tablespoon of baking soda with enough water to make a paste, and dab onto hives.

Alternatively, apply a cream of tartar paste in the same way.
- **Stress Less** Stress can aggravate allergic reactions, so anything you can do to calm your mind and body may help hives disappear more quickly.

> ⚕ **WHEN TO CALL THE DR.:** If you develop hives around your eyes or in your mouth, or have trouble breathing, seek emergency medical care immediately.

▶ | HEAT RASH

If you've ever gone hiking on a hot day, and ended up with a stinging, itchy rash on your chest, in your armpits, or on the backs of your knees, chances are good it was heat rash. Sometimes called "prickly heat" due to the stinging sensation, heat rash is the result of sweat that had nowhere to go. Tight-fitting clothing or compressed body parts can block sweat ducts and trap perspiration under the skin, leading to swelling, inflammation, and the formation of tiny bumps or blisters on the skin's surface.

A Prickly Problem

- **Chill Out** The solution to heat rash is to get cool and reduce sweating. Head for air-conditioning or a cool shower. Use cold compresses or rub an ice cube over the reddened skin. Then try a light dusting with cornstarch. This old-fashioned remedy works by drawing moisture out of the skin.
- **Have a Soda Bath** Add a cup of baking soda to a warm bath. Soak for 30 minutes.
- **Make a Paste** If a bath isn't an option, add enough water to baking soda to make a paste, and apply to the rash. Leave on for 20 minutes, and then rinse off with cool water.

good to know: ABOUT HEAT RASH

- Wear loose-fitting clothing that wicks moisture away from your skin.
- Reduce sweating when it's hot by staying in air-conditioned buildings or using fans.
- Avoid heavy creams and lotions that could block pores.

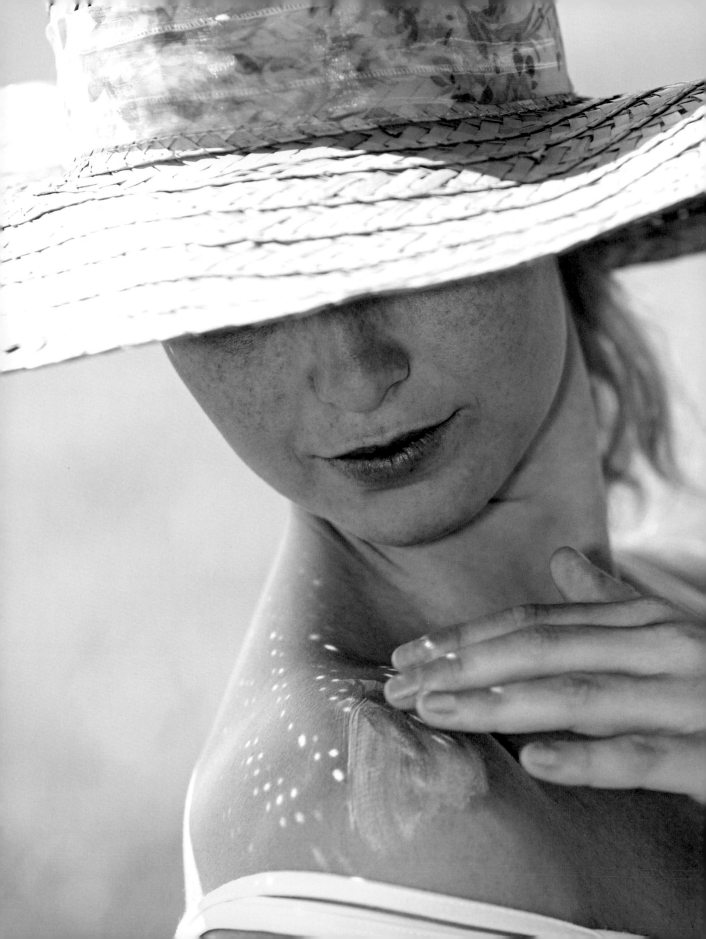

Skin Damage

18 RECIPES FOR SKIN REPLENISHMENT

Who hasn't nicked themselves shaving, smacked a knee opening a car door, or singed a knuckle flipping food on the grill? Although some of us are more accident-prone than others, minor injuries are part of everyday life. Small cuts, bruises, and burns aren't medical crises, but they do require a little first aid to prevent infection and speed healing. Every well-stocked medicine cabinet or first aid kit should have a supply of bandages and some antibiotic ointment, cream, or spray. But many simple home remedies are also very effective for treating life's little accidents. They can help stop minor bleeding, soothe a burn's heat, and keep the swelling and discoloration of a bruise in check.

▶ | CUTS & SCRAPES

When something sharp cuts the skin or something rough abrades it, a little blood may flow. The first step you should take for any cut or scrape is to stop the bleeding by applying pressure. Press down using a clean cloth or paper towel, or if nothing like that is available, simply use your hand. Hold the cut area, if possible, so it's higher than your heart. Keep the pressure on for at least 15 minutes, unless the bleeding stops sooner. Once the bleeding has stopped, clean the area around the cut or scrape gently but thoroughly with soap and water.

Smooth & Soothe

- *Try Calendula* After a cut or scrape is clean, dab on a bit of calendula salve, available at health food stores. You can also spray on some nonalcoholic calendula spray. The herb calendula has been used for centuries to help fight infection and speed healing (see page 79). Let dry and then cover the wound with a bandage or gauze.
- *Manage It With Myrrh* Studies have shown that myrrh is another useful herb for treating minor injuries, as it helps stimulate the production of white blood cells at the wound site. Make a myrrh solution by mixing a teaspoon of myrrh tincture (available at health food stores) with a half cup of distilled or filtered

water. Flush the injury and the area around it with this solution two or three times a day. Let air-dry, and re-cover.

- *Dab on Honey* If you don't have calendula, myrrh, or an antibiotic cream in your first aid kit, honey can be a quick fix for minor injuries that have penetrated the skin's surface and so pose a threat of infection. Honey has natural bacteria-fighting properties, and it also forms a soothing seal on broken skin. Dab a little onto the wound and cover with a bandage, or simply let the honey dry to form a protective coating.

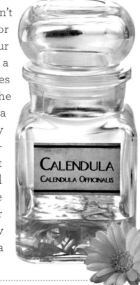

WHEN TO CALL THE DR.: If 15 minutes of steady pressure doesn't stop bleeding from a cut, especially if the blood is bright red or spurting (indicating it's coming from an artery), seek medical help quickly. • Abrasions that contain deeply embedded dirt, gravel, or metal should be treated by a doctor. • Call your health care provider if a cut or scrape becomes filled with pus, or red streaks develop around it. Both are signs of infection. • Call your doctor if the wound has ragged edges, gaps open with movement, or is on the face. Sutures may be needed in order to speed healing and prevent scarring.

MAKE YOUR OWN ICE PACK

Gel ice packs are very handy first aid kit staples. They are great for chilling bruised skin because they conform easily to the body's bumps and angles. But you can make an inexpensive substitute at home with just water and alcohol.

Simply place 2 cups of water and $1/3$ cup isopropyl (rubbing) alcohol in a freezer-strength zip-top plastic bag. Zip securely shut and place in the freezer. The alcohol prevents the water from freezing solid. After about 12 hours, you'll have a slushy, icy mix in a bag that can conform to any body part that gets bumped too hard. And, just like the store-bought versions, it's refreezable again and again.

▶ | BRUISES

Bumps and bangs often lead to bruises. Although the skin is usually still intact after these injuries, muscle and connective tissues are crushed, along with small blood vessels called capillaries. Blood leaking out of these damaged vessels pools beneath the surface of the skin, forming a red or purplish area that is tender to the touch. The palette of purples, browns, and even greens that you see as a bruise begins to heal are signs that the body is breaking down and reabsorbing the blood, bit by bit. Although bruises generally heal just fine on their own, time-tested remedies can speed the healing.

Banish the Black & Blue

- **Chill It** Ice can help constrict blood vessels and limit the release of blood from damaged vessels. Place an ice pack wrapped in a thin towel on a bruise as quickly as possible. Leave it on for 10 minutes, and then take a break for 20. Repeat this pattern—10 minutes of ice and 20 minutes of no ice—for several hours.
- **Apply Arnica** A favorite treatment for bruises in Europe, arnica has been used for centuries. Arnica gel or cream is available at health food stores and many pharmacies. Apply arnica to a bruise three to four times a day.

⚠ **CAUTION:** Use arnica for bruises, but do not apply to wounds or broken skin.

- **Try a Tea Bag** Saturate a tea bag in cold water, wring out the excess, and apply to a bruise as a quick way to soothe the injury.
- **Switch to Heat** After 24 hours, help improve circulation to the bruise by applying gentle heat. Use a heating pad, hot water bottle, or moist, warm compress for 10 to 20 minutes, two to three times a day.
- **Add an Astringent** Both vinegar and witch hazel are mild astringents. Dabbing on either of these solutions several times a day may help speed healing of a bruise.

⚕ **WHEN TO CALL THE DR.:** See your doctor if you have a bruise near a knee, ankle, wrist, or other joint that leads to swelling of the joint. • If you develop bruises that are not the result of an injury, let your doctor know.

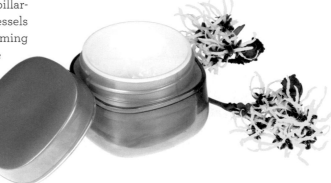

▶ | BURNS

The first step in treating minor burns is to stop the burning process as quickly as possible. Wick heat away by soaking the burned area in cool (not cold!) water or applying a cool, moist compress for five to ten minutes. Once the fiery sensation eases, assess the damage. If the skin is simply red, slightly swollen, and tender, you've probably got a first-degree burn—only the outermost layer of skin has been harmed. If you see tiny blisters, the damage went deep enough to cause a second-degree burn. Most

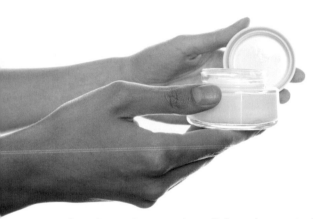

first-degree burns and small (less than an inch or two across) second-degree burns can usually be safely treated at home. For anything more serious, head to the emergency room.

Nurse a Burn or Scald

- **Clean After Cooling** After cooling the burn with water, gently pat the area dry. Clean the burned area of any grit or dirt carefully, being sure not to break the skin or any blisters that have formed.
- **Apply Aloe** Once the burn is completely cooled, apply aloe vera cream or gel to the burned area to soothe the damaged skin and speed healing. You can also snip off a leaf from an aloe plant and apply the mucilaginous gel that oozes from the leaf in the same way. Alternatively, apply calendula salve (see the section on cuts and scrapes).
- **Keep It Covered** Next, cover the burn with a sterile gauze pad or bandage to ease pain and reduce the chance of infection. Wrap or tape gauze loosely in place so that no pressure is on the burn.
- **Ease With Vitamin E** As the burn starts to heal, pierce a capsule of vitamin E and rub the liquid gently into the damaged skin several times a day to keep the healing skin from drying out and cracking and to help prevent scarring.

Soothe a Sunburn

- **Have a Soak** To relieve the pain of extensive sunburn, soak in a tub of soothing lukewarm water into which you've swirled a cup or two of aloe vera juice or two tablespoons of baking soda. Afterward, apply a thin coating of aloe gel on the burned area.

- **Cool It** Add 2 drops of peppermint oil to 1 cup of lukewarm water. Chill the mixture until cold. Saturate a cotton ball with the liquid and use to gently bathe sunburned areas.

LAVENDER & ALOE SOOTHING MIST

Adapted from Kathi Keville and Mindy Green, *Aromatherapy*. Spritz sunburned skin with this soothing combination.

½ cup all-natural, unflavored aloe vera juice
½ teaspoon lavender essential oil
1 tablespoon organic apple cider vinegar
1 capsule vitamin E

Place the first three ingredients in a small bowl. Pierce the vitamin E capsule and squeeze its contents into the bowl. Whisk everything together and pour the mixture into a small spray bottle. Refrigerate until cold. Mist sunburned skin as needed (shake before using).

- **Tame the Itch** As sunburned skin heals, it may begin to itch and flake. Tame the itch by adding a powdered oatmeal preparation such as Aveeno to a tub of cool water, or by placing 2 cups of ordinary breakfast oats in a cheesecloth bag (or tied up in a handkerchief) and adding the bag to the water as the tub fills.
- **Chill With Green Tea** Brew a strong solution of green tea by placing 3 to 4 green tea bags in a pot and adding about 2 cups of just-boiled water. Steep for 15 minutes, pour the tea into a bowl, and then refrigerate until cold. Saturate a washcloth in the chilled tea and apply as a soothing compress.

good to know: ABOUT BURNS

- Don't cool a burn with ice or ice water— exposing damaged skin to intense cold can make things worse.
- Despite what your grandmother might have said, skip the butter or bacon grease. Putting these fatty substances on a burn can slow healing and may cause an infection.

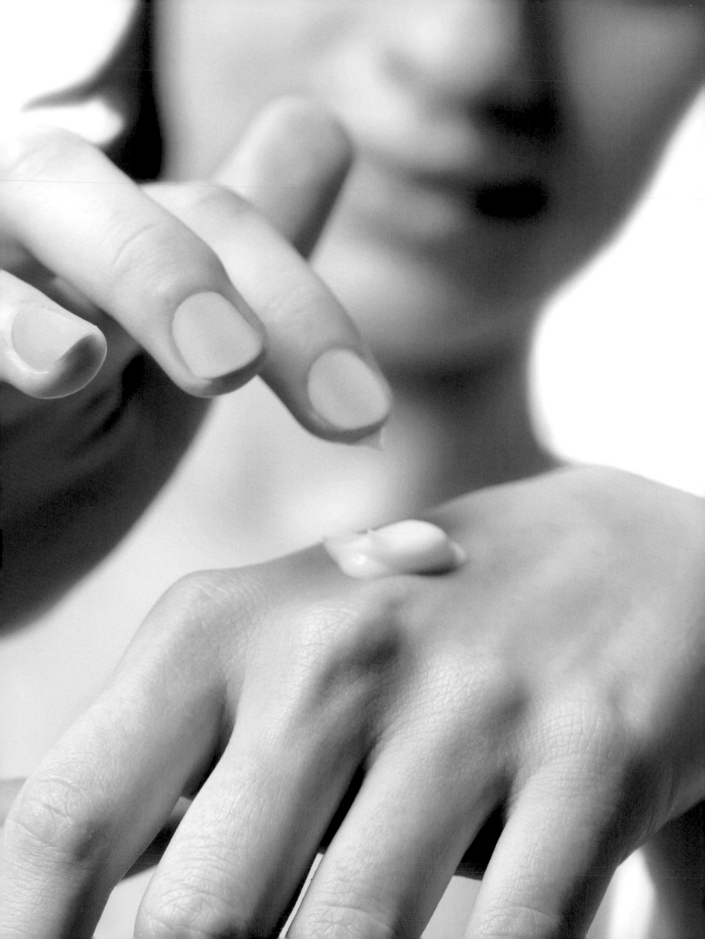

Skin Infections

15 SIMPLE WAYS TO FEND OFF INFECTION

Skin is the body's largest organ, a thin but remarkably strong and stretchy covering that protects what's inside us from the assaults of the outside world. It is our first line of defense against harmful chemicals, temperature extremes, potentially threatening disease agents, and the destructive rays of the sun. Skin is also dynamic. Cells in the outermost layer are constantly being replaced—at the astounding rate of 30,000 to 40,000 per minute—by new cells formed in underlying layers. For all its toughness, though, skin is not impenetrable. Under the right circumstances, bacteria, fungi, and viruses can gain a foothold to cause infection.

▶ | ACNE

Acne is often considered a bane of teenagers, but it can occur in people of just about any age. One cause is skin cells producing an excess of a protein called keratin, which in turn blocks oil ducts inside hair follicles, the tiny openings in skin from which hairs grow. Blocked follicles can become a breeding ground for bacteria. The result is nasty skin eruptions ranging from whiteheads and blackheads to pus-filled pimples and inflamed, painful, boil-like cysts. Over-the-counter and prescription medicines are available to treat acne. But home remedies are also worth a try.

Ban Those Blemishes

- **Try Tea Tree Oil** Tea tree oil has known antibacterial properties. One approach to treating acne with tea tree oil is to cleanse the affected area daily with tea tree oil soap or tea tree oil cleansing pads, and then apply a tea tree oil gel—all are available at many natural food stores. (A recent study showed that a gel with 5 percent tea tree oil works almost as well as 5 percent benzoyl peroxide, one of the most common over-the-counter acne treatments.) Alternatively, add 2 to 3 drops of tea tree essential oil to ½ cup of very warm water. Saturate a cotton ball with this mixture and dab onto affected areas.

⚠ **CAUTION:** Never apply undiluted tea tree essential oil to bare skin. Be careful not to get tea tree oil solution into eyes. Allergic reactions and contact dermatitis have been reported in some people using tea tree oil. If redness, itching, or oozing develops after topical application, stop using the solution and consult your doctor.

- **Spice Up the Solution** A folk remedy for treating pimples consists of mixing equal amounts of powdered nutmeg and honey to make a paste. Dab a little of this mix on a pimple, leave on for 20 minutes, and then rinse off.
- **Make a Mask** Some people find that applying a thin coating of milk of magnesia (a solution of magnesium hydroxide

good to know: ABOUT ACNE

- Don't squeeze, pick, or prick pimples or other forms of acne.
- Wash affected areas gently—don't use a washcloth, scrubbing pad, or loofah, and avoid harsh astringents and masks.
- Dirt, sweat, and bacteria can all make acne worse, so avoid touching your face or resting your chin or cheek on your hands.

usually taken as a laxative) to acne areas at bedtime can help.

■ *Ice It* At the first sign of a pimple, slip an ice cube into a small zip-top bag, or wrap in a single layer of damp paper towel. Hold the cube on the pimple for 30 to 60 seconds. Repeat several times a day.

■ *Apply a Compress* Another option to reduce acne-related redness is to soak a chamomile tea bag in cold water, squeeze out most of the water, and apply it to skin for about 30 seconds.

⚠ **CAUTION:** Avoid using chamomile if you are allergic to ragweed, asters, chrysanthemum, and other plants in the Asteraceae family.

▶ ATHLETE'S FOOT

Opportunistic fungi cause this very common infection in the skin's outermost layer. The classic symptom is itchy, reddened, flaking, or scaling skin. Athlete's foot typically takes hold in the skin between toes, but it can also appear on the soles and sides of the feet, and may even spread to toenails (or to the groin area, where it's called jock itch). Moisture is this fungus's best friend, meaning locker rooms, swimming pools, and bathrooms are likely sites of contamination. But insulated boots, thermal socks, plastic shoes, and damp sneakers can also promote infection. The fungi that cause athlete's foot are persistent; treatment can take weeks. There are many OTC antifungal creams and sprays for this skin infection, but many natural remedies as well. The following remedies are largely based on anecdotal evidence, rather than scientific studies.

Fight the Fungus

■ *Treat With Tea Tree* There is good scientific evidence that tea tree oil has relatively strong fungus-fighting properties. Soak feet for ten minutes in a pan of shallow water (about 4 cups) to which you've added about 20 drops of tea tree oil. Dry thoroughly. Repeat morning and night.

■ *Try Oil × 2* Mix 4 to 5 drops tea tree oil with about 1 teaspoon of olive, almond, or avocado oil. Rub some of this mixture onto affected areas twice a day. Caution: Oily feet can be slippery; put on socks!

■ *Attack With Herbs* In a small container, add 10 drops of lavender essential oil, 10 drops of tea tree oil, and a dab of pure aloe vera gel to about 1 ounce of calendula salve (available in health food stores or make your own, see page 81). Mix well and rub a dab of this onto affected areas several times a day.

⚠ **CAUTION:** Oils and salves may interfere with evaporation of moisture on feet, and so potentially could encourage conditions that favor fungal growth. If your athlete's foot infection worsens after applying oils or salves, discontinue use and see your doctor.

▶ WARTS

Warts are small, typically benign skin tumors caused by some of the dozens of different strains of the human papillomavirus. Common warts tend to appear on people's hands, although they can show up on feet, faces, and necks as well. Plantar warts typically

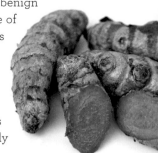

good to know: ABOUT ATHLETE'S FOOT

— Don't take baths if you have athlete's foot, because the fungus can be transferred to the groin or vaginal area as a result of tiny pieces of fungal-infected skin becoming suspended in the water.

— Avoid walking barefoot in public showers, locker rooms, and pool areas.

— After showering, use a separate towel to dry affected areas. Wash these potentially contaminated towels in hot water and dry on high heat.

HOMEMADE MASK FOR BEAUTIFUL SKIN

"Every vegetable, fruit, seed, or nut has a place in a facial or body mask," writes herbalist Jeanne Rose. All these foods add nutrients, and attributes such as texture, that work to benefit caring for the skin. Depending on the ingredients chosen, masks absorb oils, draw out impurities, treat acne, and cleanse. To make a simple mask, try peaches and cream. Combine 2 peeled and mashed peaches and 1 tablespoon heavy cream in a bowl, mash with a spoon, and stir to blend. Clean your face with a warm, wet washcloth so that you are applying the mask to damp skin. Smooth the peaches and cream mask onto your face gently and let set for about 15 minutes. Rinse with warm water.

–Annie B. Bond
Author and eco-friendly living expert

grow on the soles of the foot, and can be quite painful. Flattened plane warts often occur, like common warts, on the face, but they usually grow in clumps. OTC preparations and medical interventions such as burning, freezing (cryotherapy), and surgery often work well to get rid of these types of warts. However, many people find home remedies can be quite effective, too. The following remedies are suggested primarily for plantar warts.

War on Warts

- **Apply Oils** Soak the wart in warm water for about 15 minutes. Dry thoroughly and then apply a drop of tea tree oil diluted with a drop of almond or olive oil. Cover with a bandage. Repeat daily.
- **Try Turmeric** Scientific studies have shown that the herb turmeric contains a substance, curcumin, that inhibits certain strains of human papillomavirus. Some people have had success using turmeric to fight plantar warts. Here is a technique to try: Mix about ½ teaspoon of dried turmeric powder with enough olive or almond oil to make a stiff paste. Roll the paste into a little ball, position

it over the wart, and flatten gently to cover the wart's extent. Cover with an adhesive bandage. Replace with fresh paste once a day.

⚠ **CAUTION:** Turmeric applied to skin may cause irritation in some people. If an irritation does develop, discontinue use.

- **Soak With Vinegar** Douse a cotton ball in vinegar and tape it over the wart with an elastic bandage for one to two hours daily.
- **Treat With Duct Tape** Cover the wart with a piece of duct tape for six days (replace the tape daily). Then soften the wart by soaking it in warm water and remove the outermost layer by buffing gently with an emery board (dispose of the emery board, as it could harbor virus particles). Repeat this process for up to two months.
- **Go for Garlic** Another anecdotal home remedy for wart removal is to place a bit of minced fresh garlic onto the wart and cover with a bandage or piece of duct tape. Repeat with fresh garlic daily.

⚠ **CAUTION:** Stop treatment if garlic causes skin irritation.

- **Try Banana Peel** Some people have reported success at wart removal using banana peel. The procedure is to cut a piece of banana peel slightly larger than the wart. Place the pale, fleshy side over the wart and tape in place with duct tape. Leave on overnight. Repeat daily for several weeks, using a new piece of peel each time.

good to know: ABOUT WARTS

- Don't scratch or pick at warts. You may pick up the virus on your fingers and could possibly transfer it to other areas of skin.
- Warts tend to thrive in moist, warm environments, so keep infected areas as dry a possible.
- For warts on the face, it's best to see a doctor about removal because of potential cosmetic concerns.

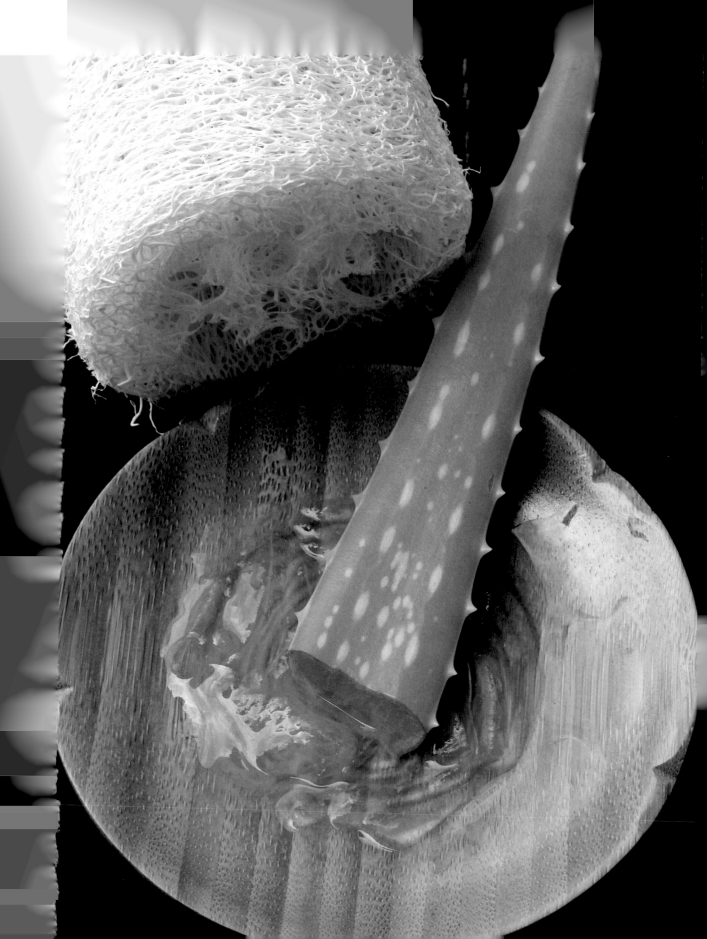

Skin Irritations

13 CURES FOR ITCHES, STINGS, & SPLINTERS

Human skin contains millions of sensory receptors. These specialized nerve endings inform you about what's happening at the body's surface and in the world beyond it. Skin has receptors that sense pressure, vibration, stretching, heat, cold, and of course, pain. Hundreds of pain receptors are packed into every square inch. Like little alarms systems, they let you know when your protective outer covering has been breached. Blisters, splinters, and insect bites and stings may seem minor, but they can cause enough pain to bring tears to your eyes. Natural remedies can help.

▶ | BLISTERS

Oh, the agony of breaking in a new pair of shoes. Stiff leather chafes with every step and, before you know it, you've got a blister. A blister is a small pocket of clear fluid, called plasma, that's been released by damaged cells and causes the skin's outermost layer to separate from underlying tissue. Friction is a common cause of blisters, but they can also form when skin is burned, frostbitten, or exposed to certain types of chemicals. Although the temptation to puncture a blister can be great, resist the urge. When blisters appear, cleanse them

gently and pat dry. Then take simple steps to help reduce pain and speed healing.

⚕ **WHEN TO CALL THE DR.:** See your health care provider if you have a blister that covers an area the size of your palm or larger. • Get medical treatment for a blister that becomes infected. Signs include inflammation, pus, and red streaks radiating from the blister. • If you have diabetes, blisters are more likely to develop without warning, take longer to heal, and become infected. Call at the first sign of infection.

Baby Those Blisters

- **Soften and Soothe** To minimize further friction and soothe the outer layer of skin on a blister, dab on a little pure aloe vera gel several times a day. Cover with a small adhesive bandage or a piece of gauze during the day.
- **Cool With a Compress** Cool a hot, painful blister with a lavender compress. Lavender (see page 99) is mildly antiseptic. Add a drop or two of lavender essential oil to a cup of

---

good to know: ABOUT BLISTERS

— If you pop a blister or it pops on its own, don't remove the loose skin that overlies it. Leave it in place to protect the sensitive (fragile) skin underneath.

— Never pop a blister caused by a burn, as this can lead to infection.

— Use moleskin—soft adhesive pads available at any drugstore—on chafed areas where a blister is likely to form if irritation continues.

— Prevent blisters on your hands by wearing work gloves.

— If you repeatedly get blisters on your feet, have your feet measured at a shoe store. You may be wearing shoes that are too tight.

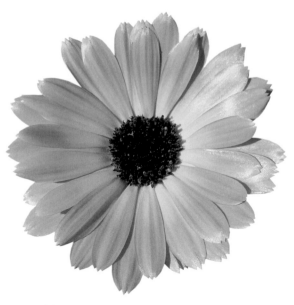

antiseptic properties. Calendula creams (available at natural food stores and some drugstores) can soothe minor skin injuries and speed healing. Follow package directions.

▶ | BITES & STINGS

Some insects bite because they want your blood. Mosquitoes and bedbugs fall into this category. Bees, wasps, and ants, together with spiders, often bite or sting only when they feel threatened or find themselves near or on you without an obvious means of escape. If you are allergic to bee or wasp stings or have been bitten by a venomous spider, seek medical help immediately. Otherwise, turn to simple remedies to soothe the irritations that result from creepy-crawly attacks.

Creepy-Crawly Counterattack

- ***Ice It*** For mosquito or bug bites, rub the bite with an ice cube for three to five minutes to help reduce swelling. Keep the ice cube constantly moving so as not to damage the skin.
- ***Rub With Onion*** A folk remedy for insect stings and bites is to cut a piece of fresh onion and apply the cut side directly to the sting for several minutes.
- ***Scrape Out a Stinger*** If you've been stung by

cold water. Saturate a soft cloth, wring out excess moisture, and apply to the blister for a few minutes. Repeat several times a day.

- ***Try Horse Chestnut*** Horse chestnut is an herb used traditionally to treat skin sores and other irritations, particularly those that involve swelling. Add about 1 teaspoon of horse chestnut tincture (available at natural food stores) to 1 cup of cool water. Fold a piece of gauze or soft cloth into pad about twice the size of the blister. Saturate it with the liquid, and apply to the blister for 20 minutes. Repeat several times a day.
- ***Heal With Calendula*** Calendula (see page 79) is an herb with anti-inflammatory and

BLISTER-SOOTHING SALVE

$^2/_3$ cup calendula oil (available at some natural food stores or online)
2 tablespoons pure beeswax, chopped fine (have a little extra on hand)
5 drops tea tree essential oil
5 drops lavender essential oil

Place the calendula oil in the top of a double boiler and warm gently over low heat. Add 2 tablespoons chopped beeswax and continue to warm the mixture, stirring occasionally, until the wax is completely melted. Remove from heat and let cool slightly. To test what the salve's final consistency will be, place 1 tablespoon of the mixture in the freezer for one to two minutes. If the cooled salve seems too firm, add a little more calendula oil to the mix. If it doesn't seem firm enough, gently reheat the oil/wax mixture in the double boiler and add a little more beeswax and heat again until completely melted. When you're satisfied, add the essential oils and stir well to combine. Pour the mixture into clean, dark-colored glass jars with tight-fitting lids. Apply the salve to blisters and other minor skin irritations.

a honeybee, chances are the barbed stinger and the little poison sac attached to it, are still stuck in your skin. Working quickly, use something with a straight, flat edge—a credit card can work well—to gently scrape the stinger out (scrape in the opposite direction that the stinger went in). Don't try to pick the stinger out with your fingernails or a tweezers, as this could put pressure on the poison sac and inject more honeybee venom into your skin. After the stinger is out, wash the area well, and ice it (see opposite).

> **WHEN TO CALL THE DR.:** If you've been stung by any insect and have difficulty breathing, a rapid pulse, or swelling in your mouth or throat, head to the emergency room or call 911.

▶ | SPLINTERS

Splinters (or slivers) are tiny fragments of a substance such as wood, metal, or glass that become embedded in the skin. Splinters can also come from handling plants with thorns, such as blackberries, or needles, such as cacti. The sharp plant part punctures the skin and buries itself under the surface. Splinters that have been driven deep into the skin—or far under a fingernail—are probably best removed by a doctor. But for minor cases, treatment at home can usually fix the problem. Although the standard technique for removing splinters in many households is to try to tease them out using sterilized tweezers—or dig them out with a sterilized needle—this is not always successful and can be more painful than the splinter itself. Consider trying some of these remedies first.

Splinter Strategies

■ *Bathe It* Warm water may help bring a splinter to the skin's surface, especially if it is made of wood (as the wood gets wet, it has a tendency to swell). Soak the skin with the splinter in warm water for 15 minutes several times a day. If the splinter begins to emerge, grab it with tweezers and gently tug it free.

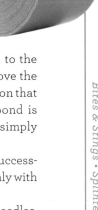

■ *Use Epsom Salts* This time-tested remedy can help draw out splinters and stingers. Add a tablespoon of Epsom salts to a bowl of water and soak the sliver for 20 minutes.

■ *Tape It* If part of the splinter is protruding from the skin, place a piece of duct tape over it. Press gently to ensure that the tape adheres well to the splinter's protruding end. Then remove the tape, pulling it in the opposite direction that the splinter went in. If the sticky bond is strong enough, you might be able to simply pull out the splinter.

■ *Cleanse It* Once a splinter has been successfully removed, clean the area thoroughly with soap and water.

■ *Glue It* For one or more tiny cactus needles, often too small to see, spread liquid white school glue such as Elmer's on the affected area. Let the glue dry and spread a second, maybe even a third, layer on the area. Let each dry completely. You should be able to painlessly lift the dried glue off the skin, and chances are good that the cactus needles will come out with it.

good to know: ABOUT SPLINTERS

— Don't ignore an embedded splinter that has become infected. Signs of infection include pus, swelling and inflammation, and red streaks radiating from the splinter site. If any of these symptoms are present, seek medical care.

— Wear gloves when working with materials such as wood or prickly plants that tend to be sources of slivers, or when picking up broken glass.

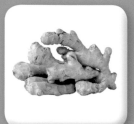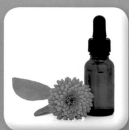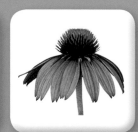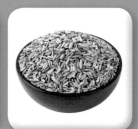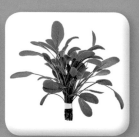

CHAPTER TWO

herbs for

healing

Healing Herbs

155 POINTERS ON MEDICINAL PLANTS

Plants are the oldest medicines, and every ancient culture developed herbal therapies based on plants that grew close at hand. Ayurveda, a largely plant-based system of traditional medicine native to India (see page 263), came into being at least 5,000 years ago. Traditional Chinese medicine (see page 295) is almost as old, and its vast collection of herbal remedies includes thousands of medicinal plants as ingredients. Australia's Aborigines, however, have the oldest system of herbal medicine, dating back some 50,000 years, and throughout that time have used many of the continent's plants for treating injuries, illness, and disease.

Natural Solutions

This chapter includes 14 herbs selected because they are well known and relatively common, they're typically easy to find in stores and online (and in some cases, easy to grow as well), and they can be used to treat a variety of minor ailments. Calendula and chamomile are native to southern and southeastern Europe; both have been used for many centuries to treat skin conditions, and chamomile is a very old remedy for digestive upsets. The intensely fragrant herbs lavender, lemon balm, rosemary, and sage all hail originally from regions bordering the Mediterranean Sea. St. John's wort also has its botanical roots in Europe and has been prized for its mild sedative effects since at least the time of the ancient Greeks. Fennel, ginger, and turmeric are indigenous

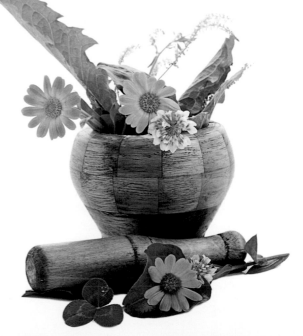

to Asia and Southeast Asia. Ginger and turmeric have both been used in traditional Chinese medicine and Ayurvedic medicine for hundreds, if not thousands, of years. Peppermint comes from England, the result of a natural cross between two other members of the mint family. North America's representatives in this chapter are echinacea, a home remedy for treating colds and flu, and slippery elm, renowned for its throat-coating, stomach-soothing mucilage. Finally, tea tree is a versatile herb from Australia, used by Aborigines for possibly tens of thousands of years, but only "discovered" in the 20th century.

Use With Care

Like the home remedies in Chapter 1, many of the herbal remedies in this chapter have been passed down from generation to generation. In some cases, their effectiveness is supported by scientific research, but in others, evidence as to how well a particular remedy works may be largely anecdotal. Some people mistakenly believe that if a remedy is "natural," there's no chance that it might have side effects. This isn't true. Herbs are plants, and certain plants—in any form—can cause allergic and other negative reactions in some people. Research has also shown that some herbs can potentially interfere with the action of various prescription medications. Before using any of the remedies in this chapter, carefully read any cautionary notes included with them. If you're not sure that a natural remedy might be safe for you, consult your health care provider.

SIMPLE TRUTHS FROM HISTORY

Christopher Columbus is not only credited with discovering America but he also initiated the transoceanic trade of plants from one continent to another. You may think of potatoes as Irish, but until Europeans' arrival in the Andes, potatoes were unknown elsewhere. The same is true of corn, now a dietary staple for much of the world's population. Columbus brought lemons to the Americas and introduced chocolate and red peppers to the rest of the world. Now the entire spectrum of the world's herbs is available either from your local natural food store or on the Internet. But with thousands of choices of herbs and herbal products, how do you begin to choose what's right for you? The answer—as you will see in this chapter—is "keep it simple."

In medieval European herbal traditions, single herbs gathered from the garden or countryside were known as "simples." These were the common herbs that most people knew and used, because they were readily available and because they worked. In this chapter, you will find information on the origin, benefits, and practical use of 14 simples—herbs that are readily available from your garden, or grocery and natural food stores. Chances are you already have some of them in your kitchen cabinets. The vast world of herbs—providing real remedies and benefits, many backed by scientific research—awaits you.

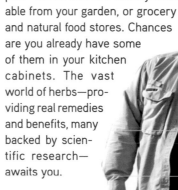

Steven Foster
Herbalist, author, photographer, and lecturer on medicinal plants around the world

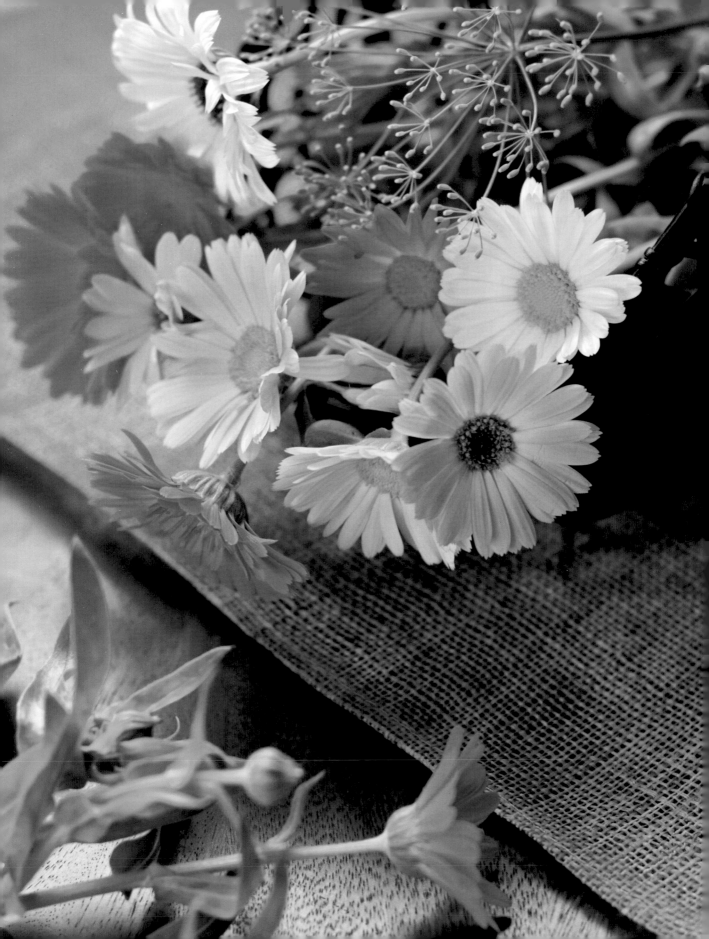

Calendula

11 WAYS TO BE KIND TO YOUR SKIN

Cheery calendula (*Calendula officinalis*) is an ancient herb native to southern Europe and North Africa that is now widely cultivated. It's sometimes called pot marigold, but don't confuse it with the pungently scented common or French marigold of the genus *Tagetes*. In the garden, calendula's blossoms are unmistakable: a single or double whorl of brilliant yellow or orange-yellow petals around a central disk, held stiffly upright above somewhat sticky foliage. In ancient times, this lovely herb was prized for its ornamental, cosmetic, and culinary properties. That's right: Calendula flowers are edible! In medieval England, the petals were dried by the barrelful, then churned into syrups and conserves, added to winter stews, and baked into breads.

Calendula has been valued as a healing herb since at least the 1100s. One of its primary uses has been as a remedy for skin ailments, ranging from minor wounds and abrasions to acne and eczema. But it also has a long track record as a remedy for fevers, stomach upsets, and ulcers. Today, calendula is used in herbal medicine to treat many of the same conditions, and with good reason. Its therapeutic properties are supported by sound scientific research. Calendula has been shown to exhibit notable anti-inflammatory properties and to promote wound healing, stimulating relatively rapid regeneration of new tissue. In clinical studies, the herb has been shown to be effective in preventing dermatitis in patients undergoing radiation therapy for breast cancer. Calendula inhibits the growth of many types of bacteria, and also provides some protection against damaging ultraviolet rays.

▶ | WOUNDS

The bacteria-inhibiting and skin-regenerating powers of calendula make it an herb to reach for when you've cut, scraped, or otherwise abraded your skin. It's very effective as an all-around topical first aid remedy that helps stop minor bleeding, ease pain, and promote rapid healing. Think of it as one of nature's remedies for life's little accidents. You can find calendula in several forms—lotions, salves, ointments, and tinctures—at most health food stores. Alternatively, use dried or fresh calendula petals to make your own skin-soothing remedies.

---

good to know: ALSO FOR WOUNDS

- Arnica (*Arnica montana*) is an herb with a long history as a treatment for bruises and swellings. Look for arnica gel or cream that contains real arnica extract (not a homeopathic dilution) at natural food stores. ⚠ **CAUTION:** Arnica is for external use only. Never use arnica on broken skin or open wounds.
- Comfrey (*Symphytum officinale*) should never be taken internally. However, comfrey ointments, creams, poultices, and liniments—applied externally to unbroken skin—can also help heal bruises and may ease the pain of injured or arthritic joints. ⚠ **CAUTION:** Use only topical preparations of comfrey that have been purified of toxic pyrrolizidine alkaloids.

Flower Power

- *Try a Compress* Bring quick relief to a scraped elbow or skinned knee by steeping 2 teaspoons of dried calendula flowers in a cup of just-boiled water. Cool, strain, and then saturate a cloth with the liquid to make a compress. Apply to the injury for about 15 minutes. Rather than discarding the herbs you've strained out of the liquid, use them to make a soothing poultice. Wrap the damp calendula flowers in gauze and place this over the injury for 10 to 15 minutes. Either the poultice or compress can be used several times daily, rewetting as needed.

- *Dab On a Tincture* Keep a tincture of calendula (see the Calendula Tincture recipe below) on hand for dabbing on scrapes, cuts, burns, rashes, and insect bites and stings. Rub a drop on sore gums or canker sores to soothe them as well. Although calendula is not an antifungal herb, this tincture could be used in combination with fungus-killing tea tree oil (see pages 127–128) to help relieve inflammation associated with athlete's foot.

> ⚠ **CAUTION:** Side effects of calendula are rare. However, if you are allergic to ragweed, chrysanthemums, daisies, and other plants in the aster family, you may develop a sensitivity to topical use of this herb. Discontinue use if a rash or other skin irritation develops. Do not use calendula internally during pregnancy.

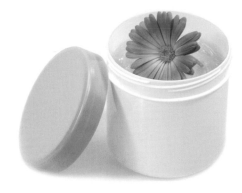

- *Smooth On Salve* Calendula salve is available at most natural food stores. It's a good item to keep stocked in your medicine cabinet or first aid kit. Follow package directions.

▶ | IRRITATED SKIN

Calendula is an exceptionally effective remedy for inflamed, chapped, cracked, and otherwise irritated skin, including diaper rash. Topical preparations of calendula are widely used in Europe, and similar formulations can be found in health food stores and pharmacies in the United States. Calendula's soothing properties are the result of it being rich in anti-inflammatory compounds called flavonoids. Take a look at the ingredients for herbal and skin care lotions, face creams, moisturizers, and similar products, and you'll find calendula listed in many of them. At least one study has shown that, applied externally, calendula can help hydrate skin, too.

RECIPE FOR HEALTH

CALENDULA TINCTURE

4 ounces dried, whole calendula petals or flower heads
Clean 1-pint glass jar with screw-on lid
1 pint grain (80-proof) alcohol (vodka works well)
Dark brown glass bottles with tight-fitting caps (available in health food stores; enough to hold roughly a pint of tincture)
Cheesecloth

1. Grind the dried herb to a powder using a mortar and pestle or a clean electric coffee grinder.
2. Place the powdered herb in the glass jar, and fill to the top with alcohol.
3. Screw on the lid and store in a cool, dark place for two weeks to steep. Shake the jar twice daily.
4. Two weeks later, strain the liquid through a sieve lined with a double layer of cheesecloth.
5. Pour the finished tincture into dark, labeled glass bottles.

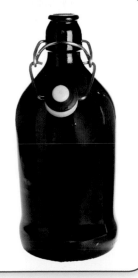

Petals for Protection

- **Soothe a Sunburn** To help protect and heal chapped or sunburned skin, it's hard to beat calendula salve. You can make your own quite easily. Coarsely chop 2 ounces dried calendula flowers in a blender or electric coffee grinder. Place the chopped herb in a pint-size, wide-mouth, screw-top jar and fill almost to the top with olive or sesame oil. Stir to make sure the chopped herb is well distributed in, and completely saturated by, the oil. Then screw on the lid and let the mixture steep for about two weeks. Pour the steeped oil through a strainer lined with two to three layers of cheesecloth. Next, in the top of a double boiler, melt about 1.5 ounces of beeswax (available from health food stores, or better yet, a beekeeper) to the strained oil. Add a few drops of tincture of bezoin (available at most drugstores) as a bacteria-inhibiting preservative. Test the salve's consistency by putting a spoonful in the freezer for a few minutes. If it's too thin when cool, add a little more melted beeswax to the oil. If too thick, add a teaspoon or so of additional olive or sesame oil; mix well. When you think you've got the right consistency, pour the salve into small, labeled jars.
- **Try a Quick Mix** If you don't have time to make a salve like the one described, you can make a reasonably effective substitute by mixing a few drops of calendula tincture with a dab of aloe vera gel. Apply this mix to irritated skin.

▶ | INFLAMMATION

In centuries past, calendula tea was a standard treatment for upset stomach, ulcers of the mouth, skin conditions, and minor wounds.

Many herbalists still recommend calendula tea for these problems. Calendula tea is palatable, gentle in its actions, and easy to brew. Simply pour a cup of just-boiled water over 1 to 2 teaspoons of dried calendula flowers. Cover the mixture and let the herbs steep for ten minutes, and then strain.

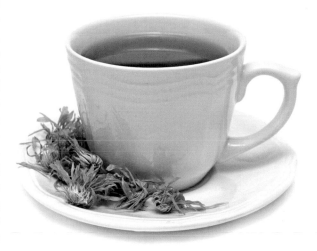

Soothing Solutions

- **Take a Tea Break** For mild indigestion, drink a cup or two of calendula tea.
- **Go for the Gargle** For a sore throat, use the cooled tea as a gargle several times a day.
- **Treat Mouth Sores** Soak the end of a cotton swab in the cooled tea and dab it on canker sores or sore areas where braces or other dental work have irritated the mouth's lining.
- **Swish and Spit** Use the cooled tea as a mouthwash to sooth swollen, irritated gums. Swish gently over affected areas and spit; repeat several times a day.
- **Dab It On** Calendula tea can also be used to treat minor wounds, in much the same way that calendula tincture (see recipe and bullet, opposite page) can be used.

good to know: ALSO FOR IRRITATED SKIN

Aloe *(Aloe vera)* is another herbal skin soother. Aloe contains a thick, mucilaginous gel inside its fleshy leaves that has been shown to be helpful in treating burns as well as other minor skin irritations (see pages 65 and 71).

Witch hazel *(Hamamelis virginiana)* has a long tradition of use as a remedy for bruises, swellings, and a wide variety of skin irritations. Make sure to choose witch hazel made from real extract derived from the bark of the herb.

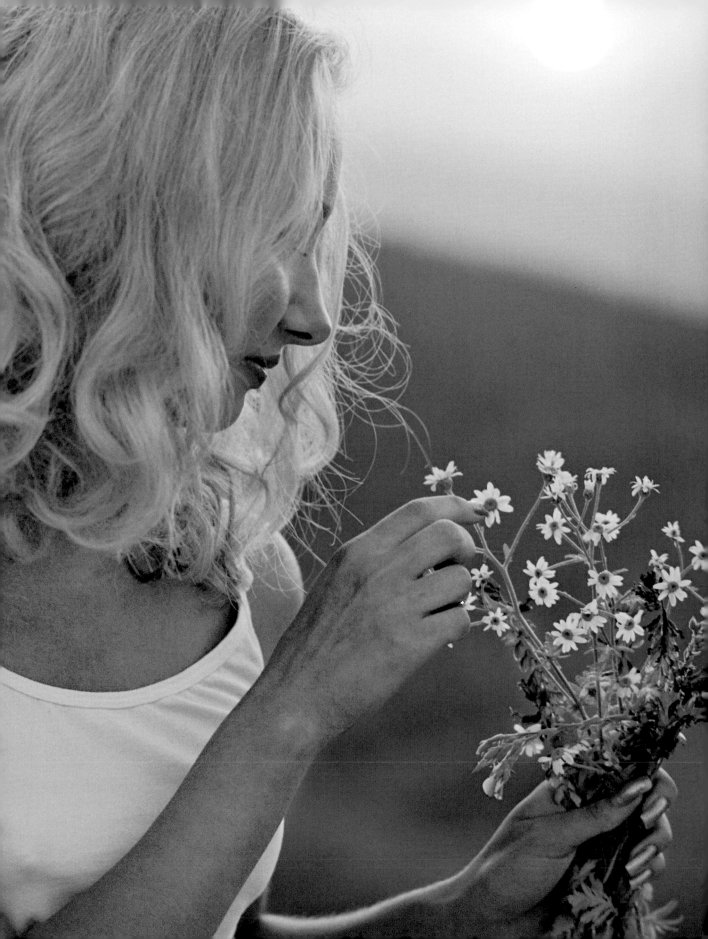

Chamomile

11 REASONS TO SMILE WITH CHAMOMILE

In medieval Europe, it's likely that chamomile grew in nearly every garden. It was a staple in the herbal medicine chest, as common to have on hand as aspirin or antacids are today. Chamomile was an herb that healers reached for to treat digestive upsets, muscle cramps, skin conditions, and nervous tension—in fact, almost any ailment. Healers gathered the cheery daisy-like flowers and apple-scented leaves and used them to create the ultimate soothing beverage: a cup of chamomile tea. When European colonists set sail for North America, they brought chamomile with them, of course. It wasn't long before the herb was rambling through American gardens and hanging to dry in great fragrant bunches from the rafters.

Over the years, chamomile hasn't lost its charm or its power to comfort and calm. It is one of the most popular and widely used herbs in the Western world. Chamomile is included in the pharmacopoeia—the official listings of approved drugs—of 26 countries.

There are two different types, or species, of chamomile used in herbal medicine. Buy a box of chamomile tea in the United Kingdom, and you'll very likely see Roman chamomile (*Chamaemelum nobile* or *Anthemis nobilis*) on the ingredient label. Almost everywhere else in Europe and in the United States, the chamomile of choice is German chamomile (*Matricaria recutita*). Although the two species differ somewhat in their chemical makeup, they are typically used in the same way to treat similar conditions. Most scientific research regarding chamomile's therapeutic effects, however, has been conducted on German chamomile.

▶ | DIGESTIVE UPSETS

In Beatrix Potter's classic *The Tale of Peter Rabbit*, chamomile tea was the prescription for Peter's tender tummy after he'd eaten too many vegetables from Mr. McGregor's garden. Modern herbalists—and many mothers and grandmothers—still consider chamomile tea a good antidote for stomach upsets in children and colic in infants. Many adults also find chamomile tea helpful for easing indigestion, bloating, and heartburn after meals. Research reveals that chamomile appears to exert protective effects on the digestive tract lining, to help relieve digestive spasms, and to soothe inflammation when taken internally. Some people also drink chamomile tea before bed to help induce sleep, but its sedative effects haven't been well studied.

good to know: ALSO FOR DIGESTIVE UPSETS

- Peppermint (*Mentha* x *piperita*) is another time-tested remedy for easing indigestion. You can brew peppermint tea easily using the dried leaf (see page 108). Research has shown that enteric-coated capsules of peppermint oil (available at some natural food stores) may ease the symptoms of irritable bowel syndrome in some people. Follow package directions.
- Goldenseal (*Hydrastis canadensis*) may also soothe the stomach and potentially aid digestion. It can be taken as a capsule or a tincture (follow package directions).

Tea Time

■ *Try the Classic Cure* When chamomile is used to treat digestive complaints, it is usually consumed as an herbal tea. Chamomile tea can be drunk either before or after meals. The recipe is simplicity itself. For a pot of tea, add 2 to 3 teaspoons of dried chamomile flowers per cup of water to the pot. Add just-boiled water and let the tea steep for five minutes. Strain, and sweeten with a little honey or other natural sweetener, if desired. Drink up to three cups a day. Children under five should not be given more than a half cup of tea a day.

■ *Add Apple* Crush a stalk of fresh chamomile and it will give off the distinct scent of apples. In fact, the Spanish name for the herb, *manzanilla,* means "little apple." Although most people enjoy the slightly fruity taste of plain chamomile tea, try this trick for adding real apple flavoring. Simply place two thin slices of apple in the bottom of a teapot. Mash slightly to release some of the juice. Add dried chamomile flowers and very hot water, as per the recipe in the previous bulleted item. Steep five minutes, strain, and sip.

■ *Go for a Combo* Ginger is another herb renowned for its ability to ease nausea, indigestion, and other stomach upsets (see pages 95–97). Combining ginger and chamomile makes for a slightly unusual chamomile tea with ginger's spicy heat. In a teapot, place 2 tablespoons of dried chamomile flowers and about a tablespoon of peeled, grated fresh ginger. Add just-boiled water and steep for five minutes. Strain and add a little honey or other natural sweetener to taste.

▶ | CANKER SORES

Canker sores (see page 45) and similar eroded areas or irritations in the lining of the mouth can be sensitive and painful. Anything that touches these sore spots, whether it's food, beverages, or a toothbrush, can make eating, drinking, and even talking difficult. Chamomile has long been a popular remedy for soothing canker sores. Herbalists sometimes recommend it as well for gingivitis, an inflammation of the gums also known as periodontal disease.

Swirl and Swish

■ *Make a Mild Mouthwash* The easiest way to use chamomile to treat canker sores is to brew a cup of chamomile tea, let it cool, and then use it as a mouthwash. Swirl a mouthful of the solution around in your mouth for a minute or so, letting it repeatedly bathe the irritated areas. Spit and repeat as often as needed.

■ *Rinse With Diluted Extract* Liquid extracts (tinctures) of German chamomile are available from health food stores and online. Make an oral rinse to soothe mouth irritation by adding 10 to 15 drops of German chamomile

---

HERBAL TEAS

In Ikaria, a longevity hot spot in Greece, locals use herbs and wild greens in teas for their diuretic effect. Steeping wild mint, chamomile, goldenrod, or other herbs in hot water is a lifelong, daily ritual in Ikaria. Diuretics encourage the kidneys to work and also expel more sodium with urine. This lowers blood pressure and can lower the risk of heart disease and dementia. Many herbal teas also have antiseptic and anti-inflammatory properties as well.

You can steep clean organic dandelion leaves, flowers, or roots in hot water for 20 minutes or steep 1 to 2 teaspoons of dried yarrow in a cup of hot water for 5 minutes. Or simply use the green tea found at your local supermarket or health food store to gain similar benefits.

–Dan Buettner
Author and lecturer on longevity

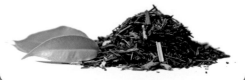

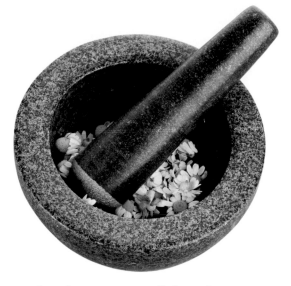

liquid extract to a small glass of warm water. Rinse with a mouthful for 30 to 60 seconds, and spit. Repeat several times a day.

- **Swab With Herbal Gel** A homemade herbal gel can help ease the pain of a canker sore. In a small glass jar, mix together a teaspoon each of echinacea liquid extract (tincture), goldenseal tincture, calendula tincture, and German chamomile tincture along with a generous tablespoon of pure aloe vera gel. Thoroughly combine the gel and the tinctures. Scoop up a dab of this mixture on the tip of a cotton swab and hold in place on a canker sore for 30 to 60 seconds. Keep the mixture refrigerated; discard after three days.

▶ | ECZEMA

The ancient Egyptians, Romans, and Greeks valued chamomile for its skin-calming properties. Chamomile is very popular in Europe for treating irritated skin, and a few studies have found that chamomile creams and lotions can help relieve the symptoms of psoriasis and eczema (see pages 59–60) in some people. In one study, a chamomile cream was shown to be helpful for relieving the itching and inflammation of eczema, although not quite as effectively as a low-dose, over-the-counter hydrocortisone cream.

Comfort With Chamomile

- **Soothe With a Soak** For eczema and other types of skin irritations, try a calming chamomile bath. Add ¼ pound of dried flowers or 10 drops of chamomile essential oil to a full tub of warm, but not hot, water.
- **Make a Poultice** Pulverize 2 tablespoons of dried chamomile flowers with a mortar and pestle or by pulsing briefly in a small food processor or clean coffee grinder. Add enough water or aloe vera gel to the ground herb to make a paste. Dab the paste over an area of inflamed skin and leave on for 20 minutes. Rinse with cool water.
- **Slather It On** A variety of chamomile ointments, lotions, and creams are available at most health food stores; they typically contain between 3 and 10 percent chamomile extract. Apply, following package directions, to help relieve symptoms of eczema.
- **Try the Tea Bag Too** Use a chamomile tea bag to make a cup of tea. Whether or not you drink the tea, use the cooled damp tea bag as a healing compress applied to a small area of eczema or otherwise irritated skin.

⚠ **CAUTION:** Chamomile is generally considered to be very safe, although rare allergic reactions have been reported in people who are allergic to ragweed, asters, chrysanthemums, and other plants in the Asteraceae family. Chamomile may make asthma worse, so people with asthma should not take it. Pregnant women should avoid chamomile because of the risk of miscarriage. Chamomile may have estrogen-like effects in the body, so women with a history of hormone-sensitive cancers, such as breast or uterine cancer, should ask their doctors before taking chamomile.

good to know: ALSO FOR ECZEMA

Witch hazel *(Hamamelis virginiana),* long prized for its astringent and antiseptic properties, may be useful for treating inflammation caused by eczema as well as other skin irritations. Look for real witch hazel that contains an extract of the herb; the witch hazel water often found in drugstores may have no witch hazel in it—read labels carefully.

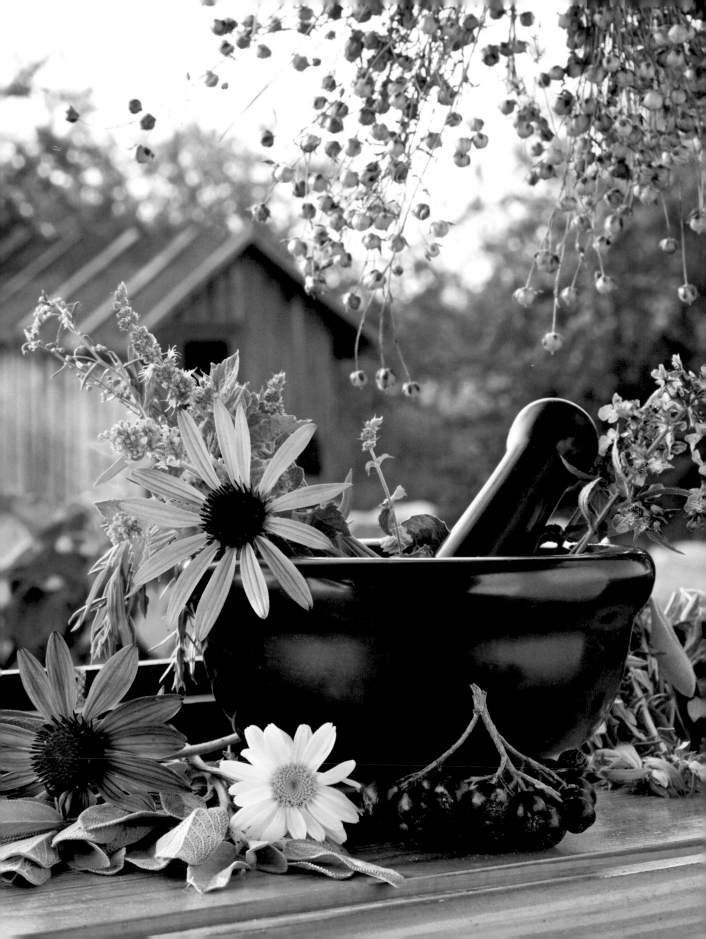

Echinacea

12 WAYS TO CURE COMMON COMPLAINTS

Native Americans were using several species of echinacea medicinally long before Europeans set foot in North America. Tribes living in the open, windswept heart of the continent considered this stately, upright plant of the prairie to be something of a universal cure-all, good for treating everything from coughs, colds, and colic to sores and sore throats. Although early settlers brought favorite herbs with them from their homelands across the sea, echinacea was a native plant they quickly adopted. By the 1800s, it was a go-to remedy for common complaints such as respiratory infections and skin conditions, as well as diphtheria, scarlet fever, malaria, and blood poisoning. With the development of antibiotics in the 1900s, use of echinacea began to decline in the United States, only to become increasingly popular in Europe—especially Germany—as an herbal remedy for colds and flu. Much of the medical research done on echinacea's effects has been carried out in Germany, and today it is one of the most well-studied plants in herbal medicine.

Laboratory studies have revealed that echinacea contains many health-promoting chemical compounds. Echinacea extracts have been shown to fight inflammation and inhibit some bacteria and viruses, and also seem to enhance the body's immune system function. Precisely how echinacea does this, however, remains unclear. Three species of echinacea are typically used in herbal medicine: *Echinacea purpurea,* the purple coneflower; *E. pallida,* the pale purple coneflower; and *E. angustifolia.* Scientists are investigating the medicinal properties of these (and other) species, but *E. purpurea* has been the focus of most research efforts.

▶ COLDS & FLU

People commonly use echinacea as an herbal remedy for colds and other upper respiratory tract ailments. Research shows the most effective way to use echinacea seems to be to start taking it at the first sign of a cold—the moment the sniffles or a scratchy throat make an appearance. There is some indication that taking echinacea at the start of a cold or other respiratory ailment may shorten its duration and lessen its severity, but more research needs to be done. Because different echinacea preparations can vary considerably in their level of active ingredients, it's a good idea to buy products made by reputable, established companies.

> ⚠ **CAUTION:** Because echinacea acts on the immune system, anyone with multiple sclerosis, HIV infection or AIDS, or other autoimmune conditions should not use this herb. Echinacea should also not be taken in conjunction with immunosuppressant drugs. If you are taking medication for any condition, including birth control pills, consult your physician before taking echinacea because the herb can affect the activity of certain drugs. People who are allergic to ragweed and other plants in the Asteraceae (daisy) family should avoid echinacea.

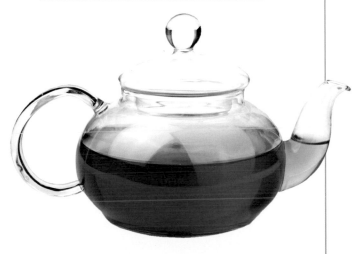

Snuff the Sniffles

- *Brew a Little Cold Care* Probably the most soothing way to take echinacea is by making echinacea tea. Add 1 or 2 teaspoons of dried echinacea to a cup and add just-boiled water. Steep for ten minutes, and then strain. Add a little honey or other natural sweetener, if desired. Drink one to three cups a day for no more than seven to ten days.

- *Spice It Up* Echinacea is not the most flavorful herb. If the taste isn't appealing, boost it by mixing it with other cold-care herbs. Here's how: Combine two parts dried echinacea, one part dried thyme, one part dried peppermint leaf, and one part dried hyssop in a small container. Steep a tablespoon of this mixture in a cup of just-boiled water for 15 minutes, and strain. Take up to three cups a day starting at the first sign of cold or flu symptoms.

⚠ **CAUTION:** Pregnant women should not use hyssop.

- *Gargle It Away* Next time you feel a sore throat or other cold and flu symptoms coming on, try a gargle using echinacea tincture, which is available in most health food stores. Add 2 teaspoons of tincture plus ½ teaspoon salt to a glass (about 8 ounces) of warm water. Stir well until the salt is completely dissolved. Take small mouthfuls, gargle, and spit. Repeat daily as needed.

- *Take a Tincture* Some herbalists recommend alcohol-based echinacea tinctures (preferably made from the root) as the most effective method for getting a dose of the herb's immune system–boosting compounds. At the first sign of a cold, add ½ teaspoon echinacea tincture to a small glass of warm water and drink. Repeat this three more times during the day so you are getting a total of 2 teaspoons tincture daily. Continue for up to a week.

▶ | WOUNDS & SORES

Echinacea is typically thought of as a cold and flu remedy. Yet it does have other therapeutic uses. Preparations of echinacea have mild antiseptic properties. When applied to minor cuts and scrapes, echinacea may help decrease inflammation and promote wound healing. Although more research needs to be done, there is also some indication that certain compounds in echinacea may help to dull or numb pain, making it a gentle remedy for soothing minor injuries.

Drips, Drops, & Dabs

- *Dab It On* Add several drops of echinacea tincture to a little warm water. Saturate a cotton ball with the solution and dab onto small cuts and scrapes or small abrasion-caused blisters that have burst and become raw.

---

good to know: ALSO FOR COLDS & FLU

— Several double-blind clinical trials have shown that the herb andrographis *(Andrographis paniculata)* may help reduce the severity of symptoms of upper respiratory infections such as the common cold. Be aware that andrographis can cause stomach upset in some people.

— Elder *(Sambucus nigra)* has a long history as a folk remedy for the common cold and other types of respiratory infections. Human studies have also found that elderberry juice may help shorten the duration of flu symptoms. Elder extracts are sometimes combined with zinc in lozenges for coughs and sore throat.

— Eucalyptus *(Eucalyptus globulus)* is an OTC ingredient in many cold remedies, including cough drops. It is also a common ingredient in ointments used to help relieve congestion due to colds and flu.

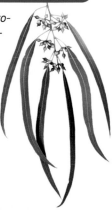

A GIFT FROM CHINA

Astragalus is an herb widely used in China to strengthen the immune system, especially during winter months when one is more prone to colds and flu. Science shows it increases substances in nasal secretions that help fight off viral infections. Astragalus is traditionally taken as a tea or added to soup. The following is a simple recipe for homemade Chinese astragalus soup:

4 cups vegetable broth
2 carrots, sliced
1 cup Chinese cabbage, sliced
4 slices astragalus root
1 teaspoon soy sauce, low sodium

Put all ingredients in a saucepan. Bring to boil, turn down the heat, and simmer covered for 20 minutes. Remove large slices of astragalus root and serve.

–Tieraona Low Dog, M.D.
Author and integrative medicine expert

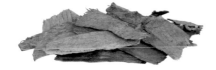

- **Make a Tea Bag Compress** Thoroughly saturate an echinacea tea bag with warm water. Use the bag as a compress to treat small skin injuries.
- **Rinse 'Em Away** Canker sores (see page 45) may benefit from a topical treatment of echinacea. Add several drops of echinacea tincture to a small glass of warm water. Swish the solution over the affected area for about 30 seconds and spit. Repeat as needed. If you don't have echinacea tincture, brew a strong cup of echinacea tea, let it cool, and then rinse your mouth in the same way.

- **Pack It In** An old folk remedy for sore or irritated gums is to grind a piece of dried echinacea root into a fine powder (use a clean coffee grinder). Wet the powder slightly and then pack it between your cheek and the sore gum.
- **Try a Double Whammy** An alternative to the previous remedy is to break open 2 echinacea capsules and mix the powder with enough aloe vera gel (make sure it is pure gel, with no additives) to make a paste about the consistency of toothpaste. Put a wad of this on a sore gum or canker sore.

▶ | BITES & STINGS

In the early 1900s, echinacea was promoted in parts of the United States as a treatment for snakebites. If you're bitten by a snake, skip the echinacea and seek immediate medical attention! But for easing the pain and swelling caused by insect bites, applying a tincture of the herb externally may help ease the discomfort.

Bite 'Em Back

- **Get a Drop on It** If a honeybee stings you, carefully remove the stinger. Then put one or two drops of echinacea tincture directly on the red, inflamed bump. Echinacea's slight pain-killing properties may ease the hurt, and its anti-inflammatory ingredients may lessen the swelling. Applying echinacea tincture is also a way to help sanitize the site of the sting. Treat insect bites in the same way.
- **Keep It Contained** Depending on the type of bite or sting, applying echinacea tincture might help keep any venom injected by the offending insect from spreading into nearby tissues. Chemical analyses on echinacea show that it seems to counteract venom's ability to slip between cells.

good to know: ALSO FOR WOUNDS & SORES

Dog rose (*Rosa canina*), the classic wild rose, has been used medicinally for centuries. In modern herbal medicine, dog rose petals are sometimes used in tonics and gargles for mouth sores. Vitamin C–rich rose hips are also used in preparations to treat colds and minor infections.

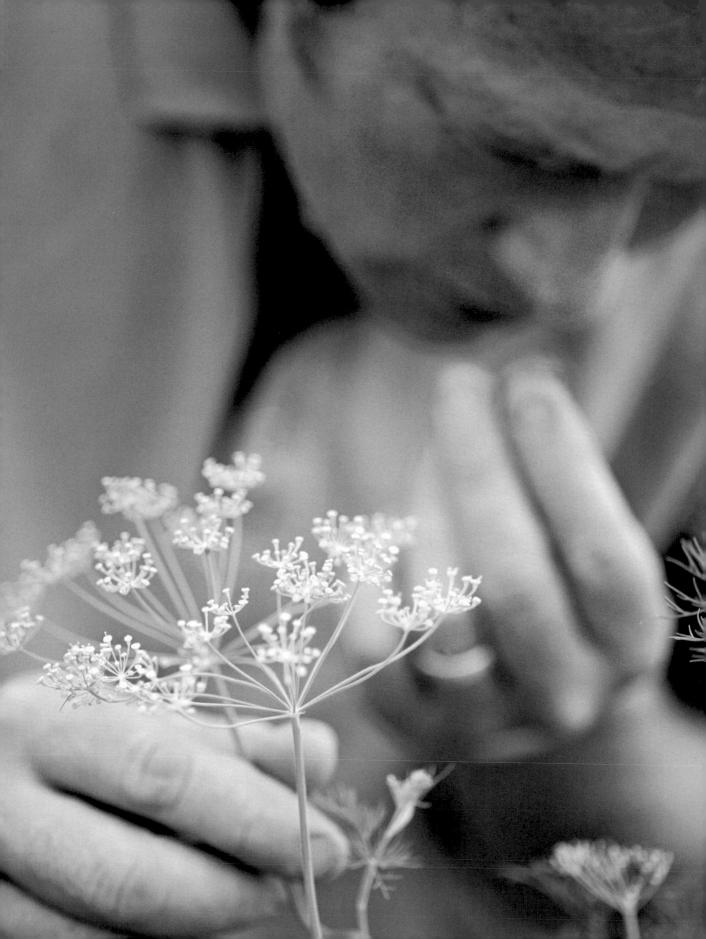

Fennel

12 WAYS TO GET A FENNEL FIX

Fennel has a rich history as a culinary herb, and a medicinal one. Closely related to anise, caraway, and dill, fennel (*Foeniculum vulgare*) produces small, hard seeds with a flavor similar to anise or licorice. If you've eaten authentic European rye breads or Italian sausages, you've probably encountered fennel seeds. The ancient Greeks may have been the first to appreciate fennel's medicinal properties. Both the Greeks and the Romans used fennel to treat a wide variety of health problems, particularly digestive upsets, including colic in infants. Practitioners of Ayurvedic medicine in India have valued fennel as a digestive aid for eons. Chewing fennel seeds to help digestion—and freshen breath—is still a tradition in India, and offering candied fennel to departing diners is a common practice in Indian restaurants worldwide.

There's good reason for fennel's enduring popularity. Medicinally, fennel seeds are considered to be a carminative, an herb that aids digestion and alleviates cramping by relaxing muscles in the digestive tract (carminatives are often added to laxatives to prevent cramping). As a carminative, fennel also helps to relieve gas. Fennel seeds also contain compounds that help thin mucus and aid expectoration, making them useful for treating coughs and congestion.

> ⚠ **CAUTION:** Consumption of fennel in food, teas, or tinctures is generally considered safe. Fennel essential oil, however, should never be taken internally. During pregnancy, limit fennel intake to what is found commonly in foods.

▶ | INDIGESTION & GAS

Fennel contains an aromatic compound called anethole that is known to inhibit spasms in smooth muscles such as those in the walls of the stomach and intestines. Gastrointestinal muscle spasms contribute to, and can even bring on, indigestion. Anethole and other compounds in fennel also have mild antibacterial properties. The digestive tract is home to billions of bacteria—many of which are involved in the gas-generating fermentation of food—perhaps explaining why fennel seems to act as a damper on gas production.

Sweet Relief

- **Chew the Seeds** Follow the tradition set thousands of years ago in India and the Far East: Chew fennel seeds after a meal. Start with about ¼ teaspoon of seeds. Chew them slowly in your mouth, like gum. When they are completely pulverized, you can either swallow them or spit them out. Another option: Sprinkle ½ to 1 teaspoon of fennel seeds on your food daily.

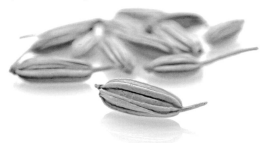

- **Brew the Tea** A tea brewed from fennel seeds has a mild, slightly sweet taste reminiscent of licorice. It's easy to make. First, gently bruise 1 to 2 teaspoons of fennel seeds. You can do this by mashing them lightly in a mortar and pestle, or spreading them on a cutting board and rolling over them lightly with a rolling pin. Place the bruised seeds in a cup, add just-boiled water, and let steep for ten minutes. Strain. If desired, sweeten with honey, stevia, or maple syrup.

THREE-SEED DIGESTIVE TEA

Fennel isn't the only "seed" that soothes an upset stomach and can help relieve gas. Anise and caraway seeds, combined with fennel seed, make for a delicious and effective digestive aid.

Combine 1 teaspoon fennel seed, ½ teaspoon anise seed, and ½ teaspoon caraway seed. Gently bruise the seeds (see the bulleted item on bruising the seeds on page 91) and place them in the bottom of a cup. Add just-boiled water and steep ten minutes. Sweeten as desired.

- **Try the Tincture** Fennel tinctures are available at most health food stores and can be used to make a simple fennel digestive aid. Add 1 or 2 teaspoons of fennel tincture to a glass of cool water. Drink up to three glasses a day between meals.
- **Mix Fennel and Milk** An old folk remedy for upset stomach or intestinal cramping is to heat 1 tablespoon of bruised fennel seeds and 1 cup milk to a gentle simmer. Strain, let cool slightly, and sip the hot liquid. Try this only if you are not lactose intolerant or have no problems with dairy products.
- **Massage With Fennel Oil** Combine aromatherapy (see page 259) with massage to ease indigestion. In a small dish, blend 3 drops of fennel essential oil in 2 tablespoons of sweet almond oil. Wet your fingertips with the mixture and apply to the bare skin of your lower abdomen. Using firm pressure, massage your lower abdomen in a clockwise pattern: up on the right side, across to the left, down the left side, and across to the right. To enhance the soothing effect, wrap a thin soft towel around a hot water bottle and hold it against your abdomen after the massage.

 WHEN TO CALL THE DR.: Everyone has occasional indigestion. But if indigestion lasts two or more weeks, see your health care provider. • Severe flatulence that isn't relieved by natural remedies or by changing your diet could be a sign of a serious medical condition.

▶ | CONSTIPATION

By relaxing the muscles in the lower intestine and encouraging their smooth, rhythmic contraction, fennel can promote normal bowel movements and ease the bloated feeling that often accompanies constipation. Increase your water intake, add more fiber into your diet, get regular exercise, and try the following fennel remedies to help resolve the problem.

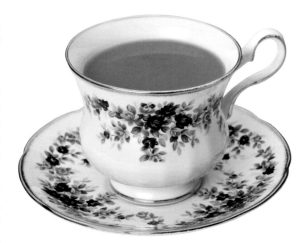

Fiber Fix

- **Drink the Tea** Fennel tea (see the bulleted item for making tea on page 91) is a safe and gentle-acting remedy for constipation relief. Drink up to three cups a day until the problem resolves.
- **Eat the Bulb** All parts of the fennel plant are edible. Fennel bulb is the white, layered, lower portion of the plant from which the leaves arise. It's typically eaten raw or cooked as a

good to know: ALSO FOR CONSTIPATION

Psyllium (*Plantago ovata, P. afra*) is an herb commonly used as a gentle bulk laxative to treat constipation. Psyllium seed husks are an excellent source of soluble fiber. When the husks combine with water, they swell to roughly ten times their original volume. Interestingly, psyllium can also be used to treat common diarrhea and may be helpful for easing the symptoms of irritable bowel syndrome.

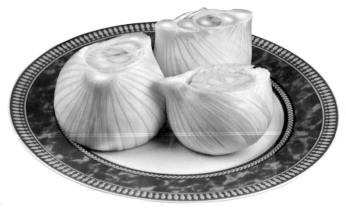

vegetable. One cup of sliced raw fennel bulb has about 115 calories and provides 2.7 grams of constipation-fighting dietary fiber, slightly more than 10 percent of the 25 grams a day recommended by the U.S. Food and Drug Administration.

▶ | COUGHS

Thanks to its pleasant taste and natural expectorant properties, fennel is an ingredient in many cough drops and cough syrups. Because it thins mucous secretions, the herb also helps clear respiratory passages so you can breathe more easily.

Fend Off a Cough With Fennel

■ *Inhale Steam* Inhaling fennel-infused steam may help alleviate coughing and help loosen phlegm. Add 2 drops of fennel essential oil to a large heatproof bowl. Add 2 to 3 cups of just-boiled water. Drape a towel over your head and shoulders to make a tent, and lean over the bowl. Take a small inhalation through your nose. If inhaling the steam feels comfortable, continue breathing the fragrant vapors for about ten minutes. Keep face at least 12 inches from the water's surface.

⚠ **CAUTION:** Inhalation therapy is not appropriate for children younger than age three.

■ *Quiet That Cough* Combine 3 tablespoons fennel seed, 2 tablespoons dried mullein flowers, and 2 tablespoons dried peppermint leaf in a container with a tight-fitting lid. Place 1 tablespoon of this mixture in a cup, add just-boiled water, and steep for ten minutes. Sweeten with honey to enhance the expectorant properties, and sip slowly.

■ *Make It With Marshmallow* To make another fennel-based herbal tea that can help even violent coughing, combine 2 tablespoons each of fennel and anise seeds, 4 teaspoons of dried marshmallow root, and 3 teaspoons dried thyme in a container with a tight-fitting lid. Place about 2 teaspoons of this mixture in a cup, add just-boiled water, and let steep ten minutes. Sip slowly to help quiet spasms.

COOK UP COUGH SYRUP

Fennel cough syrup is a natural cough-relief aid that's free of the side effects that sometimes come with many over-the-counter cough medicines. In a saucepan, combine 2 teaspoons fennel seed, 3 tablespoons organic honey, and 1 cup of water. Bring the ingredients to a boil. Reduce the heat and let the mixture simmer on low, stirring occasionally, for about 20 minutes; it will thicken slightly. Cool and strain. Take a tablespoon of syrup every three to four hours as needed. Store in the refrigerator for up to a week.

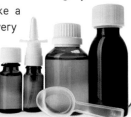

RECIPE FOR HEALTH

good to know: ALSO FOR COUGHS

Thyme *(Thymus vulgaris)* has been used medicinally—and in cooking—for many centuries. Thyme tea is another time-honored herbal remedy to help calm coughs and clear mucus.

Butterbur *(Petasites hybridus)* is used in modern herbal medicine primarily as an antispasmodic. It's often recommended to help ease chronic cough or asthma. Butterbur has also been used in treating gastric ulcers and spasms of the urinary tract. ⚠ **CAUTION:** Butterbur contains pyrrolizidine alkaloids (PA), a group of compounds that can be toxic to the liver. Only products labeled "PA free" should be used.

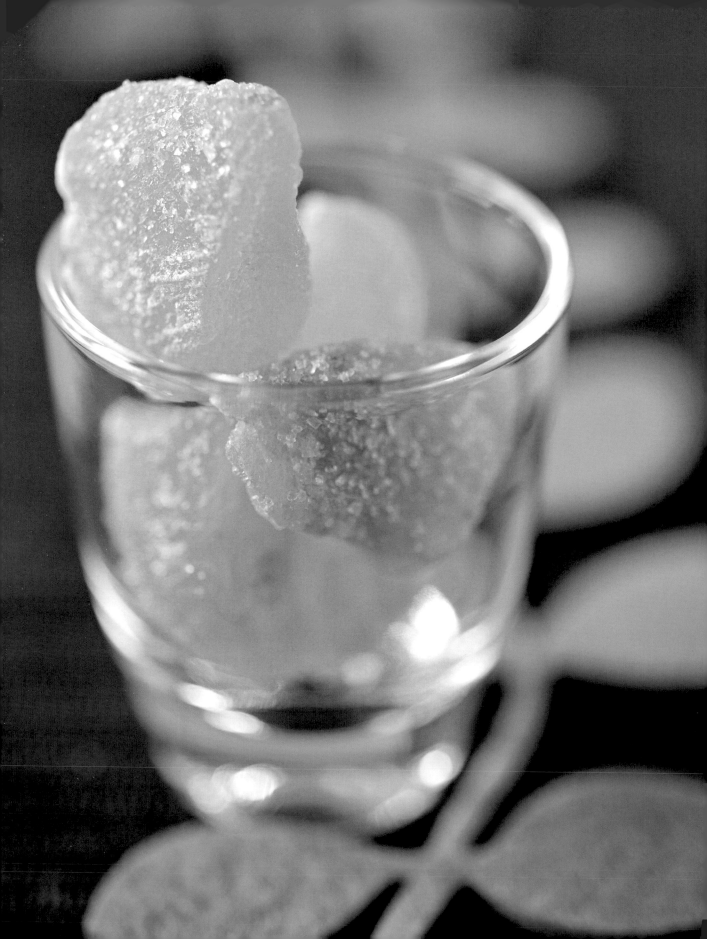

Ginger

10 WAYS TO ENGINEER RELIEF

Ginger's gnarled, knobby roots are ingredients in both cooking and herbal medicine, and have been for several thousand years. Beneath the root's tough skin is a fibrous, pale to golden yellow flesh that tastes simultaneously sweet and hot. The flavor is unmistakable, whether you encounter it in ginger snaps or Asian and Indian curries. Ginger has been an essential herb in traditional Chinese, Ayurvedic, and Arabic medicine for centuries to treat all manner of ailments. The Greeks and Romans found ginger to be an excellent cure for intestinal upsets as well as internal parasites. During the Middle Ages in Europe, noble and common folk alike held ginger in such high esteem for treating indigestion, nausea, and respiratory infections that the herb was believed to have come from the Garden of Eden.

When an herb is used consistently for thousands of years, you know there's probably something reliable behind the traditions. That's certainly true for ginger. Many scientific studies support ginger's effectiveness in combating nausea, whether it's triggered by indigestion, motion sickness, "morning sickness" during pregnancy, or chemotherapy treatments. The way ginger prevents and relieves nausea is not completely understood, but one hypothesis is that certain chemical substances in the herb bind to receptors in the digestive tract that then "turn down" the sensation of nausea. The substances also speed up digestion, so food moves out of the stomach and into the intestines, making it far less likely to "come back up." Other studies have shown that ginger can significantly reduce inflammation, which may explain why it has been used in Chinese medicine for thousands of years to reduce the pain of arthritic joints. Ginger shows some evidence of having anticancer properties as well, but more research in this area is needed.

⚠ **CAUTION:** Do not give ginger to children under two, and consult your doctor about proper dosing before giving ginger to children older than two for nausea or upset stomach. Pregnant women should not take more than 1 gram (1,000 mg) of ginger a day. People who take blood-thinning medications should not take high doses of ginger without medical supervision.

▶ | MOTION SICKNESS

If planes, trains, and automobiles leave your stomach heaving, ginger is definitely worth a try as a motion sickness remedy (see also pages 55–56). There is some research to indicate that ginger can quell nausea as well, or almost as well,

good to know: ABOUT GINGER

- Some people find taking ginger on an empty stomach is most effective for preventing nausea.
- Whenever possible, use fresh ginger or candied ginger. The powdered herb contains fewer active compounds.
- Fresh, unpeeled ginger can be stored in the refrigerator for up to three weeks. In the freezer, it will keep for about six months.
- Pregnant women should not consider ginger a go-to remedy. They should not consume more than 1 gram (1,000 mg) of ginger a day and never more than four days in a row.

GINGER TEA WITH A TWIST

Many people find plain ginger tea quite pleasant. But if you'd like a little more complexity of flavor, a citrusy ginger tea may be the solution.

Place 12 thin slices of fresh peeled ginger-root in a pan with 4 cups of water. Boil eight to ten minutes. Strain the hot liquid into a bowl. Add the juice of 1 orange and ½ lemon and sweeten with ¼ cup honey or maple syrup; stevia is another sweetener option (add as needed to reach desired sweetness). Stir well to mix all ingredients. Pour a cup (reheat in the microwave, if desired) and enjoy.

Pour a cup of just-boiled water over ¼ to ½ teaspoon powdered ginger and steep for ten minutes. Strain through a paper coffee filter, and sweeten if desired.

- **Chew Before You Go** Before you head off on a trip, peel and slowly chew a ¼-inch piece of fresh ginger (about ¼ gram). If the taste of fresh ginger is too strong, chew the same amount of candied ginger. Chew it slowly; don't just gulp it down.
- **Pop a Pill** Ginger is also available in capsule form. Follow package directions. Be sure to begin taking the capsules before you start moving and before motion sickness sets in.

⚠ **CAUTION:** Pregnant women shouldn't exceed 1 gram (1000 mg) of ginger per day (in any form) for more than 4 days.

as common over-the-counter motion-sickness medications—without the side effects of drowsiness or dry mouth. The secret is to take ginger as a preventive measure *before* you think you might get queasy. Ginger also seems to be an effective short-term treatment (taken no longer than four days) for morning sickness (see pages 56–57).

Ginger Zingers

- **Sip Ginger Tea** Peel a piece of fresh ginger about the size of your thumb. Grate or chop finely. Simmer the ginger in 2 cups water on low heat for about 15 minutes. Strain and sweeten to taste. Drink a cup, up to three times a day.
- **Make a Quick Cup** If you don't have fresh ginger on hand, or don't want to take the time to peel and chop it, you can make a cup of ginger tea using the ground spice.

▶ | INDIGESTION

Inside the stomach, ginger neutralizes acids, calms smooth muscle contractions, and boosts digestive juices. It can provide fast relief for indigestion. It's safe and inexpensive and well worth a try. Note that some people who suffer from heartburn or the symptoms of gallstones occasionally find ginger aggravates their problem. Start slowly, with small amounts.

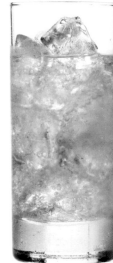

Inhibit Indigestion

- **Calm With Carbonation** A cup of ginger tea can ease many cases of indigestion. Alternatively, try this naturally carbonated ginger ale for fighting stomach upsets, bloating,

good to know: ALSO FOR INDIGESTION

- Cinnamon (*Cinnamomum verum, C. cassia*) is often recommended by herbalists as a remedy for digestive upsets and indigestion and to soothe nausea and vomiting as well. It is available as cinnamon sticks, or quills, as the powdered spice, and in capsule form.
- Parsley (*Petroselinum crispum*) is more widely used as an herbal remedy in Europe than in the United States. Herbal practitioners often recommend parsley seeds and leaves, fresh or dried, to calm indigestion. And it is a good breath freshener as well. ⚠ **CAUTION:** For pregnant women, consuming a little bit of parsley in food is fine; medicinal doses, however, are discouraged.

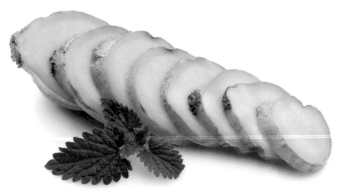

and intestinal cramps. In a saucepan, combine 1 inch fresh gingerroot, peeled and grated, with 1 cup water and ¾ cup raw sugar. Cook over medium heat until the sugar is dissolved and the mixture thickens slightly. Remove from heat and steep, covered, for an hour. Strain the syrup and refrigerate for another hour. Pour into a two-liter container with a tight-fitting lid. Add ⅛ teaspoon active dry yeast, 2 tablespoons fresh lemon juice, and 6 cups water and shake to mix. Put on the lid and let the container stand at room temperature for 48 hours, and then refrigerate. Use the ginger ale within ten days. (There may be slight yeast sediment on the bottom of the container.)

- *Go With the Sweet Stuff* Candied ginger is widely available in health food stores and many grocery and drugstores. When indigestion strikes, slowly chew a small piece of candied ginger, swallowing the juice. It's tasty, but don't eat it like candy. Take your time and let it exert its stomach-calming actions.

▶ | JOINT PAIN

Ginger is being scrutinized by medical researchers for its ability to reduce inflammation associated with arthritis. Gingerols are some of the primary active components in gingerroot and are the substances responsible for the herb's distinctive flavor. Gingerols appear to be potent anti-inflammatory compounds, able to suppress inflammation-promoting substances in the body.

Inflammation Ammo

- *Add to Your Diet* Many herbal health practitioners suggest adding fresh ginger to foods, drinking ginger tea or ginger juice, or taking ginger capsules to relieve inflammation due to arthritis pain. Follow package directions.
- *Make a Compress* Combine ¼ cup peeled, freshly grated ginger and 1 cup water in a small saucepan. Simmer on very low heat, watching closely. Remove from heat just before the water has boiled away. Remove the hot ginger with a slotted spoon and place on a piece of cheesecloth (several layers thick) or a clean kitchen towel. Fold the gauze or cloth around the ginger into the size of a compress and press down, expressing the juice and saturating the fabric. Place the compress over a painful joint and leave in position for about ten minutes.

⚠ **CAUTION:** Remove the compress promptly if you experience any discomfort.

GINGER, SPICE, & CALM

There's no easier way to add an unexpected spike to a dish than with fresh ginger! The comforting and yet exotic aroma is calming but exciting. Add fresh ginger to your butternut squash soup to add depth and warmth. Bored of regular chicken soup? Mimic the flavors of Thai-style chicken soup, *tom kha gai:* Simmer knobs of ginger, coconut milk, and fish sauce with your basic chicken stock. Finish with chicken, lots of vegetables, and some fresh cilantro—and you'll have an exciting new spin on an old classic.

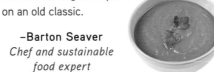

–Barton Seaver
Chef and sustainable food expert

97

GINGER

FOODS FOR HEALTH

good to know: ALSO FOR JOINT PAIN

Arnica (*Arnica montana*), rubbed on the skin as an ointment, cream, or salve, can provide relief for joint pain in some people. Arnica flowers can also be steeped in hot water and used as a base in compresses and poultices to treat arthritis pain. ⚠ **CAUTION:** Arnica should never be taken internally and should not be applied to broken skin or near the mouth or eyes.

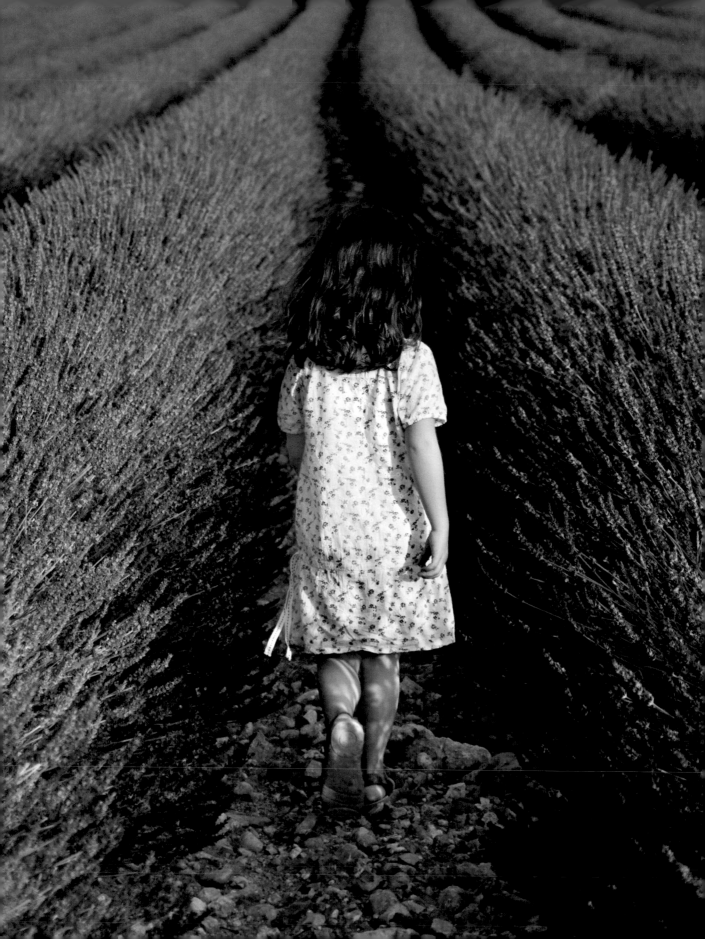

Lavender

12 REASONS TO LOVE LAVENDER

What does the scent of lavender bring to mind? Bars of fine, French-milled soap? The best therapeutic foot massage you ever had? The smell of your grandmother's skin when she gave you a hug? The powerful but intensely pleasing aroma of lavender (*Lavandula angustifolia*) is one your nose doesn't soon forget. It's a classic fragrance distilled from a truly classical herb. The ancient Romans adored lavender. They used it to perfume both their bodies and their bathwater. Even the Latin root of the herb's English name—*lavare*—means "to wash." But lavender has much more to offer than an agreeable odor. It's been used medicinally for thousands of years. Throughout the Mediterranean world, and later in India and Tibet, lavender was valued for its disinfecting and antiseptic properties and its ability to quell anxiety and clear the mind.

By the Middle Ages, the herb was a remedy of choice for dressing wounds and treating coughs, colds, infections, sleeplessness, depression, and rheumatic aches and pains. If you'd suffered from a headache in that age, a medieval healer would likely have suggested that you tuck a sprig of fresh lavender behind your ear to drive it away.

Research has confirmed what the ancients—and perhaps your grandmother—knew: Lavender does calm, soothe, and slightly sedate us when we inhale its remarkable scent. Lavender is widely used in modern herbal medicine and aromatherapy. It's commonly employed to ease tension, stress, insomnia, headaches, anxiety, and depression. And many people find that minor skin ailments, such as fungal infections, cuts and scrapes, and even eczema, respond well to lavender's therapeutic touch.

▶ STRESS RELIEF

Lavender contains many biologically active chemical compounds. Some of the most medicinally important are rapidly absorbed through the skin and mucous membranes, including the lining of the nose. Scientific studies indicate that these substances can help reduce anxiety and improve concentration. When you've had a dreadful day or feel you'll never, ever catch up on your work, try some of these lavender remedies to help your brain and body unwind.

Live Better With Lavender

- ***Sniff It*** Pure lavender essential oil is available at most natural food stores. Insert a piece of a cotton ball into a small glass or plastic vial with a tight-fitting lid. Drip 2 to 3 drops of lavender essential oil onto the cotton and cap the vial. Keep the vial with you and when you feel anxious, pop the top and inhale the fragrance slowly and deeply for 30 to 60 seconds. Or

---

good to know: ALSO FOR STRESS RELIEF

Passionflower (*Passiflora incarnata*) is another calming herb, good for combating stress and anxiety (and sleep problems, too). Its dried parts—flowers, leaves, and stems—are used to prepare infusions and tinctures and are also available in capsule and tablet form.

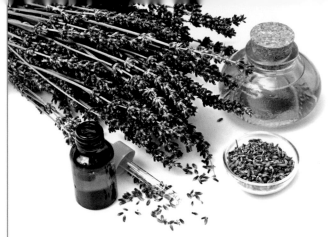

put a few drops of lavender oil on a tissue to keep accessible in a pocket for quickly and discreetly holding to your nose.

⚠ **CAUTION:** Herbal essential oils such as lavender essential oil should not be taken internally. Always dilute essential oils before applying to skin.

■ *Surround Yourself With Steam* Place 2 to 3 drops of lavender essential oil in the bottom of a large heatproof bowl. Add 4 cups of just-boiled water. Make a tent out of a towel draped over your head and shoulders, and lean over the bowl. Keep your eyes shut and your face 12 inches or more from the water's surface. Take a small inhalation. If breathing the steam feels good, continue inhaling for five to ten minutes.

⚠ **CAUTION:** If you have asthma or any other respiratory condition, consult your doctor before inhaling steam infused with lavender or other essential oils. Not appropriate for children under the age of three.

■ *Soak Away Stress* Add 5 to 10 drops of lavender oil to a full, warm bath and vigorously agitate the water to disperse the oil well. (Hint: For better dispersion, add the oil to 1 tablespoon of milk or Epsom salts first, and then put this in the water.) Scatter a handful of fresh or dried lavender flowers on the water's surface, if desired. Soak, surrounded by lavender's scent.

■ *Shower in the Scent* Mix 3 drops of lavender essential oil with about 1 tablespoon of water in a small plastic dish or container. Get in the shower, and when your hair is thoroughly wet, pour the oil and water mixture onto the top of your head. Stand under the running water again and let the oil's fragrance cascade around you for a few minutes; keep your eyes shut so as not to get oil in them. Then shampoo and rinse as normal.

■ *Dab It On* Mix 2 to 3 drops of lavender essential oil and 1 teaspoon of sweet almond oil in a small dish. Dip the tips of your index fingers in this mixture and rub your temples with small circular motions for several minutes. Alternatively, put several drops of the oil mixture on a warm moist washcloth (rub gently to distribute into the cloth). Fold the washcloth lengthwise several times, lie down, and place it along the back of your neck. Close your eyes and inhale the fragrance.

▶ INSOMNIA

Lavender is an old folk remedy for treating insomnia. Several studies have shown that lavender can help induce sleep in some people. Try the following remedies after a stressful day when sleep seems to be eluding you.

Inhale Insomnia Away

■ *Prep Your Pillow* Before you crawl into bed, put a few drops of lavender essential oil on a tissue or cotton ball and slip it between the pillow and pillowcase close to where your head will lie. Or if you have access to fresh lavender, use several flowering stalks or a small cluster of leaves in the same way.

■ *Spritz the Sheets* Mix 5 drops of lavender essential oil with 1 cup of water in a small

good to know: ALSO FOR INSOMNIA

— Skullcap (*Scutellaria lateriflora*) is another herb herbalists and naturopaths suggest as a relaxant to treat insomnia as well as anxiety. Its dried leaves (with or without stems, flowers, and fruits) can be steeped in hot water to make tea.

— Some people find valerian (*Valeriana officinalis*) an effective alternative to commonly prescribed sleep medications for treating insomnia and other sleep problems.

LAVENDER SALVE

Make this fragrant, soothing salve in minutes. Use it on minor cuts and scrapes, or patches of dry, irritated skin.

¼ cup organic shea butter
1 tablespoon organic sweet almond oil
4 teaspoons pure beeswax, grated
12 drops pure lavender essential oil
Contents of 1 vitamin E capsule

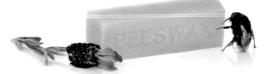

Put the shea butter, oil, and beeswax in the top of a double boiler. Warm slowly until the ingredients are completely melted. Stir well. Remove from heat and add the lavender oil and vitamin E. Stir again until thoroughly combined. Pour the mixture into a small dark brown or blue glass jar with a tight-fitting lid.

spray bottle. When you turn back the sheets at night, spray a little of this mixture into the air several feet above the bed. The mist will settle onto the fabric.

■ **Try Tea** Drink a cup of lavender-based herbal tea before bed. In a glass jar with an airtight lid, combine one part each dried lemon balm leaf, dried catnip, and dried peppermint leaf with two parts each dried lavender flowers and dried chamomile flowers. Mix together well. Put 2 teaspoons of this mixture in a cup, add just-boiled water, and let steep for five minutes. Strain and sweeten if desired.

⚠ **CAUTION:** Avoid chamomile if you are allergic to ragweed or other plants in the aster family.

▶ | SKIN IRRITATIONS

Although some of lavender's chemical constituents help pacify jangled nerves, others have antibacterial, antifungal, antioxidant, and anti-inflammatory properties. Lavender essential oil, derived from the plant's purple flowers, can be used in a variety of ways to soothe irritated skin and help heal minor injuries and infections.

The Skin-ny on Lavender

■ **Fight a Fungus** Because of its antifungal action, lavender essential oil may help in treating athlete's foot. Mix 3 drops of lavender oil with 1 teaspoon of sweet almond or grapeseed oil. Rub into the affected area twice a day. Alternatively, combine 2 teaspoons of tincture of benzoin with 5 drops of lavender oil and 5 drops of thyme oil. Massage a little of this mix into the affected area every night before bed.

■ **Make a Lavender Compress** To soothe eczema or other skin irritations, steep a tablespoon of dried lavender flowers in a cup of just-boiled water for 15 minutes. Cool and strain the liquid. Saturate a clean cloth, wring out the excess, and place this lavender compress over the affected area for 15 minutes. Repeat several times a day. You can also dab this lavender infusion on cuts and scrapes as a mild antiseptic.

■ **Stop the Irritation** To quell the itch of insect bites or stings, mix 5 drops of lavender essential oil with a teaspoon of sweet almond oil. Dab a drop of this mix on an itchy spot. You can also apply it to blisters to help soothe the irritation.

good to know: ALSO FOR SKIN IRRITATIONS

─ Aloe (*Aloe vera*) is famous for soothing a range of skin irritations (see pages 65 and 71).
─ Witch hazel (*Hamamelis virginiana*), a staple of many first aid kits, is an old and effective remedy for minor skin irritations and injuries. Look for products that contain real witch hazel extract.

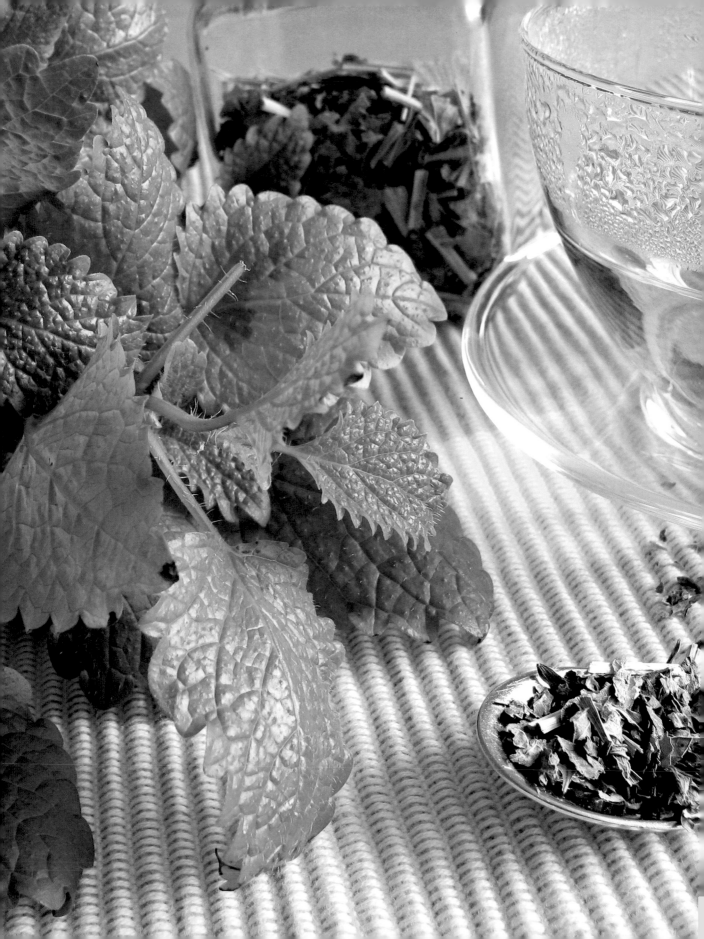

Lemon Balm

12 PATHS TO CALMING CURES

Lemon balm has healing in its name. The lemony fragrance that the leaves release when crushed is indeed a balm to the spirit. The scent is refreshing, calming, and comforting, all at the same time. Once referred to as the "gladdening herb," lemon balm has a history as a remedy for easing anxiety and lifting the spirits of troubled souls. The ancient Greeks may have introduced the herb into the Arab world, where it was praised as a cure for heart conditions and depression, and as an aid to strengthening the mind. Historically, lemon balm *(Melissa officinalis)* may have reached the peak of its popularity in the 1600s, when a group of French Carmelite nuns concocted an alcohol-infused blend of lemon balm and the herb angelica that they spiked with various spices.

What was dubbed Carmelite water became a reach-for remedy for headaches, indigestion, sleeplessness, and nerve pain as well as one of the earliest known alcohol-based perfumes.

As was the case with some other herbs, lemon balm fell out of use in the United States during the early 1900s. Yet in Europe, interest in lemon balm and its medicinal properties continued to grow. Today, herbalists in Germany and other European countries routinely suggest lemon balm to relieve tension and anxiety, and—often in combination with other herbs—to treat insomnia and indigestion. Research into lemon balm's effects has also shown that the herb has antibacterial and antiviral properties. One of the viruses lemon balm seems to inhibit is herpes simplex virus, the cause of cold sores.

▶ | STRESS RELIEF

Lemon balm's volatile oils contain antispasmodic substances that tend to reduce contractions in smooth muscles and generally have a soothing, slightly sedating effect. In short, the herb may help you relax, possibly enough to ease you gently into sleep. Research on people with dementia, including Alzheimer's disease, has shown that lemon balm extract may help improve cognition and relieve agitation and restlessness, although further studies are needed before any conclusion can be reached.

Balm for Calm

- *Make a Calming Cup* Of lemon balm tea, that is. You can brew it from either fresh lemon balm leaves (the plant is a cinch to grow in almost any sunny garden) or dried leaves, which are widely available at health food stores or online. Pour a cup of just-boiled water over 6 to 8 fresh lemon balm leaves, or 1 to 2 teaspoons of dried leaf, and steep for five to seven minutes. Add a sprig of fresh spearmint or peppermint and a little honey or stevia to sweeten.

- *Brew at Bedtime* If stress is keeping you awake at night, a variation on lemon balm tea that includes other sleep-inducing herbs may help. Mix 1 teaspoon dried lemon balm and ½ teaspoon each of chamomile flower, skullcap, and passionflower (all available at health food stores) in a cup. Fill with just-boiled water and let steep ten minutes. Strain and sweeten, if desired. Sip this slowly just before you climb into bed.

⚠ **CAUTION:** Passionflower is not recommended during pregnancy; it may also interfere with blood-thinning medications. Avoid chamomile if you are allergic to ragweed or other plants in the aster family.

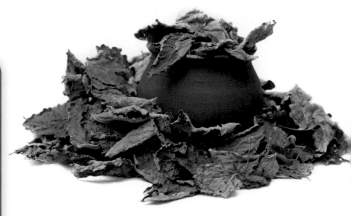

BALMY LEMON SODA

You'll need fresh lemon balm leaves for this refreshingly light and calming carbonated drink:

2 cups fresh lemon balm leaves
1 quart just-boiled water
2 tablespoons honey
1 quart of plain carbonated water
  (club soda works well)

In a heatproof bowl, add the leaves and just-boiled water. Stir to combine and steep 30 minutes. Strain and let the liquid cool. Add honey and stir well. Refrigerate until cold. When ready to serve, add carbonated water to the lemon balm mixture and pour into ice-filled glasses. Garnish with a slice of fresh lemon and a sprig of fresh lemon balm.

- *Ease Tension With Massage* You can buy lemon balm essential oil in health food stores or online. Mix 2 to 3 drops lemon balm oil with 1 tablespoon of a carrier oil such as sweet almond oil, grapeseed oil, or jojoba oil. Use this oil mixture to give your arms, hands, legs, and feet a cooling, calming massage treatment.

▶ | DIGESTIVE AID

Lemon balm is very gentle in its actions, and as a digestive aid, it's suitable for soothing stomachs, relieving bloating, and banishing gas in both children and adults. Although it's fine to use lemon balm alone as a digestive aid, it also combines well with other herbs that are good for easing indigestion (see pages 83 and 107).

Settle the Stomach

- *Combat the Upset* A cup of lemon balm tea (presented previously in the section titled "Balm for Calm") is a good choice when your stomach is knotted up with anxiety or your last meal simply didn't sit well.
- *Cool It* As a warm-weather alternative to a hot cup of lemon balm tea, try this: In a large heatproof bowl, add 1 tablespoon dried lemon balm leaf, 1 tablespoon dried peppermint leaf, and 1 tablespoon dried chamomile flowers. Add 3 cups of just-boiled water. Let steep 15 minutes. Cool and strain into a pitcher. Sweeten with a little honey, stevia, or maple syrup, and then add 2 to 3 cups of ice. Let chill a few minutes and serve.

⚠ **CAUTION:** Avoid chamomile if you are allergic to ragweed or other plants in the aster family.

- *Quiet the Colon* If your digestive upset feels like an intestinal problem, this soothing recipe might help: Combine 1 teaspoon dried lemon balm leaf, ½ teaspoon dried organic dandelion leaf, and ¼ teaspoon crushed fennel seeds (fennel is helpful for easing intestinal gas; see page 29). Put these in a cup, cover with a scant cup just-boiled water, and let steep for about ten minutes.

good to know: ALSO FOR STRESS RELIEF

- The herb ashwagandha *(Withania somnifera)* is also used in herbal medicine for combating stress. Its species name, *somnifera,* means "to induce sleep."
- Hops *(Humulus lupulus)* are the conelike fruits of this widely grown hardy vine. Hops have been valued for centuries for their stress-relieving, sedative effects. A sachet of hops, slipped beneath the pillowcase before bedtime, can be a calming sleep aid.

- **Cook With It** The mild, lemony taste of lemon balm combines nicely with fruits that can also be used as an aid to digestion. If you have a source of fresh lemon balm leaves, steep several handfuls of leaves in 2 to 3 cups of just-boiled water for about 20 minutes. Cool and strain the liquid; discard the leaves. Add fresh or dried fruit (think plums, apples, figs, or prunes) to the lemon balm liquid and simmer gently on low heat until the fruit is softened and plump. Good for breakfast or as a dessert.

▶ | COLD SORES

As long ago as A.D. 1000, an Arab physician and philosopher prescribed lemon balm for ulcerated sores. How interesting that recent research on lemon balm's antiviral properties shows that it can speed healing and reduce symptoms of cold sores, which are caused by a type of herpes simplex virus. Something in lemon balm hinders viral replication. In one study, people who applied lemon balm extract cream to cold sores on their lips experienced significant improvement in just two days. It also seemed to help prolong the interval between cold sore outbreaks in some people.

Coping With Cold Sores
- **Soothe the Sore** Lemon balm ointments are available at many health food stores and pharmacies. Look for a lip balm containing one percent lemon balm extract to help shorten healing time, prevent infection spread, and reduce symptoms of recurring cold sores. Follow package directions. Note that oral herpes (cold sores) and genital herpes are caused by very similar types of herpes simplex virus. If genital sores are a problem, try applying lemon balm ointment to treat them, too.
- **Try the Essential Oil** At the first characteristic tingle of a cold sore, mix 5 drops of lemon balm essential oil with 1 teaspoon of olive oil or sweet almond oil. Dab a little of this mixture on the tingling spot three times a day.
- **Drench It** Prepare a very strong cup of lemon balm tea by brewing 2 tablespoons of dried lemon balm leaf in a cup of just-boiled water. Let it steep for at least 30 minutes. Strain and discard the herbs. Refrigerate the liquid until cold. Saturate a cotton ball and dab on the cold tea—at the first tingle or sign of a sore—for a minute or two. Repeat often throughout the day, for as long as the breakout lasts.
- **Fight Back With Cold** Make some strong lemon balm tea, as described previously. After you've cooled and strained the tea, pour the liquid into an ice cube tray and freeze. Use the cubes like miniature ice packs. Moisten a cube in water (so it won't stick to your lip) and apply it directly to the "tingly" spot (or the sore, if it's developing) for 30 seconds—keep the ice cube constantly moving, though, so the skin on your lip doesn't get too cold. Repeat this procedure several times a day.

good to know: ALSO FOR DIGESTIVE AID

Lemongrass *(Cymbopogon citratus)* has long been used in Ayurvedic medicine, and more recently in Western herbal medicine, to treat digestive disorders. Lemongrass leaves can be used to make a stomach-soothing, lemony tea. They are also common ingredients in many Thai and Vietnamese dishes.

Devil's claw *(Harpagophytum procumbens)* doesn't sound like it could improve much of anything, but there is some evidence that substances in this herb stimulate digestion. Devil's claw's root and secondary tubers contain bitter compounds that stimulate secretion of saliva and digestive juices, potentially enhancing digestion and relieving indigestion, gas, and bloating. ⚠ **CAUTION:** Because devil's claw stimulates the production of stomach acid, avoid it if you suffer from peptic ulcers or heartburn.

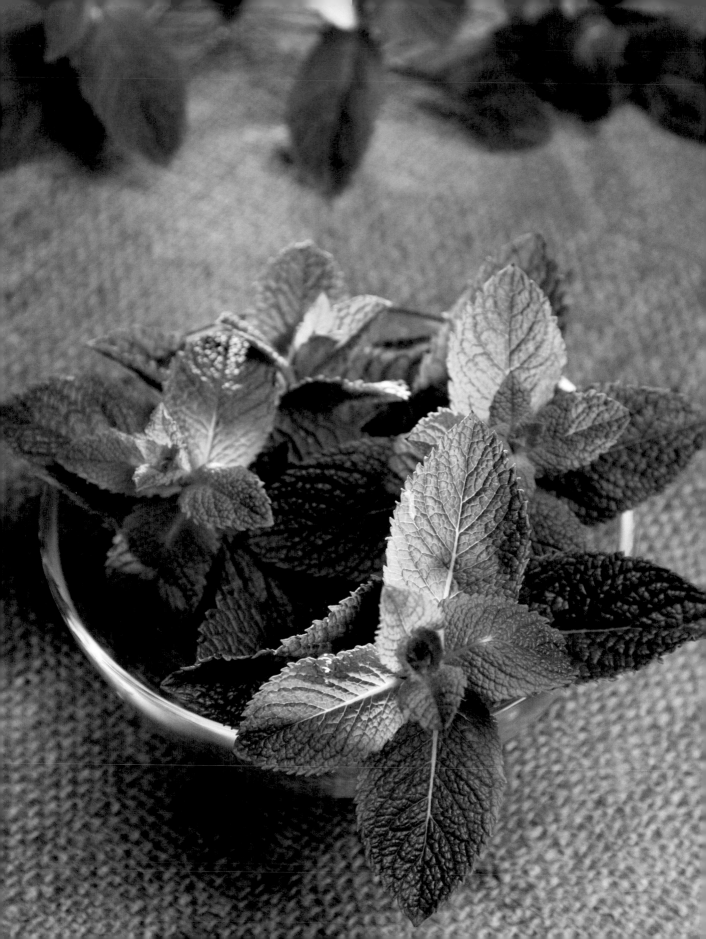

Peppermint

13 WAYS MEANT TO MEDICATE

Peppermint *(Mentha x piperita)* was a happy accident of nature, the result of cross-pollination between spearmint and water mint. Someone stumbled upon this new mint hybrid in the English countryside in 1696. Roughly 50 years later, fields of peppermint were under cultivation near London in one of England's most famous mint-producing regions. What makes peppermint so remarkable is the high percentage of menthol in its essential oil. That menthol punch gives the herb its warm peppery fragrance and cool, crisp flavor. Today, peppermint is one of the world's most popular flavorings, found in everything from chewing gum and toothpaste to candy canes and after-dinner mints.

Mints of many varieties have been used in herbal medicine since antiquity, mostly for treating ailments of the digestive tract. Peppermint is no exception. Peppermint's active constituents have antispasmodic and carminative (gas-relieving) actions. Peppermint appears to soothe digestive upsets by relieving spasms in the smooth muscle of the intestinal wall, and also helping to expel gas. The herb is also quite effective for reducing nausea. The herb's menthol produces a cooling effect on the skin that makes it a natural choice for soothing minor skin irritations and providing relief from tension headaches.

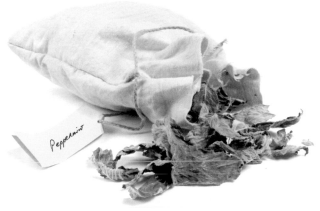

▶ INDIGESTION & IBS

When your belly is roiling, cramping, or swelling with gas, peppermint is a good herb to reach for. Thanks to its antispasmodic effects, peppermint calms overactive muscles in the digestive tract. It eases stomach churning, and helps relax the ring of muscle separating the esophagus and stomach, thus allowing gas in the stomach to escape upward, as belches. As muscles further down the digestive tract relax, trapped intestinal gas can move down, out, and away. Peppermint also appears to stimulate the flow of bile, a substance produced by the liver that aids in the digestion of fats. Research has shown that peppermint can also help relieve the symptoms of irritable bowel syndrome (IBS), a miserable intestinal difficulty characterized by cramps, gas, and alternating bouts of diarrhea and constipation.

⚠ **CAUTION:** Consult your health care provider before using peppermint if you have gastroesophageal reflux disease (GERD), hiatal hernia, or gallbladder problems. Be aware that peppermint may make heartburn worse in some people. Pregnant women and nursing mothers should consume peppermint only in moderation.

---

good to know: ALSO FOR INDIGESTION & IBS

└ Psyllium *(Plantago ovata, P. afra)* is another herb shown to be effective in treating mild to moderate cases of IBS and inflammatory bowel disease. Psyllium husk (the seed coating) is the main ingredient in many bulk laxatives.

FRESH LEAF & FENNEL TEA

Try this recipe for settling an upset stomach when you have access to fresh peppermint and lemon balm leaves:

½ cup fresh peppermint leaves
½ cup fresh lemon balm leaves
2 teaspoons crushed fennel seed

Put the leaves and seeds in a large teapot or saucepan. Add 3 cups of just-boiled water and steep, covered, for ten minutes. Strain and sweeten if desired. Drink hot or cold with ice. Refrigerate leftovers.

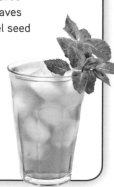

Meant for Intestinal Ills

- **_Try Tea_** Peppermint tea is a classic stomach settler. You can make it with fresh or dried leaves, or commercial tea bags. To make a basic cup of peppermint tea "from scratch," place a heaping teaspoon of dried peppermint leaf in the bottom of a cup. Fill with just-boiled water and steep for 10 to 15 minutes. Strain and sweeten, if desired. Enjoy up to four cups a day.

⚠ **CAUTION:** Do not give peppermint tea to infants and very young children, as menthol may cause a choking reaction.

- **_Do a Combo_** Try mixing peppermint with other antispasmodic and carminative herbs for relief of indigestion, especially indigestion accompanied by bothersome intestinal gas. Mix a tablespoon each dried peppermint, catnip, chamomile, basil, and fennel seeds in a glass jar with an airtight lid. Put a heaping teaspoon of this mixture in a cup, add just-boiled water, and steep for ten minutes. Strain and sweeten as desired.

⚠ **CAUTION:** Avoid chamomile if you are allergic to ragweed or other plants in the aster family.

- **_Try Tinctures_** Make an indigestion aid by stirring 10 to 20 drops of peppermint tincture (available at most health food stores) into about 8 ounces of cool water. Sip slowly. Repeat three to four times a day, between meals.
- **_Choose Capsules for IBS_** Although peppermint tea is good for stomach upsets, the remedy of choice for irritable bowel syndrome is enteric-coated capsules of peppermint oil, available at health food stores and some pharmacies. The coating allows the capsule to pass intact through the stomach (where it could cause heartburn) so it is released only in the intestines. Follow package directions.
- **_Give Yourself a Stomach Massage_** In a small dish, mix 5 drops of peppermint essential oil with 1 tablespoon of sweet almond oil. Lie down, and apply some of the oil to the skin of your abdomen. Using relatively firm pressure, give yourself an abdominal massage, working in a clockwise direction: up the right side of your abdomen, across just under the diaphragm, down the left side, and across above the pubic bone. Such a massage can be very soothing for indigestion and gas.

▶ SKIN IRRITATIONS

Pop a peppermint after-dinner mint into your mouth, and you'll instantly feel its cooling effect. Peppermint is a common ingredient in many muscle rubs and skin creams as a way to provide temporary relief from muscular aches and to soothe skin irritation. Applying peppermint infusions (teas), diluted peppermint essential oil, or commercially made peppermint-based creams to irritated skin can bring quick, cooling relief.

good to know: ALSO FOR SKIN IRRITATIONS

- Evening primrose (*Oenothera biennis*) is also suggested by modern herbal practitioners to treat skin conditions, including eczema.
- Patchouli (*Pogostemon cablin*) is an herb with a balsamic, woody scent that is commonly used in aromatherapy (see page 259). Patchouli is sometimes suggested by herbalists for skin irritations such as dermatitis and eczema.

Go for the Cool Aid

- **Create a Compress** To soothe minor skin irritation, saturate a clean washcloth with a cooled solution of peppermint tea (in the previous section titled "Meant for Intestinal Ills"). Squeeze out the excess and fold the moist cloth to roughly the size of the affected area of skin. Apply as a compress for 15 to 20 minutes. Repeat as needed.
- **Massage for Relief** Add ½ teaspoon peppermint oil to ½ cup sweet almond oil or a similar neutral carrier oil. Wet your fingertips with this mixture and gently massage it into an area of chapped, irritated, or sunburned skin.

⚠ **CAUTION:** Never apply peppermint oil to the face of an infant or small child, because it can cause spasms that interfere with breathing.

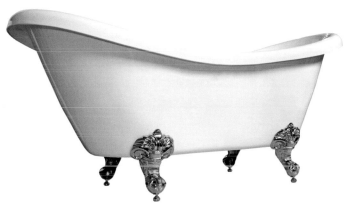

- **Add to the Bath** Add a pot of peppermint tea to bathwater to ease stress and soothe minor skin irritation. Steep 6 heaping tablespoons of dried peppermint in 1 quart of just-boiled water for 15 to 20 minutes. Add the tea to the bathwater as the tub fills. Alternatively, add 10 drops of peppermint essential oil to a full tub of bathwater.

▶ | HEADACHE

When a headache strikes, you can choose to pop an aspirin or other over-the-counter headache medication. But peppermint is a time-tested approach to headache relief that's simple and without side effects.

Chill "Pills"

- **Cool It** Pour 3 cups just-boiled water over 3 peppermint tea bags. Steep, covered, for about ten minutes. Remove the tea bags and add 1 cup ice cubes. When the ice melts, dip a washcloth into cold tea and apply to your forehead for ten minutes. Repeat as needed.
- **Massage Away the Pain** Mix 2 drops of peppermint essential oil with 1 teaspoon of sweet almond oil or olive oil in a small dish. Wet the tips of your fingers with the oil, and massage your temples with small circular motions. Massage across your forehead as well. Be careful not to get the oil in your eyes.
- **Breathe It In** Place a drop or two of peppermint essential oil on a cotton ball and hold it under your nose (do not touch the oil to the skin). Close your eyes and inhale the scent for 30 to 60 seconds to promote relaxation and help ease headache pain.
- **Try the Steam Treatment** In a large heatproof bowl, add 5 drops of peppermint oil to about 4 cups of just-boiled water. Drape a towel over your head and shoulders and lean over the bowl. Keep your eyes closed and your face at least 12 inches above the water's surface. Make a small inhalation. If this feels comfortable, inhale the peppermint vapors for ten minutes.

⚠ **CAUTION:** Infants and children should not inhale peppermint vapors.

good to know: ALSO FOR HEADACHES

- Skullcap (*Scutellaria lateriflora*), another member of the mint family, is used in herbal medicine as a mild relaxant appropriate for relieving tension headaches.
- Willow bark (*Salix alba, S. purpurea, S. fragilis*) has long been used to alleviate pain. Willow bark contains salicin, which the body converts to salicylic acid, the same pain-killing substance that is in aspirin. Herbal practitioners often suggest willow bark teas for relieving headache and arthritis pain.

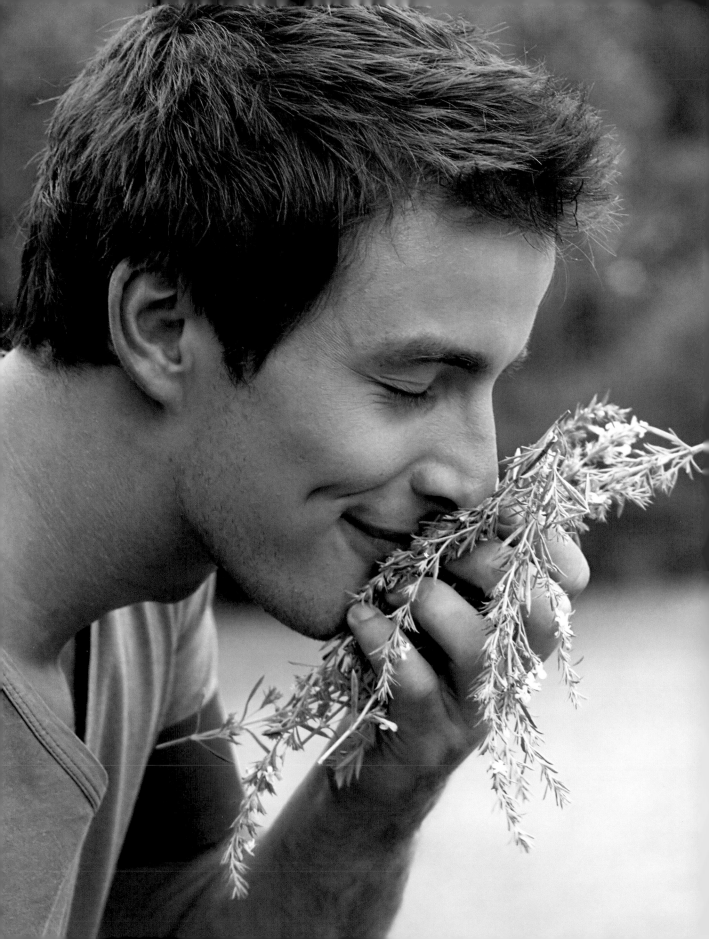

Rosemary

10 WAYS TO APPLY GOOD SCENTS

"There's rosemary; that's for remembrance." So says the lovely Ophelia in *Hamlet*, the tragedy Shakespeare penned more than 400 years ago. The link between rosemary and remembering—loved ones, loyalties, vows—has deep roots in a number of cultures. Mourners in some European countries still carry sprigs of rosemary in funeral processions and cast the herb into the grave during the burial. Rosemary's fragrance is as memorable as some of the customs associated with it. It's a peculiar mix of pungent pine and spicy, bittersweet mint that is a surprising complement to many foods, which is why rosemary has been prized as a culinary spice for centuries.

Rosemary's roots in herbal medicine are equally old. Traditionally, *Rosmarinus officinalis,* as botanists call it, was used to improve memory, fight depression, ease muscle and joint pain, treat indigestion, clear skin infections, heal wounds, stimulate hair growth—and ward off bubonic plague. Protection from plague aside, modern herbal medicine still employs rosemary as a natural remedy for many of the same complaints. Today, herbalists recommend rosemary topically to soothe aching muscles and joints and to treat a variety of skin conditions. They suggest taking it internally—typically by brewing the leaves into rosemary tea—to calm minor stomach upsets. Rosemary essential oil is used in aromatherapy (see page 259) primarily as a physical and mental stimulant, for pain relief of sore muscles and joints, for easing headaches, and to relieve symptoms of colds and flu. Interestingly enough, there is also data supporting the use of rosemary aromatherapy for improving mental function and—yes—memory.

▶ SKIN INFECTIONS

Scientists have discovered that rosemary extracts can inhibit several types of bacteria and fungi, including a number of pathogenic bacteria, such as *Staphylococcus aureus,* which can cause skin infections. Try some of the following remedies to harness rosemary's antiseptic properties.

⚠ **CAUTION:** Rosemary extracts with concentrated essential oils can cause a rash in some people when skin is exposed to sun. If that happens, discontinue use. Never apply undiluted rosemary essential oil to skin.

Ah, There's the Rub

■ *Inhibit Bacteria Naturally* Many commercial antibacterial soaps contain bacteria-killing chemicals such as triclosan and triclocarban. These substances are effective, but they are environmental hazards and may put your health at risk. For example, triclosan—currently under review by the U.S. Food and Drug Administration—can

good to know: ALSO FOR SKIN INFECTIONS

Myrrh *(Commiphora myrrha)* is the fragrant resin of the myrrh tree. Certain chemical compounds in myrrh have been shown to exhibit antimicrobial, antiparasitic, and antifungal activity and to help relieve inflammation and heal wounds.

combine with chlorine in tap water to form a potential carcinogen. You can make a natural, plant-based alternative to these commercial products in just a few minutes. Simply add 10 to 20 drops of rosemary essential oil to 1 cup of pure, unscented liquid castile soap (see page 208), available at health food stores and many drugstores. Mix thoroughly and pour into a pump soap dispenser.

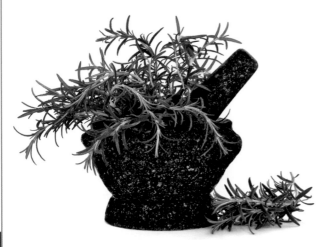

■ **Rinse Away Dandruff** Those little white flakes of scalp skin that settle embarrassingly on your shoulders have many possible causes, including stress, overactive oil glands, a hormone imbalance, dermatitis, and possibly a yeastlike fungal infection. Rosemary may help reduce the flaking. Make a rosemary hair rinse by pouring 2 cups of just-boiled water over 2 heaping teaspoons of fresh or dried rosemary leaves. Let it steep for 15 minutes, and then strain. When cool, transfer to a plastic squeeze bottle. After you wash your hair, squeeze out excess water, and then slowly drizzle the rinse into your hair. Let it sit for a minute or two, then rinse with warm water.

⚠ **CAUTION:** Stop using this remedy if it irritates your skin.

■ **Banish Lice** Head lice are more of an invasion than an infection. These tiny, wingless insects live close to the skin surface and lay eggs around hair follicles. Medicinal shampoos kill head lice, but beware: Some contain pesticides known to cause nervous system damage. Try a natural approach instead. Mix 10 drops rosemary oil, 15 drops each of thyme and lavender oils, and 20 drops tea tree oil into ¼ cup grapeseed or sweet almond oil. Pour this mixture over hair (and lice!) and massage deeply into the scalp for two minutes. Pile hair on top of head and cover with a plastic shower cap. Wrap your head in a towel, make a cup of calming herbal tea, and relax for an hour. Then shampoo and rinse well.

▶ **MUSCLE & JOINT PAIN**

Many herbalists recommend applying preparations of rosemary to the skin's surface to ease minor aches in muscles and joints. Health food stores carry a variety of creams, ointments, and salves that contain rosemary extracts. You can use these products to soothe whatever is sore, or make your own pain-and-ache relievers.

⚠ **CAUTION:** Never apply undiluted rosemary essential oil to skin.

Muscle Meds
■ **Get a Jump on the Ache** Before heading to the gym, going running, or engaging in any kind of vigorous exercise, try this rosemary sports rub to stimulate muscles and help prevent inflammation. In a small bowl, combine 2 drops rosemary essential oil, 1 drop lavender essential oil, and 1 drop eucalyptus essential oil. Add 4 teaspoons of grapeseed, sweet almond, or

good to know: ALSO FOR MUSCLE & JOINT PAIN
Horse chestnut (*Aesculus hippocastanum*), available as a gel, ointment, or cream at many health food stores, is a topical treatment for muscle strains and minor sprains—one that's very popular in Germany. Follow package directions. ⚠ **CAUTION:** Preparations containing horse chestnut extracts should not be applied to broken skin.

MORNING WAKE-UP HAIR RINSE

Vinegar helps balance the pH of skin and hair, and leaves hair naturally shiny. Try this simple hair rinse recipe using rosemary:

½ cup fresh rosemary leaves
1 quart organic apple cider vinegar

Put the herbs in a quart glass jar with a tight-fitting lid and fill almost to the top with vinegar. Secure the lid and place the jar in a sunny window; leave for one to two weeks. Strain out the herbs and pour the strained liquid into a plastic squeeze bottle. To rinse hair after shampooing, add 1 to 2 tablespoons of rinse to about ¼ cup water. Pour through your hair, massaging well into the scalp. Rinse well with warm water.

apricot kernel oil. Blend well, and apply the mixture to skin over muscles and joints that are most likely to get a hard workout.

- **Soak Away Pain** Add 5 to 10 drops of rosemary essential oil to a full tub of hot water for an invigorating and muscle-relaxing bath. Or tie sprigs of fresh rosemary (or a handful of dried rosemary leaves) in a muslin bag and hang it under the faucet while running a hot bath. Alternatively, soak the bag in the bath while you are in it yourself.

- **Make Your Toes Happy** If you spend a lot of time standing, or you wear high heels, you know how much your feet can ache at the end of the day. A rosemary-infused foot soak can help. In a plastic tub large enough to accommodate your feet, add 4 drops each of rosemary, eucalyptus, and peppermint essential oil. Add enough hot water (not so hot it could burn you, though) so you can submerge your feet to just below the anklebone. Soak for at least ten minutes.

▶ | MEMORY

The ancients believed that rosemary could uplift the soul and strengthen the memory. Several preliminary studies suggest that they were on to something. One study, for example, noted that when volunteers underwent rosemary aromatherapy for several minutes, their anxiety levels dropped, their alertness increased, and they showed increased speed in doing mathematics. Although inhaling rosemary's unique fragrance won't guarantee you a passing grade on your next calculus exam, it might help you stay more focused while you study.

Stimulating Scents

- **Surround Yourself With Scent** If you need to concentrate, add 5 to 10 drops of rosemary oil to 2 cups of water in a spray bottle. Shake well to mix. Spritz a little into the air every hour.

- **Have a Cuppa!** Rosemary tea is an invigorating brew. Add just-boiled water to 1 teaspoon crushed dried rosemary leaves (or 1 heaping teaspoon chopped fresh leaves). Steep for ten minutes and sweeten, if desired.

- **Fight Fatigue** For a quick pick-me-up, put a few drops of rosemary oil on a handkerchief or cotton ball. Hold it under your nose and inhale the fragrance for 30 to 60 seconds (don't touch the oil to your skin). Repeat as needed to stay alert.

good to know: ALSO FOR MEMORY

- The herb bacopa *(Bacopa monnieri)* has been shown to enhance mental function and memory in laboratory tests and animal studies and in a few human trials. It may affect the levels and metabolism of acetylcholine, a key neurotransmitter in the brain and central nervous system.

- Rhodiola *(Rhodiola rosea)* is an herb that's fairly new to herbal medicine in the United States, though researchers in Russia and Scandinavia have researched its effects for more than 40 years. Herbalists recommend it—as tea, tincture, or extract—to enhance attention span and memory. Its role in stress reduction and countering mental fatigue seems promising.

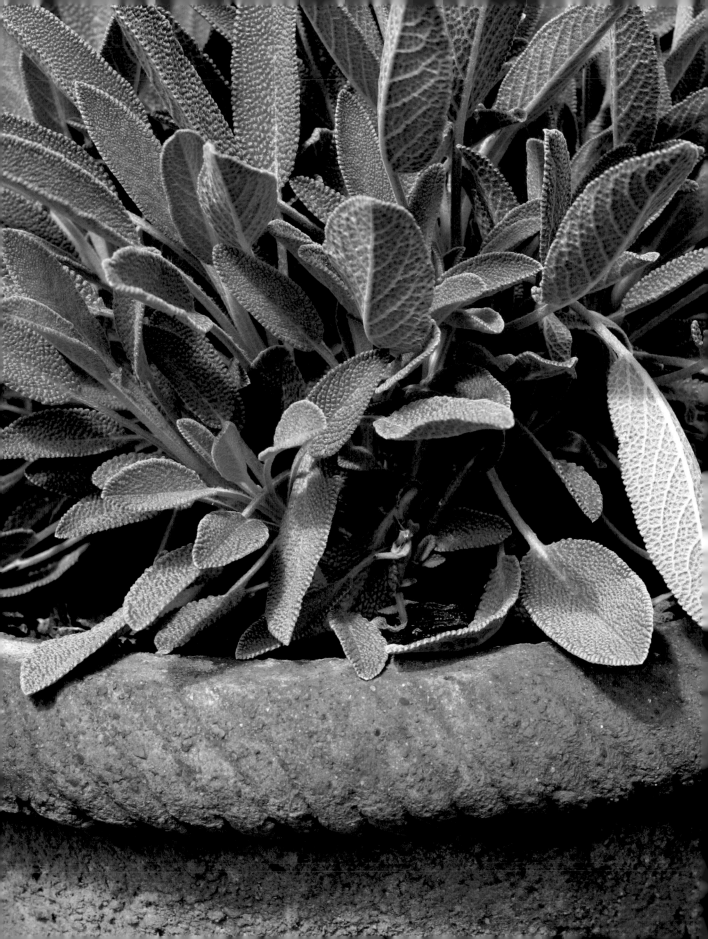

Sage

8 WAYS TO MAKE SAGE CHOICES

Many people know sage only from Thanksgiving, when they chop the herb's gray-green leaves to flavor the stuffing for the holiday bird. Sage is a classic, aromatic seasoning for poultry and many other foods. But it's also a medicinal herb, and has been linked with good health and long life for many centuries. Sage was so sacred to the ancient Romans that they gathered it with great ceremony, in white tunics and bare feet, having first offered sacrifices of bread and wine to the god Jupiter, to whom the herb was dedicated. When the Roman legions marched across Europe and Britain, they brought sage with them. In the centuries that followed, sage became a staple in medieval herbal and kitchen gardens.

It was used to treat hoarseness, coughs and lung conditions, indigestion, liver disease, fever, and to clean wounds and stop bleeding. Sage was also a remedy for helping reduce secretions such as sweat, watery eyes, and runny nose, and to aid in drying up breast milk in mothers ready to wean their babies. Sage was also thought to slow the decline of mental faculties that often accompanies old age.

Recently, the link between sage and mental health has been getting some modern, scientific support. Researchers have shown that the essential oil of common sage, *Salvia officinalis,* may improve mood and mental performance in young adults and boost memory and attention span in older adults. One small study showed that an extract of sage was helpful to people with mild to moderate Alzheimer's disease. Modern herbal practitioners typically recommend sage for treating coughs, colds, and bronchitis, for easing sore throat pain and tonsillitis, calming indigestion, and relieving excessive sweating, including night sweats associated with

menopause. You're likely to encounter sage in natural deodorants and mouthwashes, too. Laboratory studies suggest that essential oils in sage have antimicrobial properties.

> ⚠ **CAUTION:** Sage is generally regarded as safe if used in small amounts for short periods. Some species of sage contain thujone, a chemical that can affect the nervous system. Extended use or taking large amounts of sage leaf preparations may result in restlessness, vomiting, vertigo, rapid heart rate, tremors, seizures, and kidney damage. It also may lead to wheezing. Pregnant women and nursing mothers should not take sage internally.

▶ | COUGH

Coughs due to colds and flu are as common as the over-the-counter cough medications supposedly good for treating them. Yet in recent years, it's been shown that few, if any, of these products are all that effective. Sage, on the other hand, has a long history as a cough remedy. Try sage—for short periods—for natural cough relief.

Combos for Coughs

■ *Stop the Tickle* People have been brewing sage tea to help treat coughs

COUGH COMFORT TEA

Honey, lemon, thyme, and sage combine in this cough-calming tea.

2 teaspoons grated organic lemon rind
1 teaspoon fresh sage, chopped fine (can substitute
  1 teaspoon dried sage leaf)
½ teaspoon fresh or dried thyme leaf
Juice from ½ fresh organic lemon
Organic clover honey

Add the lemon rind and herbs to a cup and fill with just-boiled water. Cover and steep 15 minutes. Strain the tea, and then add the lemon juice and enough honey to sweeten to your taste. Stir well to mix. Drink up to three cups daily for cough relief; limit use to three days.

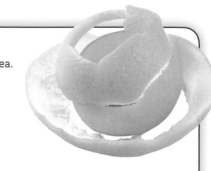

for many centuries. A basic recipe is to steep 1 heaping teaspoon chopped sage (either fresh or dried leaf) in 1 cup just-boiled water for ten minutes. Strain and sweeten, as desired. Sip slowly, letting the hot liquid trickle down your throat. Drink up to three cups a day, but for no more than three days. For a variation on this basic sage tea, see the recipe for Cough Comfort Tea above.

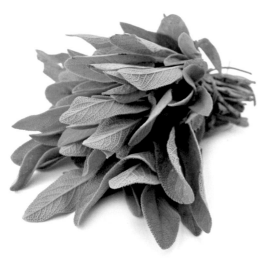

- **Stir Up Some Syrup** Sage and honey can combine to make a soothing and great-tasting natural cough syrup. Add 2 ounces (about ¼ cup) dried sage to 4 cups of water in a large saucepan. Simmer over low heat until the liquid is reduced to 2 cups. Strain and discard the herbs. Combine the 2 cups of sage liquid with 1 cup honey and simmer very gently, uncovered, for about 20 minutes. The mixture should take on the consistency of syrup. Optional: Add 1 tablespoon of brandy or vodka to help preserve the syrup. Cool, pour syrup into a glass jar with a tight-fitting lid, and refrigerate. Take ¼ to ½ teaspoon every two to three hours to relieve cough; limit use to three days.

⚠ **CAUTION:** Never give honey to infants or children younger than age one.

good to know: ALSO FOR COUGHS

- The herb eucalyptus (*Eucalyptus globulus*) has been used to treat both coughs and sore throats for many years in the Western world and for thousands of years by Australian Aborigines. Eucalyptus is an ingredient in many OTC cough drops and chest rubs.

- Thyme (*Thymus vulgaris*) has been prescribed since the Middle Ages as an herbal remedy for coughs and respiratory complaints of all kinds. Modern herbalists recommend it—as tea, capsule, or syrup—for spasmodic coughs. Several volatile oils in thyme, including carvacrol and thymol, account for its expectorant as well as potent antimicrobial properties.

- Herbalists sometimes recommend bee balm (*Monarda didyma*) for treating coughs and sore throats. Bee balm (along with other herbs such as thyme) contains thymol, a chemical compound with strong antimicrobial properties. Thymol is an ingredient in some antiseptic mouthwashes and toothpastes.

▶ | SORE THROAT

Sage has been used to soothe sore throats for centuries, and recent research confirms that it's quite effective—especially when combined with other inflammation-fighting herbs—for relieving the scratchy, painful, back-of-the-throat irritation that so often accompanies colds and flu.

good to know: SORE THROAT

└ Hibiscus *(Hibiscus sabdariffa)* is rich in vitamin C as well as throat-soothing mucilage that can ease the pain of a sore throat.

Sage Advice for Scratchy Throats

- **Try Sage Tea Variations** Plain sage tea (see recipe on opposite page) is fine for sore throats, but try experimenting with variations to see what works for you. For example, put 1 teaspoon dried sage leaves and ¾ teaspoon bruised fennel seed into a cup and add just-boiled water. Steep ten minutes and strain. The fennel imparts a natural sweetness, and also has antimicrobial and antispasmodic properties. For another option, combine 1 teaspoon each dried sage, dried lemon balm leaf, dried echinacea aerial parts, and freshly grated organic orange peel. Steep in just-boiled water for ten minutes.
- **Gargle Away Pain** Make this vinegar-based gargle to have on hand before the cold and flu season hits. Combine 2 tablespoons dried sage leaves and 2 tablespoons dried thyme leaves in a clean coffee grinder or small food processor. Grind well, and place the powder in a clean quart mason jar. Cover with 2 cups of organic apple cider vinegar, stir to completely wet and distribute the herbs, and secure the lid. Keep at room temperature for two weeks, shaking once a day. Strain the liquid into a dark-colored bottle and refrigerate. To use as a gargle for a sore throat, mix 1 to 2 tablespoons of this vinegar mixture into a small glass of warm water. Gargle and spit; repeat three to four times a day.

- **Try the Tincture** Make an instant sore throat gargle by adding 5 to 10 drops of sage tincture (available at most natural food stores) to a small glass of warm water. Gargle and spit. Repeat three to four times a day.

▶ | SWEATING & ODOR

Chemical compounds in sage act to reduce perspiration and some other body secretions. Germany's health authorities approve the use of sage as a treatment for excessive sweating, including sweating brought on by night sweats and hot flashes, based on traditional use and human studies. Many herbalists recommend sage tea as an occasional night sweat–taming natural remedy.

Some No-Sweat Solutions

- **Keep Sage Tea on Hand** To remedy occasional night sweats, brew a concentrated version of sage tea to keep on hand in the fridge. Steep 4 heaping tablespoons of dried sage in 2 cups boiling water. Cover tightly and let stand four hours. Strain, discard the herbs, and refrigerate the tea concentrate. When you need relief, mix some of the concentrate with water to make a cup of regular-strength tea, and heat.

⚠ **CAUTION:** Drink small amounts as needed, rather than routinely. Consult your health care provider about persistent or regular night sweats.

- **Blend a Body Powder** For a natural approach to controlling heavy perspiration and body odor, thoroughly blend ½ cup baking soda, ½ cup cornstarch, 1 tablespoon ground sage, and 1 tablespoon ground rosemary in a small glass jar with an airtight lid. Using a cotton ball or powder puff, dust this mixture under your arms or wherever dampness or odor is a problem.

good to know: SWEATING & ODOR

└ Astragalus *(Astragalus membranaceus)* is an herb used in traditional Chinese medicine (see page 295) to treat many conditions, including night sweats (often in combination with other herbs).

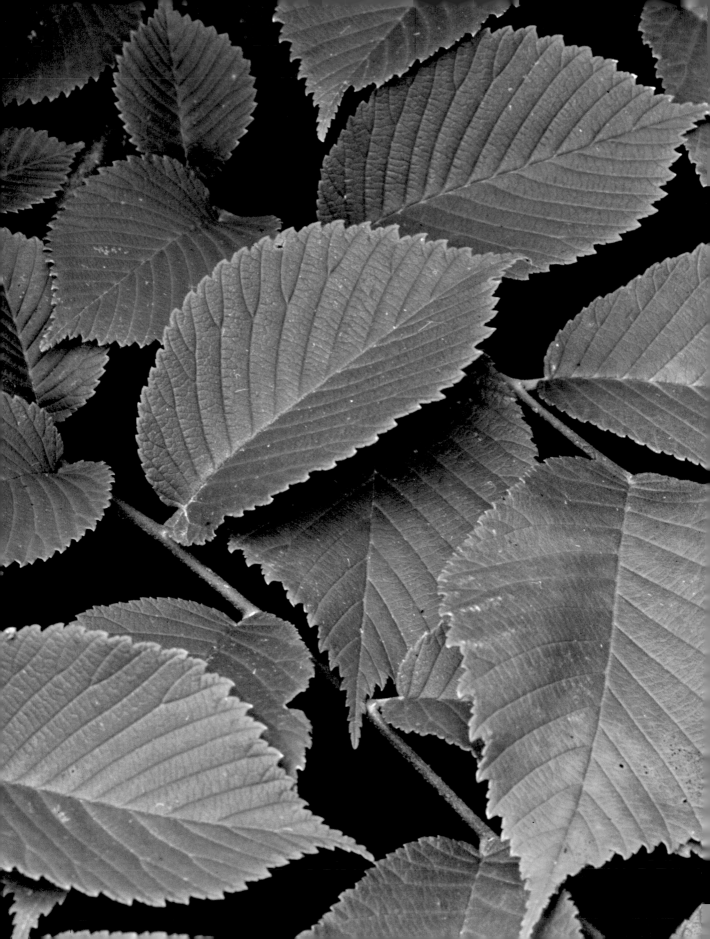

Slippery Elm

10 WAYS TO SOOTHE THROATS & TUMMIES

Native Americans were the first to discover that the reddish inner bark of the slippery elm tree *(Ulmus rubra)* contains mucilage, a substance that turns slippery when wet. This slick gel proved to be a remarkably versatile natural remedy. Indians mixed the powdered bark with fats or oils to make healing salves for minor wounds, burns, boils, and skin irritations. They brewed it into drinks given to cure stomach and bowel complaints. And they created thick, soothing slippery elm tonics for quieting coughs, easing sore throats, and calming hoarse voices. American colonists quickly adopted slippery elm and used it for many of the same ailments. Poultices made of slippery elm bark were a standard treatment for gunshot wounds during the American Revolution.

Slippery elm settled comfortably into the American pharmacopeia during the 1800s and has been a popular natural remedy ever since. It is one of the few herbs approved by the U.S. Food and Drug Administration, and is sold as a nonprescription (over-the-counter) drug. Slippery elm's unique properties make it particularly good for soothing and healing inflamed mucosal (lining) tissues of the digestive tract, from the throat on down. Herbalists recommend it for coughs and sore throats as well as heartburn and a variety of intestinal ailments. Slippery elm powder and products are widely available, but wild trees have been overharvested in many parts of their range to supply the herbal medicine market. If you have a choice, choose brands that use slippery elm powder derived from cultivated trees.

> ⚠ **CAUTION:** Consumption of slippery elm preparations and products may slow the absorption of oral medications. Therefore, take oral medications either an hour before or several hours after consuming slippery elm. Although slippery elm is generally considered very safe, avoid this herb if you have, or suspect you have, any bile duct obstruction or gallstones.

▶ | COUGH

Many herbs are good for soothing coughs, but slippery elm is unique in the way it coats and protects the back of the throat. You'll find slippery elm in a number of forms in health food stores, including easy-to-use capsules, lozenges, extracts, and tea bags. But don't shy away from making your own slippery elm remedies using the finely powdered bark and a few other basic ingredients. It's simple and fun.

Cough Control

- ***Stir and Sip*** Make basic slippery elm tea to quiet a cough by placing ½ teaspoon of powdered bark in a cup. Slowly add just-boiled water, whisking gently with a fork. Let the mixture stand for five to ten minutes, stir again, and sip slowly. Drink two to three cups per day.
- ***Spice It Up*** By itself, slippery elm has a pleasant, mild taste. To create a cup of cough-controlling tea with a little more flavor and zip, make the recipe above and

then add 2 tablespoons light coconut milk or almond milk and a hearty dash of cinnamon, cardamom, and nutmeg. Stir well to combine all ingredients and sweeten to taste with honey or stevia powder according to your preference.

- **Mix Your Own Cough Medicine** Stir 1 ounce (about 2 tablespoons) of slippery elm bark powder and 3 tablespoons honey into 2 cups of just-boiled water. Let cool 30 minutes; stir again. Take 1 tablespoon dose as needed to help quiet coughing.

Before the arrival of Europeans, at least six Native American tribes, including the Cherokee and Iroquois, used slippery elm bark to treat sore throat. Slippery elm lozenges have been sold in the United States since the late 1800s, and are available today in many health food stores and pharmacies. You can make your own at home, too.

good to know: ALSO FOR SORE THROAT

— Cayenne *(Capsicum annuum)* hardly seems like an antidote for sore throat. But herbalists sometimes suggest using a small amount of the powdered herb (a good-size pinch) mixed into a small glass of water as a gargle.

— Licorice *(Glycyrrhiza glabra)* root provides a trifecta of relief. Since ancient times, this sweet tasting root with tissue-coating properties has been used to treat cough, sore throat, and digestive problems such as gastritis and heartburn. It is available as lozenge or tablet and soothingly effective as a tea. ⚠ **CAUTION:** Licorice is safe if taken for less than a week.

— Hibiscus *(Hibiscus sabdariffa)* is rich in vitamin C as well as throat-soothing mucilage that can ease the pain of a sore throat.

GINGER & SLIPPERY ELM THROAT SOOTHERS

These "lozenges" are actually thin, honey-soaked slices of parboiled fresh ginger, coated in slippery elm and licorice root powders. They won't actually dissolve in your mouth, so they last a long time (until you chew and swallow them), and they are good for sore throat, cough, and indigestion. You'll need the following to make them:

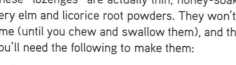

A piece of fresh gingerroot about the size of your hand
Water
½ cup honey
8 to 10 drops each of thyme, mint, and bitter orange essential oil
3 tablespoons (approximately) slippery elm powder
3 tablespoons (approximately) licorice root powder

Peel the ginger root and cut into ¼-inch slices. Cut large slices in half. Put the slices in a small saucepan, cover with about two inches of water, and simmer on low heat until they begin to soften, about 20 to 30 minutes. Drain off the water and lay the slices on a paper towel; use another paper towel to pat dry.

Place the honey in a small bowl and add the essential oils. Stir well to combine. Add the ginger pieces and stir gently, making sure the pieces are well coated by the honey mixture. Cover and let sit for an hour.

Mix together the slippery elm and licorice powders in a small, shallow dish. Cover a cookie sheet with a piece of waxed paper. Remove the ginger pieces from the honey mixture one by one, allowing excess honey to drip off. Dip each slice in the powder, coating both sides well. Place on waxed paper. Repeat the powdering procedure several more times over the next day, until the powder is no longer absorbed. Store finished "lozenges" in an airtight container in the refrigerator. ⚠ **CAUTION:** Pregnant women should consume no more than 1 gram (1,000 mg) of ginger daily.

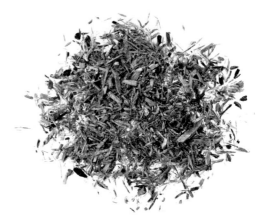

Thwart a Sore Throat

- **Gargle and Swallow** Make a cup of plain slippery elm tea (see the previous section titled "Cough Control"). Take a mouthful, gargle with it for 15 seconds, and then swallow slowly, letting it trickle down your throat. Repeat until you finish the cup.

- **Simmer and Strain** For variety, try this version of slippery elm tea, which also contains marshmallow root—another throat-soothing herb. In a glass jar with a tight-fitting lid, mix together thoroughly ½ cup each of coarsely ground slippery elm bark (not powder), marshmallow root (not powder), cinnamon bark (broken into pieces), fennel seed, and dried organic orange peel. Measure a heaping tablespoon of this mixture into a teapot, add 2 cups of boiling water, stir, cover, and steep for 20 minutes. Strain into a cup, and sweeten with honey or stevia if desired. Take up to three cups daily.

- **Roll Your Own** In a small bowl, combine 2 tablespoons slippery elm powder and 2 teaspoons honey. (As an option, add 1 drop of anise seed essential oil for flavor.) Mix gently but thoroughly with a fork or your fingers to make a firm dough. Divide the dough into 20 small pieces and roll them into little balls. Roll the balls in additional slippery elm powder and flatten them slightly into a lozenge shape. Allow the lozenges to air-dry for several hours. Store in a covered container in the refrigerator. For a very different sore throat and cough lozenge—one that can also ease indigestion—see the recipe on the opposite page.

▶ | DIGESTIVE UPSETS

Slippery elm contains soothing mucilage that coats the lining of the digestive tract; it also contains antioxidant compounds that help fight inflammation. Herbalists recommend slippery elm for indigestion, heartburn, gastroesophageal reflux disease (GERD), Crohn's disease, irritable bowel syndrome (IBS), ulcerative colitis, and diarrhea. Check with your doctor, however, before combining any of the natural remedies below with medications you may already be taking for these conditions.

Upstage Digestive Upsets

- **Sip for Relief** When occasional heartburn flares, sip a cup of plain slippery elm tea (see the previous section titled "Cough Control").

- **Calm IBS** Stir ½ to 1 teaspoon of slippery elm powder into a cup of hot water. Flavor with 1 teaspoon of maple syrup and a dash of cinnamon. Drink once or twice a day.

- **Try a Gruel** When indigestion or bowel troubles strike, mix up this soothing "gruel." Measure 1 tablespoon of slippery elm bark powder in a small bowl. Slowly add ½ cup boiling water, stirring constantly, to make a thick paste. Add about ½ cup more boiling water while continuing to stir, until the mixture takes on the consistency of cream of wheat. Add a pinch of cinnamon or pumpkin pie spice, and a little maple syrup to sweeten. This mixture can also help soothe sore throats and ease coughs.

---

good to know: ALSO FOR DIGESTIVE UPSETS

- Catnip *(Nepeta cataria)* is another herb that herbal practitioners sometimes recommend to help settle upset stomachs.
- Cat's claw *(Uncaria tomentosa, U. guiaensis)* has anti-inflammatory properties and is sometimes suggested for treating gastritis and colitis (intestinal inflammation).
  ⚠ **CAUTION:** Don't use cat's claw if you have an autoimmune disease or are taking immunosuppressive or blood pressure medications.

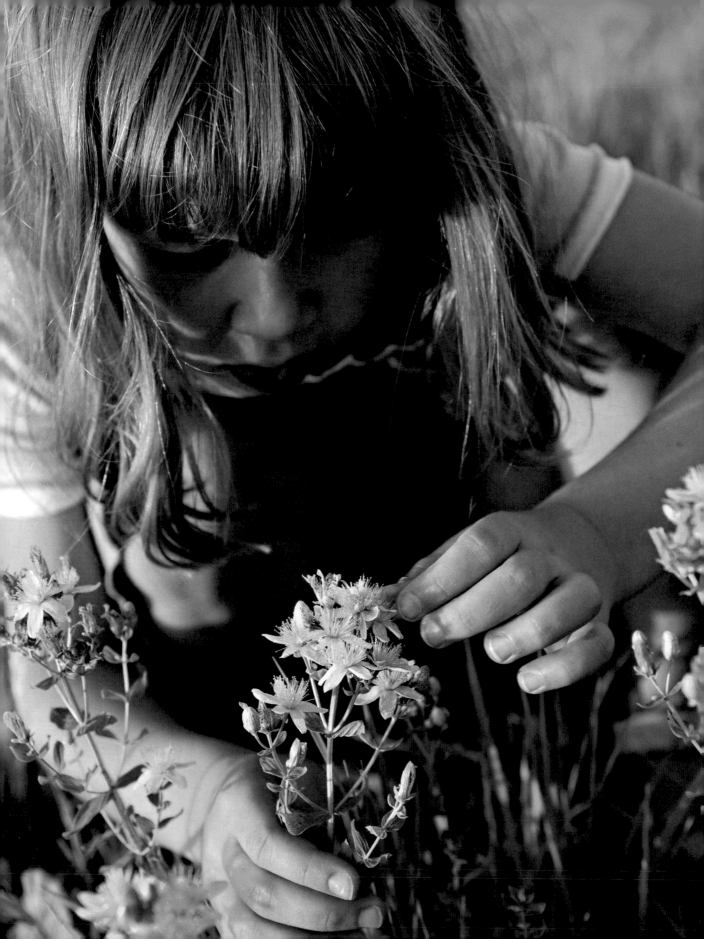

St. John's Wort

9 WAYS TO MEDICATE MIND & BODY

You have to wonder about a plant that bleeds. Yet that's what St. John's wort seems to do. Touch the delicate yellow flowers of this common meadowland herb, and beads of blood red liquid appear on the petals. It's not really blood, of course, but an oil oozing from tiny glands. The effect is a little eerie, though, so it's not surprising that the ancients believed St. John's wort was a plant of great importance and powerful magic. It was hung over doorways to keep evil spirits at bay, and burned in ceremonies to cleanse, protect, or sanctify a place. During the rise of Christianity, the bleeding plant became associated with St. John the Baptist. It was believed to bloom on the saint's June birthday, and bleed on the late August anniversary of his beheading.

Blood, evil, and symbolism aside, St. John's wort was also a respected healing herb. The Greeks and Romans used it to treat wounds, snakebite, and nerve pain, and to ease the minds of people who were troubled or dispirited. By the Middle Ages, St. John's wort was considered a remedy for many things, not the least of which were afflictions such as anxiety, melancholy, and nervous disorders. During the 1700s, the herb became firmly entrenched in American herbal medicine. Its popularity faded in the early 1900s—as many herbs did—and then it experienced a remarkable revival in the late 20th century. Today, St. John's wort is the most widely used herb in modern herbal medicine for treating mild depression.

A number of studies have demonstrated that St. John's wort may be as effective for treating mild depression in some people (about 70 percent of cases) as some selective serotonin reuptake inhibitors (SSRIs) that doctors routinely prescribe—and with fewer side effects. Other studies are less conclusive. Nevertheless, many European doctors widely prescribe St. John's wort for treating mild depression. In the United States, there is considerable interest in St. John's wort as a natural remedy (the herb is among the best-selling dietary supplements in mainstream retail stores), but it is not a prescription medication. Research has revealed that St. John's wort also has notable anti-inflammatory, antibacterial, and antiviral properties, making it useful for treating minor injuries and skin irritations, as well as muscle and joint pain.

▶ | DEPRESSION

St. John's wort contains a host of biologically active chemical substances, including the compounds hypericin and hyperforin. How the herb's compounds work to help relieve mild depression isn't clear, but several theories have been put

---

good to know: ABOUT ST. JOHN'S WORT

- St. John's wort can make skin overly sensitive to sunlight. If you are taking the herb and have fair skin, avoid tanning beds and wear sunscreen (see page 224), a hat, and sun-protective clothing when out in the sun.
- If you are taking St. John's wort and decide to stop, do so gradually and under the supervision of your health care provider. Stopping abruptly may cause unpleasant side effects.

ST. JOHN'S WORT TINCTURE

It's a month-long project to make this homemade herbal tincture, but well worth the effort:

About 2 handfuls dried St. John's wort (aerial parts)
About 1½ cups 40% (80-proof) vodka (good quality, but it doesn't need to be the most expensive vodka on the shelf)

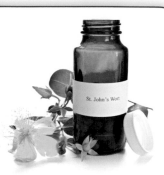

Fill a clean, dry, pint-size glass jar with a tight-fitting lid about half full with dried St. John's wort. Add enough vodka to cover the herbs completely. Wait 15 or 20 minutes and check the alcohol level. Dried herbs typically swell as they soak up liquid, so add more vodka to make sure the herbs are completely submerged (there should be an inch or two of liquid above the herbs).

Let the tincture sit for four weeks. Shake the jar daily. After a month, line a strainer with several layers of cheesecloth and pour the liquid slowly through the strainer into a pitcher. After straining, squeeze the herb-filled cloth to wring out any remaining liquid. Discard the herbs. Pour the liquid—this is the tincture—into another clean, dry glass jar with a tight-fitting lid. Amber-colored glass jars (available at herb stores or online) work well.

To use on skin, simply apply the tincture with an eyedropper or saturate a cotton ball and dab on.

forward. For instance, some studies suggest that St. John's wort might act by preventing nerve cells in the brain from reabsorbing the chemical messenger serotonin, or by reducing levels of a protein involved in the body's immune system functioning. One thing that is clear from clinical studies, however, is that St. John's wort acts more slowly than prescription drugs such as SSRIs, taking from two to four weeks to exert its effects. In herbal medicine, practitioners recommend St. John's wort as a remedy for anxiety, premenstrual syndrome (PMS), seasonal affective disorder (SAD), certain symptoms of menopause, and insomnia, in addition to mild depression.

⚠ **CAUTION:** Research has shown that St. John's wort interacts with many commonly used prescription and over-the-counter medications in ways that can interfere with their intended effects. Consult your doctor before using St. John's wort in any form if you are taking contraceptives, antidepressants, allergy drugs, immunosuppressants (such as cyclosporine), digoxin (a heart medication), indinavir and other drugs used to control HIV infection, warfarin and related blood thinners.

Derail Depression

- **Consider Capsules** Many who take St. John's wort for mild depression, anxiety, PMS, SAD, menopausal symptoms, or insomnia take capsules or tablets. These are standardized to contain 0.3 percent hypericin or 2 to 5 percent hyperforin. Before using, consult your doctor.

- **Investigate the Extract** St. John's wort is also available as a liquid extract, taken in divided doses during the day. Consult with your health care provider to determine the right dose. Be aware that simple teas made from dried St. John's wort won't help mild depression or some other conditions, because as it dries, the herb loses much of its potency.

▶ SKIN DAMAGE

In modern herbal medicine, St. John's wort is considered a worthy natural remedy for minor skin problems, including acne, sunburn, minor first-degree burns, boils, and bruises. It is also a simple treatment worth

good to know: ALSO FOR SKIN DAMAGE

Aloe *(Aloe vera)* gel—ideally from the fresh leaf—is an effective herbal remedy for minor burns, insect bites, dry and chapped skin, and other minor skin irritations.

reaching for the next time you've got an insect bite or sting, or a minor cut or scrape. Here's what to do.

Save Your Skin

- *Apply a Tincture* A St. John's wort tincture (available at natural food stores) can help disinfect damaged or irritated skin and so speed the healing process. Use it to cleanse cuts and scratches. To make your own tincture, see the St. John's wort recipe, opposite.
- *Take the Sting Out* St. John's wort's anti-inflammatory properties can help ease the pain of bee stings. After you've removed the stinger (see pages 72–73), dab on several drops of St. John's wort tincture. Repeat as needed until irritation and swelling subside.

DEPRESSION

Depression is a serious and common condition—and raises the risk of many other serious illnesses. According to the National Institute of Mental Health, nearly 7 percent of Americans suffer from depression in any given year. Only half receive treatment.

The hallmark symptoms of worthlessness, guilt, and shame often cause sufferers to feel they don't deserve treatment and to worry about the stigma. Depression challenges coping skills for even minor hassles. These factors and others create barriers to professional care, leading sufferers to delay or forgo help. If you had diabetes, would you self-treat or tell yourself to buck up and get over it? Among the depressed, far too many do.

That's sad, because several treatment options exist. Although St. John's wort is one of them, it's nonetheless wise to work in partnership with a health care practitioner.

–Linda B. White, M.D.
Educator and author

- *Cool a Cold Sore* Hypericin, one of the active ingredients in St. John's wort, has been shown to inhibit herpes simplex virus, the cause of cold sores. Next time a cold sore threatens to erupt (see page 44), begin dabbing on St. John's wort tincture at the first sign of tingling. Continue applying throughout the episode to dry and heal the affected area.
- *Ban the Burn* For minor burns and sunburns, you'll find salves, creams, and ointments containing St. John's wort extract at most health food stores.

▶ | MUSCLE PAIN

St. John's wort oil is highly regarded as a healing balm. It's made by infusing the flowering tops of the herb in oil for several weeks. The resulting infusion can be massaged into skin to relieve aching muscles and painful joints.

Rub It In

- *Make Your Own* Making your own St. John's wort oil is quite simple. It's best to use fresh flowers, picked when the herb is just coming into bloom in early summer. Gather enough flowers to fill a clean, dry pint-size glass jar (with a tight-fitting lid) almost to the top. Pour in enough olive oil to completely cover the flowers. Affix the lid and place the jar in a sunny windowsill; the oil will gradually turn a rich ruby red color. After three weeks, strain the oil through several layers of cheesecloth and store it in a dark glass container, tightly capped, for up to one year.
- *Soothe Irritations* You can use St. John's wort oil to ease the pain of minor skin irritations, boils, sunburn, and stings as well as muscle and joint pain. It's as easy as dabbing on a drop or two.

good to know: ALSO FOR MUSCLE PAIN

Arnica (*Arnica montana*) is an old folk remedy for treating a variety of skin conditions. Endorsed by German health authorities' Commission E, arnica salves and ointments (available at most natural food stores) can help ease the pain of bruises and muscle strains and may speed healing.

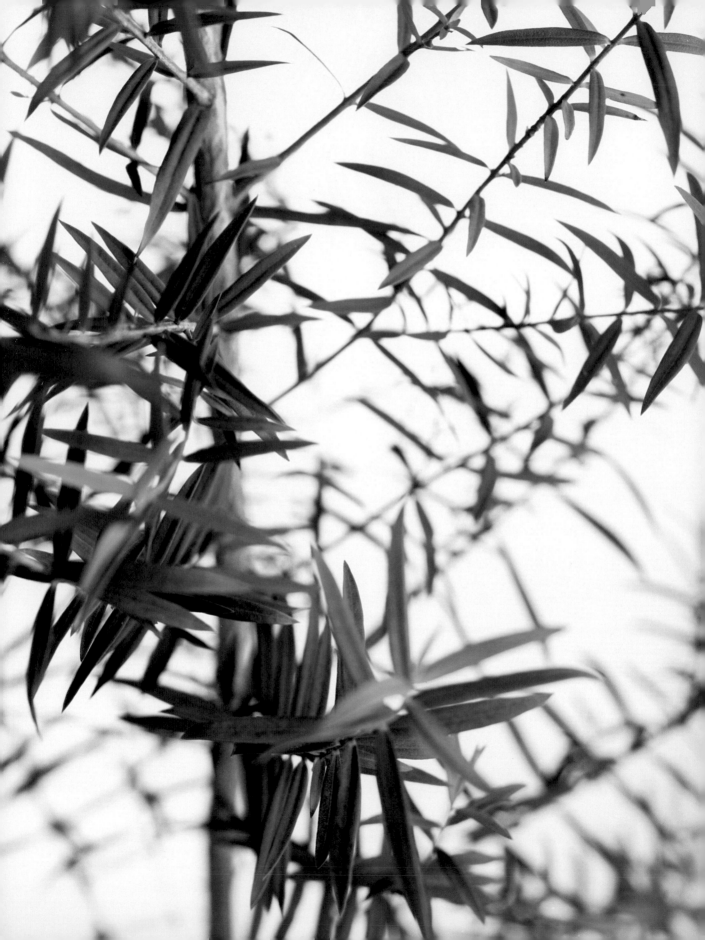

Tea Tree

14 WAYS TO INHIBIT INFECTION

Sometimes promoted as the "wonder from down under," the oil of Australia's tea tree *(Melaleuca alternifolia)* is a fairly recent addition to Western herbal medicine. Long before Europeans reached Australia's shores, Aborigines were chewing the lance-shaped leaves of this small, shrubby tree to ease coughs and sore throats. They also inhaled the aromatic oil from crushed leaves for respiratory ailments, and drank tea brewed from the leaves—the source of the English name, "tea tree"—to treat general sickness. However, the herb was pretty much ignored outside of the Aboriginal community until the 1920s, when lab tests revealed that tea tree's strong-smelling oil was a surprisingly powerful and effective antiseptic.

After the Australian medical community adopted tea tree oil for cleaning wounds and surgical incisions, its popularity grew considerably. It wasn't long before every well-equipped first aid kit or medicine cabinet in the country sported a small bottle of tea tree oil.

Throughout the 1920s and 1930s, wild tea trees were harvested for commercial production of tea tree oil. But with the rise of antibiotics, interest in harvesting the leaves waned. By the 1970s, wild harvesting had all but ground to a halt. Then a decade later, an enterprising Australian farmer set up a small tea tree plantation in northern New South Wales. The idea caught on. Establishing plantations allowed for an efficient leaf harvest, and helped to greatly increase the supply of raw material for making the oil. Tea tree oil made a comeback, and soon Europeans and Americans were trying the oil, too. Laboratory research and clinical trials support tea tree oil's effectiveness in preventing and treating minor skin infections caused by bacteria, fungi, and even some viruses. Tea tree oil has also become a familiar ingredient in many creams, ointments, soaps, shampoos, and toothpastes.

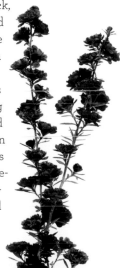

⚠ **CAUTION:** Tea tree oil, which is very concentrated, is toxic and should never be taken internally; do not apply the undiluted oil to skin. Avoid getting tea tree oil in your eyes. Allergic reactions and contact dermatitis have been reported in some people who have used tea tree oil. If redness, itching, or oozing develops after topical application, stop using the oil and see your doctor.

▶ FUNGAL INFECTIONS

At least two of the compounds found in tea tree oil are known to actively inhibit the growth of fungi—including those that cause athlete's foot. For treating athlete's foot fungus, a relatively strong solution of tea tree oil seems to work almost as well as most over-the-counter fungal ointments and creams, although it may take a little longer to notice results and completely eliminate the infection.

Formidable Fungal Fighter

- ***Attack Athlete's Foot*** Combine 2 drops of tea tree oil, 1 drop lavender oil, and 1 teaspoon of sweet almond or grapeseed oil in a small dish. Dip the end of a cotton swab in the oil and dab it on affected areas, then massage in well. Apply twice daily. Lavender also has antifungal properties, so it may help boost the power of the mix. Be aware that oily feet can be slippery feet. After applying, wear socks.

PEDICURE

Our feet are so often neglected that once you actually do something for them, you discover how much better you feel. All you need for a natural pedicure are essential oils of choice, soap, sea salt, toenail clippers, a pumice stone or loofah skin scrub, and vegetable oil. Rinse your feet and then soak them for 15 minutes in a tub of warm water and 10 drops of essential oil. Wash your feet in soap. Cut your toenails and then exfoliate with the loofah or pumice stone. Scrub the calluses next, when the skin is soft. Then pour a teaspoon or less of oil onto your cupped palm and massage into your feet. Massage into toenails. Naturally buffed nails look shiny, so use a pumice stone, sand stick, and smoothing files if desired.

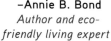

–Annie B. Bond
Author and eco-friendly living expert

- **Mix With Aloe** Mix equal parts tea tree oil and aloe vera gel. Rub into skin infected with athlete's foot fungus, morning and night.
- **Try a Combo** For more athlete's foot natural remedies that you might use in combination with tea tree oil approaches, see page 80.
- **Get the Jump on Jock Itch** Jock itch can be caused by the same fungus that causes athlete's foot, or a closely related species. Treat this common fungal infection naturally by mixing 10 drops of tea tree oil with 2 tablespoons of calendula cream or ointment (available at health food stores). Apply a thin coating on affected skin twice a day.

- **Nail That Fungus** Nail fungus is notoriously difficult to cure with over-the-counter antifungal creams, and prescription medications can have serious side effects. If fungus has invaded a nail, use a cotton swab to place a drop of pure tea tree oil directly on the nail's hard surface. Avoid the surrounding skin. Alternatively, add several drops of tea tree oil to an OTC fungal cream, and apply this to the nail area, working well into the nail bed. Continue treatment for two to three months, or until the nail has grown out completely from the time you began treatment.

- **Control Those White Flakes** Dandruff can have many causes, but one of them is a fungal infection of the scalp. Mix equal parts tea tree oil and grapeseed oil (about a teaspoon each). Apply this to the roots of your hair and massage into the scalp. Leave on overnight (wear a shower cap to bed and wrap your head in a towel). Shampoo well in the morning. Another option is to add 1 or 2 drops of tea tree oil to a capful of your regular shampoo. Try this daily until you see improvement.

▶ | MOUTH INFECTIONS

Tea tree's natural antiseptic properties can be helpful for treating minor irritations inside the mouth or on the lips; it may also help prevent gum disease, or gingivitis. Although tea tree oil should never be taken internally, it can be safely used in diluted form in and around your mouth—as long as you don't swallow it.

good to know: ALSO FOR FUNGAL INFECTIONS

- Garlic (*Allium sativum*) has been used as both food and medicine for millennia. Garlic has proven antibacterial, antifungal, and antiviral properties, making it useful for treating everything from wounds, acne, and athlete's foot to diarrhea and the common cold. When using garlic in cooking, mince well and add just at the end of cooking to preserve its infection-fighting substances.
- Thyme (*Thymus vulgaris*) contains two essential oils, thymol and carvacrol, that inhibit bacteria, fungi, and viruses. Thyme can be taken as tea, capsule, or syrup.

Mouth Meds

- **Fight Gum Disease** When gums are looking red or feeling a little irritated, don't risk letting gum disease get a foothold. Squeeze some toothpaste onto your toothbrush and add one drop of tea tree oil to the paste. Brush as usual, spit, and rinse well. If gum inflammation persists for more than a week or two, contact your doctor or dentist.
- **Treat a Cold Sore** Put 1 drop of sweet almond oil or olive oil onto a cotton swab. Add 1 drop of tea tree oil. Dab the mixture onto a cold sore. Repeat several times a day.

▶ SKIN INFECTIONS

Tea tree oil has been shown to inhibit many types of infection-causing bacteria. It's even effective against virulent, drug-resistant bacterial strains, such as methicillin-resistant *Staphylococcus aureas* (MRSA). Put the power of tea tree oil to work for a wide variety of common skin ailments and minor injuries.

Treat With Tea Tree

- **Help Heal Boils** A boil is an infection beneath the skin's surface, often in an oil gland or the result of an ingrown hair. The infection-causing agents are typically strains of *Staphylococcus* bacteria. Boils may go away on their own or rupture and drain. If a boil pops, add a few drops of tea tree oil to about a teaspoon of real witch hazel extract. Saturate a cotton ball with this mixture, and dab onto the area several times a day until healing begins.
- **Clean a Cut** Use tea tree's antiseptic properties for minor cuts and scrapes by mixing several drops of the essential oil with a tablespoon of almond oil and applying some of this mixture to the injury.
- **Make a Poultice for Shingles** If you had chickenpox or the live chickenpox virus vaccine as a kid, the virus can reactivate when immunity declines years later and appear as a painful rash, usually on the torso. Home remedies can provide some relief from the discomfort, including this tea tree oil and clay poultice (see the recipe below).
- **Make Other Skin Remedies** Using tea tree oil, you can make other remedies, including acne treatments (see page 67).

---

good to know: ALSO FOR SKIN INFECTIONS

Heal-all or self-heal *(Prunella vulgaris)* is a lesser known herb in herbal medicine, used historically to treat wounds and throat infections. Modern herbalists sometimes recommend heal-all teas for inflamed gums and sore throats, and ointments for skin ulcers, infections, bites, blisters, abrasions, and slow-healing wounds.

RECIPE FOR HEALTH

SEA CLAY & TEA TREE OIL POULTICE

Sea clay, also known as French green clay, is a fine-grained absorbent clay that can be used to clear weeping blisters and other skin problems.

In a small glass bowl, combine 2 to 3 tablespoons of sea clay with enough water to make a thick paste. Add 4 to 6 drops of tea tree oil and mix well. Cover and let stand two hours. Apply the paste in a layer about ¼-inch thick on a two-layered piece of gauze large enough to cover the affected area. Lift the poultice onto the skin, gauze side out, and secure in place with surgical tape. (You may want to wear latex gloves to avoid contaminating your fingers with virus particles.) Leave the poultice on for up to two hours. If it begins to dry out, spritz the gauze lightly with distilled or filtered water. Remove and gently clean away any clay with a warm, moist, disposable cloth. Discard the poultice. Wash or discard any other materials that may have touched the blisters. Repeat once a day.

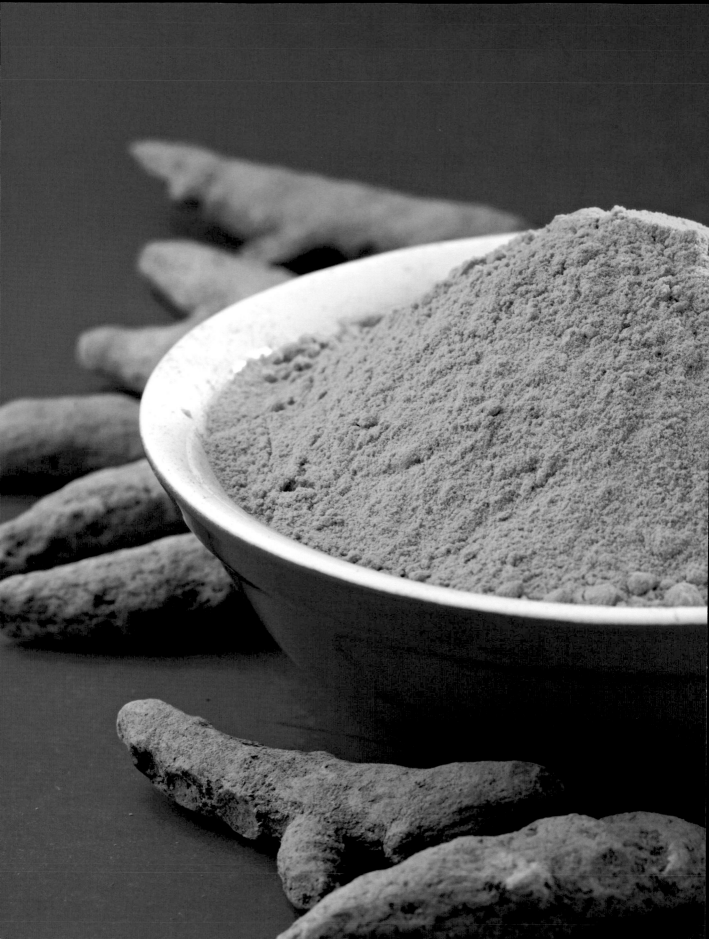

Turmeric

11 REASONS TO TURN TO TURMERIC

If you like spicy curries—or mustard on hot dogs—you know turmeric. Most likely native to India, turmeric (Curcuma longa) is a member of the ginger family. It's a plant with large, elegant leaves and very inelegant, knobby underground stems called rhizomes. Slice open a rhizome and you'll expose a fleshy, brilliant orange interior. It's this orange flesh that is dried and powdered to produce the yellow-orange spice. Turmeric is an essential ingredient in Indian and Asian curries and adds color and flavor to foods from mustard and Worcestershire sauce to butter and cheese. Although a relative newcomer to Western cultures, turmeric has been important in India and Asia for a very long time.

It is mentioned in the Vedas—ancient sacred texts of Hinduism that date to at least 1000 B.C.—as an herb linked with purity. Orthodox Hindu brides and bridegrooms still take part in an ancient ceremony called *haldi,* in which their faces are coated with turmeric paste before they take their vows.

Turmeric has been used medicinally for a remarkably long time. It's been used in Indian Ayurvedic medicine (see pages 263–265) and traditional Chinese medicine (see pages 295–297), for at least 2,500 years as a remedy for digestive and liver disorders, relieving arthritis pain, regulating menstruation, and treating skin problems. Turmeric is currently one of the most intensely studied herbs in alternative medicine. Its primary active ingredient is curcumin, a substance that exhibits strong anti-inflammatory and antioxidant properties. Curcumin is being studied for its ability to fight a wide range of human ailments—including autoimmune diseases such as rheumatoid arthritis and inflammatory bowel disease, cancer, and Alzheimer's—and possibly even to postpone the onset of age-related diseases. More research is needed to show what turmeric does and doesn't do. But add up what's known already, and you've got an herb with significant potential to fight infections (possibly even prevent some types of cancer), curtail inflammation, and promote healthy digestion. It's a hard combination to beat.

> ⚠ **CAUTION:** Turmeric added to foods is considered very safe. So is taking turmeric supplements according to package directions, although pregnant women and nursing mothers should not take turmeric supplements.

▶ INDIGESTION & IBD

Turmeric's ability to prevent inflammation manifests itself particularly well in the digestive tract by easing stomach and intestinal upsets. By promoting the release of bile into the intestinal tract, the herb is thought to encourage normal digestion as well. Germany's herbal regulatory agency, the German Commission E, has given its approval for turmeric to be prescribed by doctors for digestive problems. A number of studies have shown that turmeric also helps reduce symptoms and prevents remission of ulcerative colitis, a type of inflammatory bowel disease (IBD). You can take turmeric capsules (follow package directions) for gastrointestinal complaints, but there also are easy and delicious ways to include turmeric in your daily health regime and diet.

Terrific Turmeric

- **Brew a Zingy Tea** This ginger/turmeric tea is good for soothing upset stomachs and other digestive ailments. Ginger has natural nausea-fighting properties (see page 95) so it's a good combination with turmeric. Simply bring 2 cups of water to a boil in a small saucepan. Reduce heat to low and add ¾ teaspoon turmeric powder and ¾ teaspoon powdered ginger. Stir well and simmer ten minutes. Strain tea into a cup and add a tablespoon of freshly squeezed lemon juice. Sweeten as desired with honey or maple syrup. Drink a cup or two as needed to treat indigestion.

- **Or Try a Soothing One** Simmer 2 teaspoons turmeric powder in 2 cups water for ten minutes, stirring until the powder is thoroughly dissolved. Turn the heat to low and add 2 cups

cow's milk (or almond, soy, or coconut milk), 1 tablespoon almond oil, and 1 teaspoon of honey or maple syrup. Refrigerate the leftovers and try it cold.

- **Add to Foods** The easiest way to take turmeric is to add it to foods. It has a warm, peppery, slightly bitter flavor reminiscent of ginger. Add a little to egg salad, rice and lentil dishes, and bottled salad dressings. Add a teaspoonful to enhance take-out curries. Or try the following recipe as a rub for meats, fish, and poultry; it's delicious on veggies too.

good to know: ABOUT TURMERIC

- The body is better able to absorb turmeric/curcumin in the presence of piperine, a compound found in black pepper. When cooking with turmeric, add a little black pepper to the dish as well.
- Make sure you're getting fresh turmeric powder. Buy from reputable stores that do a brisk business in sales of bulk herbs.

▶ JOINT PAIN

For centuries, doctors trained in Ayurvedic medicine have used turmeric to treat inflammatory conditions such as arthritis. In modern herbal medicine, this yellow spice is still recommended to relieve joint pain. When applying turmeric to your skin, be sure to protect furniture and clothing because the yellow stain is difficult to remove.

Tame Pain With Turmeric

- **Fight Pain With Paste** When arthritis pain strikes, make a paste of 1 tablespoon of turmeric with enough olive oil or sweet almond oil to make a paste. Spread over the joint and cover loosely with gauze.

CLASSIC INDIAN SPICE MIX
Combine the following in a small bowl:

8 teaspoons dry mustard
4 teaspoons ground fenugreek
2 teaspoons ginger
2 teaspoons coriander
½ teaspoon ground cinnamon

4 teaspoons ground cumin
3 teaspoons turmeric
2 teaspoons cloves
1 teaspoon ground black pepper

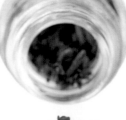

Mix well and store in a small glass container with a tight-fitting lid. Use as a base for curries, a rub for meats, and a seasoning for fish, vegetables, and eggs—almost anything!

- **Treat a Sprain** For a sprain, combine 1 teaspoon turmeric and 1 teaspoon salt with enough aloe vera gel to make a paste. Spread this over the affected area and cover to reduce swelling and inflammation.

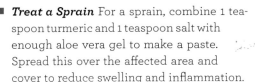

▶ | SKIN CONDITIONS

Turmeric's antimicrobial properties have been well documented. It's also been shown in studies to promote wound healing. That may be one reason why this herb has been used for so many centuries as a remedy for common skin conditions. Turmeric salves and ointments are available at many health food stores. You can make your own remedies, too.

Treat It With Turmeric

- **Banish a Boil** These skin eruptions (see page 129) can be very painful. Antibiotics may help get rid of the infection that causes a boil, but turmeric can be a very effective natural alternative. Mix a teaspoon of turmeric with a teaspoon ginger and enough aloe vera gel to make a thick paste. Spread this over the boil and cover well with a bandage or gauze. Leave on 30 to 60 minutes. Repeat once a day until the boil begins to heal.
- **Bathe a Sore Throat** A saltwater gargle is a classic remedy for sore throat (see page 25). Add turmeric's germ-killing properties by mixing ½ teaspoon salt and 1 teaspoon turmeric powder in a cup of hot water.

Stir well until the powder is completely dissolved. Gargle and spit. Repeat as needed.

- **Treat Athlete's Foot** Although your feet will turn yellow for a while, turmeric is an effective remedy for athlete's foot fungal infections. Mix ½ teaspoon turmeric powder with 1 tablespoon of calendula ointment (available at health food stores). Rub well into affected areas twice a day. Wear socks to prevent staining carpets and bedding.
- **Soothe a Burn** Aloe vera gel can help heal minor burns (see page 65). Boost its soothing effects by adding a pinch of turmeric to the fresh aloe gel you spread on a burn. Reapply the mix three to four times a day. Keep the burn covered between applications.
- **Fight Psoriasis** Some people find that turmeric can help ease the itching and irritation of psoriasis. Turmeric capsules (available at health food stores) are one option—follow package directions. Alternatively, apply a turmeric poultice. Mix a tablespoon of the powdered herb with enough olive oil or sweet almond oil to make a thick paste and spread over the infected area. Cover with gauze and wrap with a towel to prevent staining. Leave on one hour and then rinse off with cool water. Repeat three times a day.

good to know: ALSO FOR JOINT PAIN

- Comfrey (*Symphytum officinale*), once known as knitbone and boneset, is another herbal remedy used to soothe injured or arthritic joints. Comfrey preparations—ointments, gels, and creams—are available at most natural food stores. Follow package directions. ⚠ **CAUTION:** Never apply comfrey to broken skin.
- If you've ever brushed up against a stinging nettle plant (*Urtica dioica*), you know that its tiny bristles result in fiery pain. Oddly, though, nettle has been used for centuries to fight pain with pain. Applying fresh nettle leaves to skin to dull joint, muscle, or back pain is an old folk remedy. The stinging sensation acts as a counterirritant to dull the pain deeper in the body. Recent research shows that applying nettle leaves to arthritic joints can indeed ease pain. Further, nettle extracts, taken internally, reduced arthritis pain about as much as nonsteroidal anti-inflammatory drugs (NSAIDs).

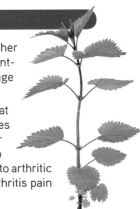

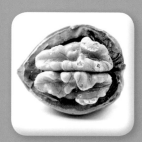 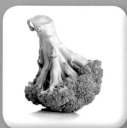 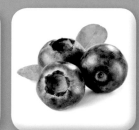 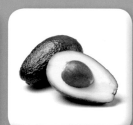 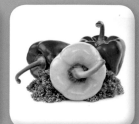

foods fo

r health

Healing Foods

20 FOODS TO BOOST HEALTH

"Let food be thy medicine and medicine be thy food." These words of wisdom are credited to the ancient Greek physician Hippocrates, often called the father of Western medicine. The concept of food as medicine may seem foreign to those of us raised on the idea that treatments for illness come in the form of pills and prescriptions. But using food to achieve better health is a recurring theme in many non-Western cultures.

Eat Well to Be Well

Somehow, here in the West, the idea of food as medicine got lost in the 20th century. The good news is we seem to be finding it again. Part of the reason is that medical research is teasing out the underlying causes of numerous diseases. Arthritis is a good example. Twenty or thirty years ago, doctors chalked up the cause of arthritis to simple wear and tear on joints. This may be true for osteoarthritis, but rheumatoid arthritis—affecting roughly one percent of the U.S. population—turns out to be an autoimmune-triggered inflammatory disease. Inside our bodies, unstable particles called free radicals promote inflammation. They can also destroy cell membranes and disrupt DNA. Substances known as antioxidants can neutralize free radicals, and suppress inflammation.

Where can you find these inflammation-fighting antioxidants? In plant foods such as leafy greens, orange and yellow veggies, and fruits that blush red, violet, and blue. Regular consumption of antioxidant-rich fruits and vegetables is associated not just with reduced risk of rheumatoid arthritis but also certain types of cancer, cardiovascular disease, stroke, Alzheimer's disease, and other declines linked to aging.

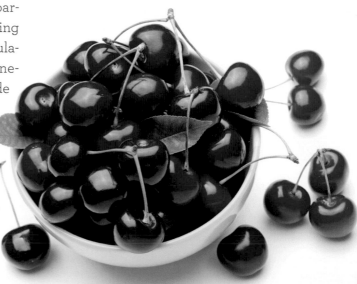

You Are What You Eat

And that's just the beginning. Simple, basic foods such as beans are not only rich in vitamins and minerals but also high in protein and packed with soluble fiber good at lowering cholesterol. Whole grains also help regulate cholesterol levels. Because they are slowly digested complex carbohydrates, they help tame blood sugar spikes, which in turn keeps insulin levels low and diabetes at bay. Cruciferous vegetables (think broccoli, cauliflower, and cabbage) contain sulfur-rich substances that can cleanse our bodies of potential carcinogens. The fats found in foods such as walnuts, salmon, olive oil, and avocados—foods once considered unhealthy and "fattening"—actually fight inflammation, lower the risk of heart disease, and may even protect against cancer. Red wine and grape juice, rich in antioxidants and other plant chemicals, foster a healthy cardiovascular system. Even chocolate, considered candy for more than a century, contains high levels of antioxidants thought to help lower the risk of coronary heart disease.

As you explore the world of health-giving foods, whenever possible, choose organically grown produce. By buying organic, you'll avoid toxic pesticide residues. But that's not all. Studies show that organically grown fruits and vegetables contain greater amounts of certain vitamins and minerals as well as higher levels of antioxidants and other plant chemicals that are fundamental to maintaining good health and helping to fight disease.

FOOD FOR THOUGHT

Through food, we seek to feed a complicated hunger. Our tables nourish us with far more than calories. Here we find joy and laughter, family, friends, and communion; the table is a place to share, to give and receive. Food, and all of its pleasures, is the centerpiece of nearly every relationship—not only with our friends and our family but also with the planet and biosphere and ecosystems that sustain and fill our tables.

Cooking, whether for our family or ourselves, is an opportunity. After a long day of work, there's nothing better than kicking off your shoes, pouring a glass of wine, and getting in the kitchen. All of the day's stresses can be transferred to the onion you're chopping—even giving occasion to shed a tear if that's how your day went.

Taking the time and making the effort to care for ourselves and our loved ones is one of the best gifts we can get or give. The dinner table is a place to share our love and thoughts, along with our broccoli or beans.

Eating well for our bodies and the planet doesn't involve sacrificing deliciousness. When we pay attention to ingredients, eating them at the peak of their season, we find new joy and nutrition in the foods we know so well.

Eat with care and be mindful of the environmental impacts of your choices. Eat with joy that we may continue to enjoy the bounty of nature. And eat together to remember what truly unites us all on this beautiful planet.

Barton Seaver
Chef, cookbook author, National Geographic fellow, and sustainable eating expert

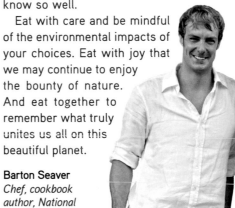

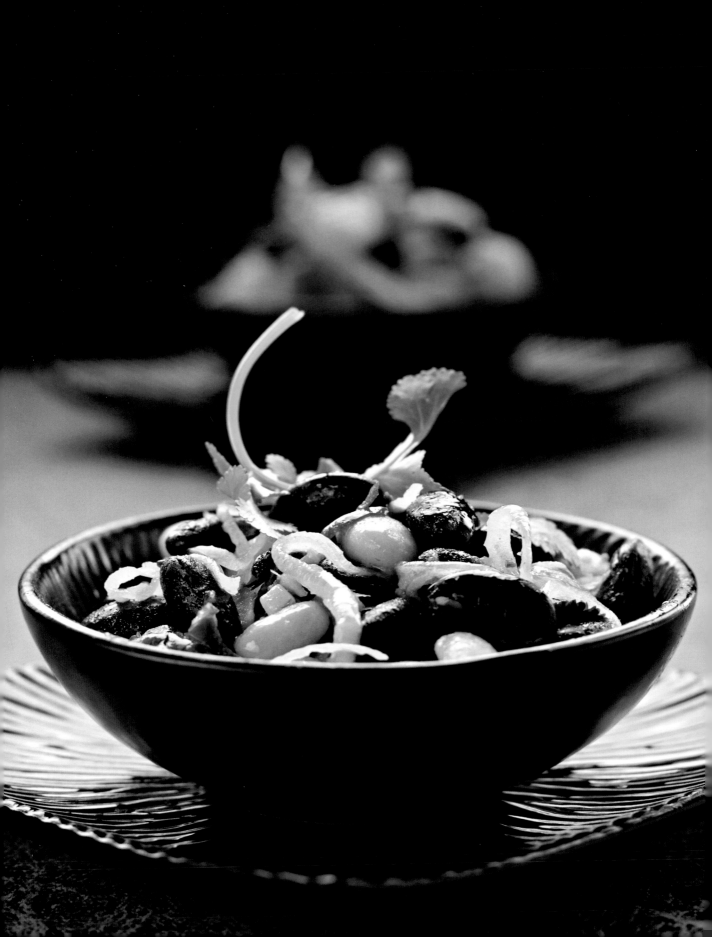

Beans

12 REASONS TO BE KEEN ON BEANS

What we call beans are actually the seeds of legumes, which are among the oldest cultivated plants. The kidney beans, black beans, pinto beans, lentils, and other bean varieties you see on grocery store shelves or in natural food store bins grew inside pods until they were mature and dry enough to harvest. Beans are not flashy foods. Nutritionally, though, they're powerhouses. Beans offer a bonanza of vitamins, including vitamins A, B_6, folate (B_9), and C, and minerals such as copper, potassium, iron, and magnesium. They are very low in fat but surprisingly rich in protein. Just a cup of cooked lentils, for example, boasts more than 17 grams of protein.

Beans are also packed with soluble fiber. In the digestive tract, soluble fiber forms a sort of gel that binds to cholesterol, blocking its absorption into the bloodstream where it can stick to artery walls. Studies have shown that some people can cut their cholesterol levels by 10 percent in six weeks simply by eating a cup of cooked beans every day. There's another benefit to beans' fiber: It appears to help stabilize blood sugar levels, keeping levels from rising too rapidly after a meal. That's good news for anyone with diabetes, insulin resistance, or hypoglycemia.

Beans may help protect against cancer, too. They contain chemical compounds shown to inhibit cancer cell growth. If you're still not impressed, consider this: The U.S. Department of Agriculture has ranked more than a hundred different foods based on their inflammation- and disease-fighting antioxidant content. Humble beans, including red, kidney, and pinto beans, placed in the top five.

▶ | RED BEANS

Red beans are nutrient superstars, a delicious, versatile, high-protein food that not only fosters good health but also helps keep weight in check. That's because the fiber in red beans and other varieties makes you feel full and satisfied—and less tempted by less healthful foods. Red beans complement many ingredients and pick up the flavor of seasonings in almost any recipe.

A Cook's Dream

- *Make 'Em the Main Dish* Red beans—really, any beans—can be a hearty, filling entrée. Cooked or canned red beans work well with ground beef, spicy sausage, chicken, and pork. They make a versatile base for vegetarian dishes, combining well with almost anything.

THE POWER OF ORANGE

Turmeric, the spice that gives curry its beautiful golden orange color, is rich in compounds that enhance digestion, reduce inflammation, and may even give your body an edge against colon cancer. The ways in which this ancient spice can improve our health is being intensely researched by scientists at leading academic centers. Here are a few simple ways that you can add turmeric to your diet:

- Mix ½ teaspoon turmeric powder in 8 ounces plain yogurt and use it as a sandwich spread or on a baked potato.
- Perk up that can of tomato soup by adding ½ teaspoon turmeric powder. Delicious!
- Enhance the flavor and health benefits of beans or macaroni and cheese by adding ½ teaspoon turmeric for every 2 cups cooked food.

–Tieraona Low Dog, M.D.
Author and integrative medicine expert

HEALING TRADITIONS

- **Combine With Rice** Beans contain a lot of protein, but it's incomplete due to the fact it's missing a few essential amino acids. That problem, though, is easily solved by eating beans with a grain, like rice, or corn. Combining beans and seeds, or beans and nuts, works well, too.
- **Add to Soup** Nothing could be simpler than adding beans to soup. Almost every culture has created recipes for some kind of bean soup. And don't stop at homemade. You can add beans to canned soups to pump up their nutrient load—and make them stretch a little further.

▶ | BLACK BEANS

Black beans are sometimes called turtle beans, which could be a nod to their shiny, dark, shell-like appearance. During cooking, black beans develop a creamy, almost velvety texture and a rich flavor reminiscent of mushrooms. Black beans share the same healthful characteristics as red, kidney, and other beans.

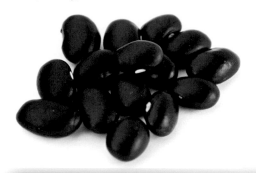

BLACK BEAN HUMMUS

Black beans stand in for traditional chickpeas in this hummus variation:

2 cups cooked black beans, drained
¼ cup tahini
2 teaspoons lime juice
1½ tablespoons extra-virgin olive oil
1 garlic clove, minced
1 teaspoon ground cumin
½ cup fresh cilantro, chopped
¼ teaspoon cayenne pepper
Salt to taste

Combine all the ingredients in a food processor and blend until smooth. Add more lime juice and olive oil as needed to achieve the desired consistency.

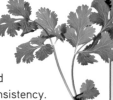

A Bean Supreme

- **Try a Breakfast Burrito** Spread a scrambled egg in the center of a warm flour tortilla. Add 2 to 3 tablespoons of cooked black beans, mashed to a paste with a pinch of cumin. Top with 1 or 2 tablespoons of salsa and a little shredded cheese and roll up burrito-style.
- **Toss Together a Lunch** Make a quick, healthful lunch by tossing together cooked or canned black beans (rinsed well), fresh or frozen corn

RED BEAN & CLEMENTINE SALAD

1 tablespoon extra-virgin olive oil
1 small garlic clove, minced
1 15-ounce can red beans, rinsed well and drained
1 teaspoon minced fresh cilantro
3 clementines, peeled and separated into segments
¼ cup crumbled queso fresco (if this cheese is not available, substitute mild feta)
1½ cups young kale leaves or baby spinach

½ medium red onion, thinly sliced
¼ teaspoon ground cumin
1 tablespoon red wine vinegar
Salt and pepper

1. In a skillet, heat oil over medium heat. Add onion and sauté one minute. Add garlic and cumin and stir until fragrant, about 30 seconds. Add the beans and heat until just warmed, about a minute.
2. Transfer the bean mixture to a bowl. Add the vinegar, cilantro, clementines, and cheese and toss together gently. Season with salt and pepper to taste. Serve immediately on a bed of kale or spinach.

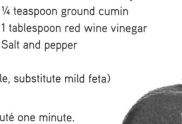

kernels, sliced black olives, chopped cilantro, chopped onion, and chopped tomato. Drizzle with olive oil and a dash of red wine vinegar. Salt and pepper to taste.

- **Go for a Quick Supper** Heat cooked or canned black beans with fresh chopped tomatoes. Toss in a pinch of chili flakes and add a squeeze of fresh lime juice. Season with salt and pepper and serve over hot brown rice.

▶ | LENTILS

Like their bean cousins, disk-shaped lentils are bursting with fiber, nutrients, and disease-fighting plant compounds. Unlike their relatives, lentils cook relatively quickly, without the need for presoaking. Native to the Mediterranean, lentils come in an array of colors. Mild brown lentils make a great addition to soups because they become quite soft when cooked. Green lentils, aka French lentils, retain their shape and firmness with cooking, and develop a nutty, peppery flavor. Red lentils turn a golden color and have a mild, slightly sweet taste. Black and orange lentils are both small—you'll often find them in Indian and Middle Eastern dishes.

A Good Thing in a Small Package

- **Boil and Serve** Make a quick vegetarian meal by boiling lentils for 15 to 30 minutes and then adding curry powder, a little fresh ginger, turmeric, and other spices, along with sautéed vegetables. Serve over rice.
- **Stretch Ground Meat** Add cooked brown lentils to ground beef or other ground meats to stretch your meat budget and add fiber to meals. You can also sneak them into meatballs and spaghetti sauces.
- **Make Soup** There are countless recipes for lentil soup, from many different cultures. Lentil soup is a classic—nutritious, delicious, and inexpensive, too.

good to know: ABOUT BEANS

- To get the best bean flavor, start with dried beans. Preparing dried beans takes time, so plan ahead. Begin by sorting the beans, and picking out damaged and shriveled ones as well as small stones and debris. Rinse the beans well under cold running water. Put in a pot, add enough water to cover, and let the beans soak for six to eight hours or overnight. (Many of the gas-causing substances in beans leech out during soaking. To prevent gas, change the soaking water several times.) Discard any floating beans, pour off the soaking water, rinse the beans, and add enough fresh water to cover well. Bring to a boil, cover, and simmer until tender, usually about two to three hours.

- Using canned beans can save a lot of time. Nutritionally, they are on a par with dried beans of the same variety, except they are high in sodium because they are canned with salt. Draining and rinsing well will remove much of the salt. (Be aware, though, that like other canned foods, canned beans may contain small amounts of a hormone-disrupting compound known as bisphenol A [BPA] found in the resin-based can liners used to reduce spoilage of can foods; look for cans labeled BPA-free.)

- In many recipes, don't hesitate to experiment with different kinds of beans. Kidney beans, for instance, can be substituted for red beans in almost any dish.

- Buy dry beans in bulk from a busy store to ensure freshness. Avoid dusty bags of dried beans that look forgotten on grocery store shelves.

- Store dry beans in a glass jar with a tight-fighting lid in a cool, dark place.

- If stored properly, dried beans should last for a year or more.

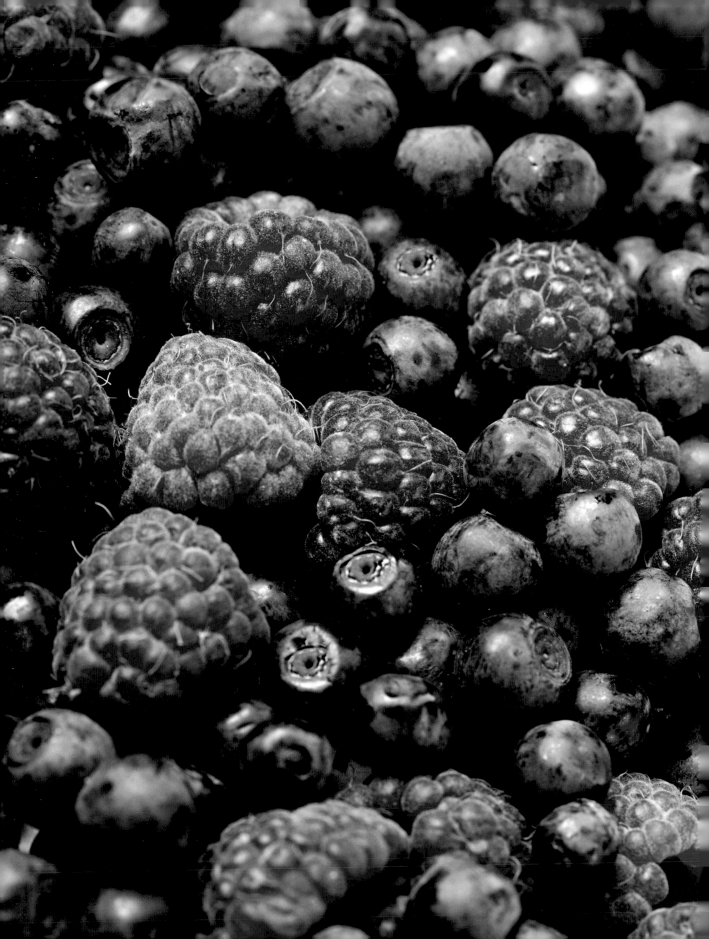

Berries

16 WAYS TO VARY YOUR BERRIES

Don't let their size fool you. Ounce for ounce, berries are some of the most healthful foods you can eat. Blueberries, raspberries, strawberries, cranberries, and other varieties of these plump, diminutive fruits have enormous nutritional and medicinal value. They're pretty, tasty, fuss-free fare. And eating just a handful a day may provide powerful natural protection against cancer, cardiovascular disease, diabetes, and a host of other maladies. The secret to berries' healthful clout lies largely in the antioxidants they contain. Antioxidants are chemical compounds that neutralize unstable molecules called free radicals. As free radicals course through our bodies, they can harm healthy cells.

Antioxidants act like bodyguards. They come between cells and destructive free radicals to ensure that no damage is done. Some of the most potent antioxidants in berries—or in any food—are anthocyanins. These purple pigments give berries their lovely red, blue, and purple hues. As antioxidants, anthocyanins protect against the types of cell damage thought to lead to cancer, heart disease, and age-related memory loss.

Other weapons in berries' disease-fighting arsenal include ellagic acid, an antioxidant shown in laboratory studies to prevent cancers of the skin, bladder, lung, esophagus, and breast; vitamin C, another familiar antioxidant; and dietary fiber, known to decrease the risk of colorectal cancer.

▶ | BLUEBERRIES

A North American native, blueberries are one of the world's few authentically blue foods. They are also one of the richest sources of disease-fighting antioxidants you can find at the grocery store. In addition to being packed with anthocyanins, blueberries are bursting with vitamin C. One serving—just one cup—provides nearly 25 percent of the daily requirement. Blueberries contain the same antioxidant that cranberries do that helps prevent urinary tract infections (see the section on cranberries). And recently, scientists reported the first evidence from human research that blueberries may improve memory. A group of volunteers in their 70s with early signs of memory decline showed significant improvement on learning and memory tests after drinking blueberry juice every day for just two months.

True Blue Berry

- ***Get 'Em Fresh*** Fresh or frozen blueberries have the highest amounts of healthful antioxidants (cooking destroys some of the valuable vitamin C). Toss a handful of fresh blueberries in your breakfast cereal and stir them into oatmeal. Sprinkle some on pancakes—along with some real blueberry syrup.
- ***Try 'Em Frozen*** Eat frozen blueberries for a snack. They make a great low-calorie alternative to less healthful frozen desserts or sugary treats.
- ***Mix It Up*** Blueberries combine wonderfully with other fruits. And they add a touch of blue color. Add them to fruit salad or as a fun blue layer to a yogurt and fruit parfait.
- ***"Season" a Salad*** Stir 1 or 2 tablespoons of blueberries into vinaigrette and pour

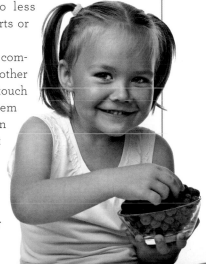

BLUEBERRY RELISH

Try this fresh blueberry combination with soft cheeses such as Brie or Camembert:

1 cup fresh blueberries
1 8-ounce can organic whole-berry cranberry sauce
1 teaspoon fresh lemon juice
½ cup roasted, chopped pecans
A pinch of cinnamon

Warm the cranberry sauce in a pan over low heat until it begins to soften and "melt." Remove from heat and stir in the blueberries, lemon juice, nuts, and cinnamon until well combined. Serve warm or cold.

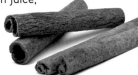

over a variety of lettuces. Top the salad with a sprinkling of freshly roasted chopped almonds (see pages 167–168).

- **Cover With Chocolate** Chocolate is another antioxidant-rich food (see page 151), and it complements blueberries' zesty fruitiness very well. Put a handful of blueberries in a small bowl. Melt about 1 tablespoon of good quality dark chocolate in a double boiler or gently in the microwave. Drizzle the melted chocolate over the berries and enjoy. Or pop the bowl in the refrigerator until the chocolate cools and rehardens to create a very different but equally delectable treat.

- **Swirl Up a Smoothie** Begin your day with blueberries by adding ½ cup milk (or soy or almond milk), ½ cup plain yogurt, and 1 cup of blueberries. Blend until smooth.

- **Add to Baked Goods** What could be better than a fresh, homemade blueberry muffin? Blueberries make a healthful addition to all sorts of baked goods, even if the cooking process does reduce their antioxidant punch.

▶ | RASPBERRIES

Delicate, cup-shaped raspberries are renowned for their succulent, sweet flavor. Like blueberries, raspberries are low in fat and high in fiber, and are antioxidant standouts. They contain vitamin C and several other compounds that can help fight heart and circulatory disease, infection and inflammation, diabetes, and age-related decline. Recent research suggests that the body readily absorbs ellagic acid from raspberries, and laboratory studies have shown that ellagic acid causes cell death in many different types of cancer cells. Other substances in raspberries appear to reduce the body's production of fat, and are currently being marketed in Japan as a weight loss aid.

Berry Berry Good for You

- **Just Love 'Em** For many people, eating a handful—or a bowl—of fresh raspberries is one of summer's most delicious experiences. Choose organic whenever possible, though, as nonorganic raspberries can be laden with high levels of pesticides.

- **Add to Yogurt** Raspberries are a favorite with yogurt. Try blending together ½ cup raspberries with ½ cup Greek yogurt and 1 teaspoon freshly chopped mint. Drizzle with a little honey, if desired.

- **Forget PB&J** You many never go back to peanut butter and grape jelly sandwiches after you try this: Mash a handful of fresh raspberries with ½ teaspoon honey to make "jam." Spread freshly ground almond butter on a slice of your favorite bread and spread the raspberries on top. Eat open faced.

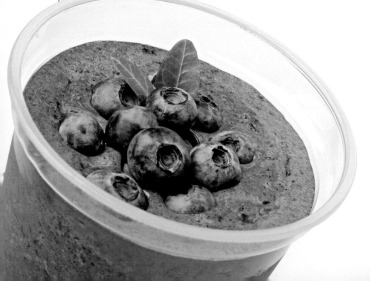

CRANBERRIES

Cranberries are the tart, scarlet cousins of blueberries, and natives of North America too. Cranberries still grow wild in parts of the eastern United States and Canada, but most are cultivated on large commercial cranberry farms. Rich in anthocyanins, vitamin C, and other disease-preventing antioxidants, cranberries gained fame in the 1980s as an effective preventive for urinary tract infections (UTIs). Antioxidants give cranberries their UTI-preventing power. The antioxidant mix in cranberries inhibits bacteria such as *E. coli* (responsible for 90 percent of all UTIs) from sticking to the cells that line the walls of the bladder and urethra. No sticking, no infection. Other research has shown that cranberries may help protect against stomach ulcers, heart disease, periodontal disease, and some forms of cancer.

Tart Treat

- *Whip Up a Cranberry Dressing* Just as vinegar sparks up salad dressing, tart cranberries can too. Crush or coarsely chop a handful of cranberries, and whisk them together with a tablespoon of olive oil and a teaspoon of honey or maple syrup. Use this mix to dress a salad of fresh greens.
- *Mix With Nuts* Dried cranberries may contain sugar, but unsweetened varieties are available, so check the ingredients label. Mix dried, unsweetened cranberries with freshly roasted almonds, walnuts, and pecans (see pages 167–169). Sprinkle on a little salt and a pinch of cayenne pepper.
- *Add to Oatmeal* If you add sugar, maple syrup, or honey to sweeten your morning oatmeal, add a handful of unsweetened dried cranberries to balance the sweet taste. Or skip the sweeteners altogether and enjoy the berries' tangy flavor.
- *Try a Green and Orange Combo* Cranberries complement many brightly colored vegetables, including leafy greens, winter squash, sweet potatoes, Brussels sprouts, and carrots. Experiment by adding fresh or dried cranberries to your favorite recipes for these foods.

WILD GREENS

In Ikaria, in Greece, where longevity is common, wild greens—with more antioxidants than green tea or wine—are abundant in fields and along roadsides. The greens are tasty both fresh and cooked, in salads with other steamed greens, or baked in a vegetable pie. They're often cooked with savory sweet foods like onions, squash, and garlic to help cut the bitterness of the greens.

In your own backyard or fields nearby, look for chickweed *(Stellaria media)*, dandelion *(Taraxacum officinale)*, and garlic mustard *(Alliaria officinalis)* in the spring. Even just a few greens with your meal will encourage your whole digestive process to work better.

–Dan Buettner
Author and lecturer on longevity

good to know: ABOUT BERRIES

- Blueberries should have a soft, powdery blue coating, called a bloom. It's natural and a sign of fresh berries.
- To minimize your intake of agricultural toxins, choose organic blueberries.
- Shake the little plastic containers in which most blueberries are packed. The berries should tumble around freely. If they don't, it's a sign that some of the berries could be smashed, moldy, or otherwise undesirable. Also look for plump berries that aren't dented.
- Raspberries can be storied in the refrigerator for a day or two, but they are highly perishable. For the greatest health benefit, eat soon after picking or purchase.
- Avoid cranberry juice cocktail, which can be loaded with sugar or high-fructose corn syrup. Look for stevia-sweetened cranberry juice.

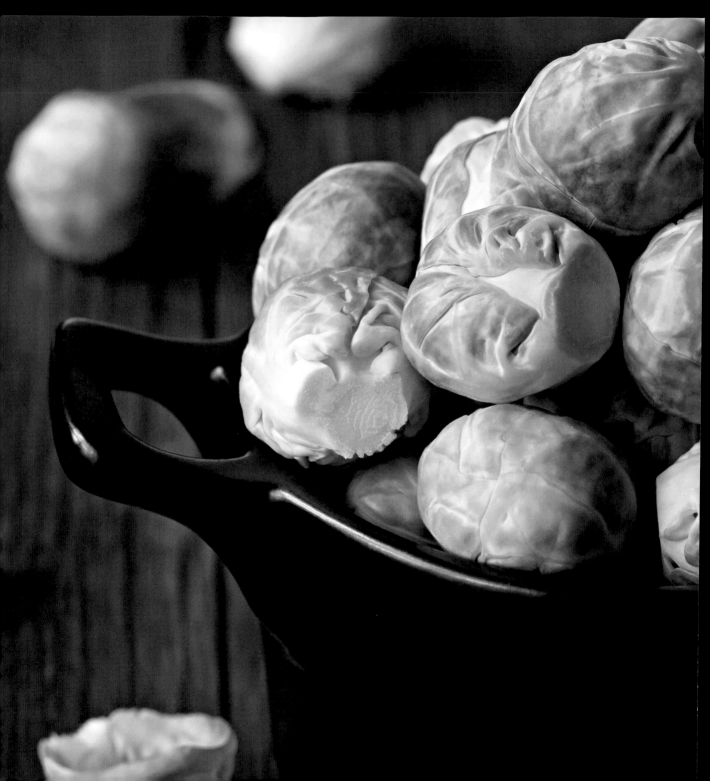

Broccoli & Related Veggies

15 WAYS TO GO GREEN

In family photos, it's usually pretty easy to spot distinctive traits that hint at common ancestry. A widow's peak here. An upturned nose or dimpled chin there. Close relationships are easy to spot in the cabbage, or Cruciferae, family too. That's the botanical group that includes broccoli, cauliflower, Brussels sprouts, kale, cabbage, collard greens, kohlrabi, bok choy, and many other vegetables. Cruciferous vegetables, as they're called, all have flowers with four petals that resemble a cross (hence the name). All exhibit a slightly sulfurous scent, too, and are also mostly crisp and crunchy and tinted in various shades of green.

But what really binds these vegetables together as a family are the health-promoting substances they contain. In addition to being rich sources of vitamins, minerals, and soluble fiber, cruciferous veggies are powerhouses in terms of anticancer compounds. Research shows that sulfur-containing chemicals called glucosinolates—together with chemical derivatives of these chemicals that form in our bodies—help eliminate potentially cancer-causing substances (carcinogens) before they get a chance to wreak havoc in cells. These compounds appear to act in ways that prevent normal cells from being transformed into cancerous ones. According to the American Institute for Cancer Research, a number of laboratory studies have shown that these "cruciferous compounds" can halt the growth of cancer cells making up tumors in the breast, lungs, colon, liver, and cervix. Other studies have revealed that diets high in cruciferous vegetables are linked to lower rates of prostate cancer, too. With all these good things to recommend them, it's no wonder health and nutrition experts suggest that we eat lots of cruciferous veggies. Aim for four or five servings a week or more.

▶ BROCCOLI

Broccoli may be the most well-known and widely consumed member of the Cruciferae family. And it's easy to see why. This tasty, dark green, crunchy crucifer is in many respects the real standout of the family. Compared with its relatives, broccoli contains the most vitamin C (165 percent of the recommended daily value in just one cup). It's also unusually rich in vitamin A (in the form of beta-carotene), vitamin K, folate (a water-soluble B-group vitamin), and a variety of antioxidants. Combine all that with broccoli's anticancer properties, and it's a vegetable that's hard to beat. Just a half cup of broccoli a day—only 22 calories' worth—is enough to provide measurable health benefits.

Bring On the Broccoli

■ *Eat It Raw, or Nearly So* The secret to preserving nutrients in cruciferous vegetables is to cook them gently and lightly, or not at all. Dark green broccoli florets, either raw or slightly blanched, are classic crudités. Add some to every veggie platter.

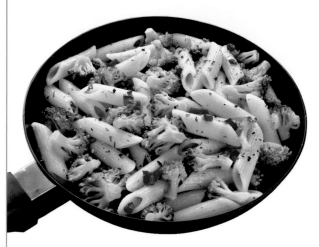

- **Chop It Up** Add chopped fresh broccoli to soups, stews, and casseroles. Although cooking causes broccoli to release some of its nutrients, they aren't lost in this case—they just become part of the dish.
- **Stir and Splash** Try stir-frying broccoli in toasted sesame oil, with a bit of garlic. Add a splash of soy sauce and a little fresh ginger and you've got a quick and easy side dish with an Asian flair.
- **Go Green Anytime** Chop a stalk of broccoli into tiny florets and very small pieces and add to an omelet. To create a quick weekday supper, steam stalks of broccoli and toss together with cooked pasta, a little olive oil, a handful of pine nuts, salt and pepper, and some freshly grated Parmesan cheese.
- **Tempt Your Kids** Your kids won't eat broccoli? Try this: Cut broccoli florets into tiny "trees." Steam lightly for a minute or two and then broil for a few minutes until the florets become crunchy (they'll get a little sweeter, too). Serve at once.

▶ | KALE

Kale is a leafy, cruciferous vegetable with deep green, ruffled leaves. The dark green hue hints at the goodness inside. Kale is loaded with antioxidants and is high in vitamins and minerals. Including kale in your diet may help reduce the risk of cancer and heart disease, protect vision, and control blood pressure. The problem with kale, however, is that many people just don't know how to eat it. Try these tips to unlock kale's tasty nature.

Tales of Kale

- **Skip the Stems** To prepare kale for cooking, use a sharp knife to cut away the leaf from the stem and central rib. Then cut the leafy parts into narrow ribbons or small pieces. They will cook and tenderize more quickly.
- **Simply Sauté** One of the easiest ways to prepare kale is to simply sauté sliced or chopped leafy parts in olive oil for about five minutes. Add a little garlic, some salt and pepper, and you're done.
- **Try a Braise** Braising is a cooking technique in which the main ingredient is seared or sautéed and then simmered in liquid on low heat. Combine chopped kale with chopped apples in a skillet with a little olive oil. Sauté for several minutes, and then add ½ cup or so chicken broth. Cover, reduce the heat to low, and let the mixture cook until the liquid is absorbed. To serve, sprinkle with balsamic vinegar, salt and pepper, and chopped, pan-roasted walnuts.

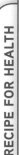

RECIPE FOR HEALTH

ROASTED KALE CHIPS

Be warned—these can be addictive:

1 large bunch organic kale

1 to 2 teaspoons kosher or sea salt

3 tablespoons (roughly) extra-virgin olive oil

Preheat oven to 350°F. Tear kale into potato chip–size pieces (discard the ribs and stalks). Rinse well and spin-dry in a salad spinner. Put the dried kale pieces in a bowl. Drizzle the olive oil over them and toss well so that all the pieces are lightly coated with oil. Spread the kale pieces in an even layer on a baking sheet lined with parchment paper. Sprinkle with salt. Bake 10 or 15 minutes until kale is crisp and edges are beginning to brown. The chips are best eaten warm.

- **Add to Soup** Kale is the perfect leafy green vegetable to chop into small pieces and add to soup. It doesn't get mushy like spinach, and the flavor intensifies as it cooks.
- **Broil It** Broiling kale is also a good way to prepare it, and because it isn't cooked in water, it retains much of its nutrients. Crisply broiled or roasted kale (see the recipe opposite) may tempt kids, too.

▶ | BRUSSELS SPROUTS

Brussels sprouts look like miniature cabbages. But although many of us love cabbage, far fewer of us are enthusiastic about Brussels sprouts. Yet these much maligned crucifers contain many of the same healthful compounds as broccoli and kale. Eating Brussels sprouts can help reduce the risk of cancer and heart disease, lower cholesterol, and prevent constipation. A half cup provides the same amount of fiber as two slices of whole grain bread. Remove the tough outer leaves and trim bottoms of sprouts before cooking.

The Blessings of Brussels Sprouts

- **Steam 'Em** Steam Brussels sprouts in a basket steamer until tender (test by poking with a fork). Toss with olive oil, a squeeze of fresh lemon, and a dash of salt. Or drizzle with a little maple syrup instead.
- **Roast 'Em** Cut sprouts in half lengthwise, rinse, and drain dry. Toss with 1 tablespoon olive oil for every 2 cups sprouts, spread in a single layer on baking sheet, and sprinkle with sea or kosher salt and freshly ground pepper. Roast in a 375°F oven for 15 to 20 minutes.
- **Shred Into a Salad** You don't have to cook Brussels sprouts. After all, we eat cabbage raw. Simply shred or slice them very thin and add to salads. The fresher the sprouts, the better their flavor. Store fresh in the fridge for no more than a day or two.
- **Chill and Dip** Cut sprouts in half lengthwise. Steam four to five minutes and then plunge into cold water to stop the cooking process. Chill completely and serve with hummus or your favorite vegetable dip.

good to know: ABOUT BROCCOLI & RELATED VEGGIES

- People with hypothyroidism should eat moderate amounts of broccoli and other cruciferous veggies. Compounds they contain can interfere with how the body uses thyroid hormones.
- Broccoli can produce intestinal gas. If this is a problem, try sipping fennel or peppermint tea (see pages 90 and 108) after a meal that includes broccoli.
- Don't overcook broccoli. Steam or sauté for just five minutes.
- When choosing broccoli at a farmers market or grocery store, look for firm florets with a purple, dark green, or bluish color, which indicates a higher beta-carotene and vitamin C content.
- Store broccoli unwashed and wrapped in paper towels in the crisper drawer; alternatively, cut off about a half inch from the bottom of each main stalk and stand upright in a small bowl or glass with enough water to cover the cut stem. The stalks will take up water like flowers in a vase, keeping the vegetable crisp and fresh.
- The broad leaves of broccoli plants are very nutritious and can be stewed like collard greens or added to soups. Next time you buy broccoli at a farmers market, ask growers about getting the leaves, too. Many may happily just give them to you.
- Wash kale thoroughly. Swish the leaves repeatedly in bowl of water. Then transfer to a colander to drain or spin-dry in a salad spinner.
- Conventionally grown kale has been shown to contain considerable pesticide residues. Reduce your potential exposure by buying only organic kale.

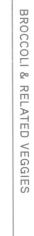

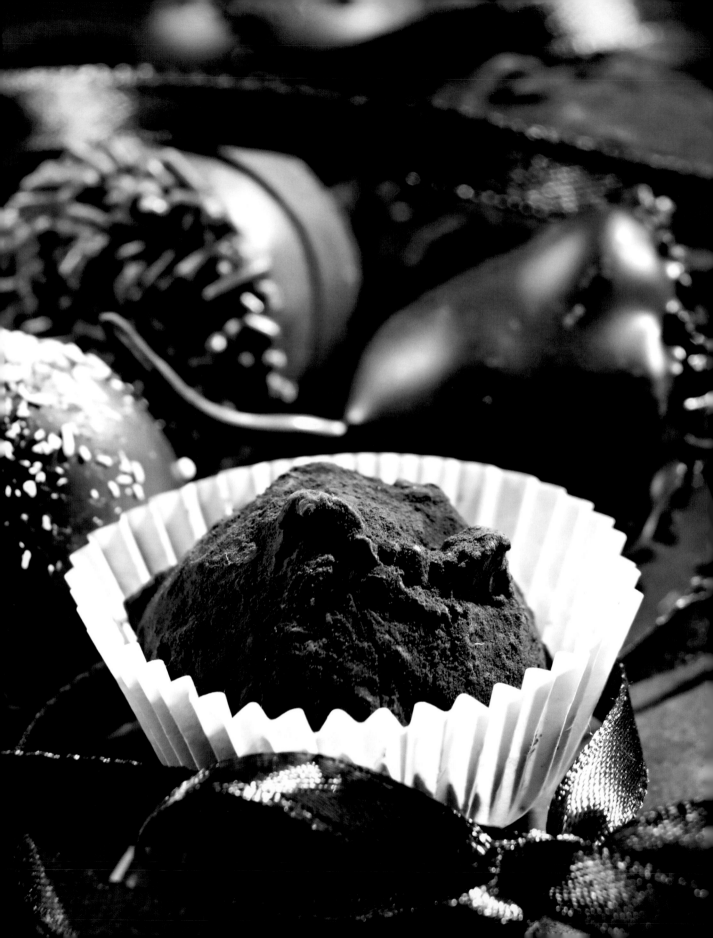

Chocolate

11 REASONS TO ROCK WITH CHOCOLATE

For many of us, just saying the word conjures up feelings of comfort and contentment, and perhaps even bliss. Chocolate is one of the world's favorite foods, one that is linked with indulgence, extravagance, and celebration. Chocolate's source is cacao, a small tree native to Central and South America. It's a strange tree in that its flowers—and later the large ribbed pods that develop from them—grow directly out of the trunk and main branches. The pods are filled with a fragrant, mucilaginous pulp that surrounds rows of dark brown seeds. Chocolate is produced from these seeds. So is cocoa and creamy cocoa butter.

European explorers didn't quite know what to make of cacao or the frothy, bitter beverage spiced with chili peppers that the Aztec and other indigenous people made from it. Introduced into Europe in the late 1500s, this chocolate drink underwent a transformation when someone hit on the idea of replacing chili peppers with sugar. Sweetened chocolate, drunk hot or cold, became all the rage, at least for those wealthy enough to afford it. But it was more than just a popular food. Europeans also used chocolate as the Aztec had: as medicine. People drank it as a healthful tonic and took preparations of it as remedies for everything from fever to fatigue. Chocolate was also used as a palatable binder or coating for administering unpalatable cures such as "powder of millipede" or "liver of eel"!

It wasn't until the 1800s that chocolate as we know it today—the sweet, solid concoction of cocoa, sugar, and cocoa butter—came to be. Although the medicinal use of cacao and chocolate persisted into the 1900s, most people in the United States and Europe came to view chocolate as candy, and things made with chocolate as dessert. That view held sway until the 1990s, when scientists discovered that chocolate contains high levels of antioxidants thought to help lower the risk of coronary heart disease by preventing fatlike substances in the blood from clogging arteries. Evidence of chocolate's value as a healthy food has been accumulating—oh, so sweetly—ever since.

▶ | DARK CHOCOLATE

The darker the chocolate, the better. Dark chocolate contains robust amounts of antioxidants called flavonoids. Similar compounds are also found in many fruits and vegetables (see page 183), red wine (see page 191), and green tea (see page 156), although research has shown that chocolate appears to have more of these disease-fighting antioxidants than any other food. The antioxidants in dark chocolate do a number of things. They help lower blood pressure; improve the flexibility of blood vessels; lower low-density lipoprotein (LDL), or "bad" cholesterol; raise high-density lipoprotein (HDL), or "good" cholesterol; and keep blood platelets from sticking together to form clots. Chocolate's antioxidants also tend to make cells more responsive to insulin (important for people with type 2 diabetes) and reduce inflammation, which is thought to contribute to many chronic diseases, including heart disease, cancer, and Alzheimer's. Finally, one study, which followed more than 1,000 heart attack survivors, showed that consuming chocolate significantly reduced the risk of having a second attack. Getting a small amount (think one small square) of dark chocolate in your diet several times a week is easy to do. Be careful about eating more than that: Due to its fat content, chocolate is a high-calorie food.

Darkly Delicious

- **Dip Some Berries** Both chocolate and berries (see page 143) are rich in disease-fighting antioxidants. Place about ⅓ cup chopped dark chocolate (or dark chocolate chips) in a microwave-safe bowl. Microwave at 50 percent power for intervals of 15 seconds, stirring in between, until chocolate is melted and smooth. (Alternatively, melt chocolate with gentle heat in a double boiler.) Add a pinch of cinnamon to the melted chocolate and blend well. Dip the lower half of fresh strawberries or raspberries into the warm chocolate and place on a plate covered with wax paper. Refrigerate until the chocolate is firm.

- **Add to Savory Sauces** Chocolate intensifies the flavors of many savory dishes. Spike your favorite barbecue sauce recipe by adding an ounce of grated bittersweet chocolate. Do the same thing when making Mexican mole or meat marinades.

- **Go Mocha** Make a delicious mocha cappuccino at home by grating a tablespoon of semisweet dark chocolate into a cup, fill with hot coffee and hot milk, and stir until the chocolate dissolves.

- **Concoct a Frozen Confection** Drizzle a little melted dark chocolate over a ripe banana, roll it in a tablespoon of chopped walnuts, wrap, and freeze.

- **Fix a Different Trail Mix** A handful of dark chocolate chips in a healthful trail mix adds variety and antioxidants.

CHOCOLATE-DIPPED ORANGE MERINGUES

4 large egg whites

¼ teaspoon salt

¼ teaspoon natural orange extract

½ cup semisweet dark chocolate chips

¼ teaspoon cream of tartar

½ cup sugar

2 ounces dark, bittersweet chocolate, finely chopped

With a mixer, beat the egg whites at high speed until foamy. Add cream of tartar and salt, and continue beating until soft peaks form. Gradually add the sugar, a tablespoon at a time, continuing to beat after each addition until stiff peaks form (the mixture should have the consistency of marshmallow cream). Gently fold in the orange extract and chopped chocolate until just blended. Drop rounded tablespoonfuls of the batter onto a baking sheet covered with parchment paper. Bake at 200°F for two hours or until the surface of the meringues is dry. Turn off heat, but leave meringues in the oven for at least another hour or until completely cool and crisp. Remove meringues from paper and arrange on a wire rack while preparing chocolate for dipping.

Place semisweet chocolate chips in a medium microwave-safe bowl. Microwave at 50 percent power for intervals of 15 to 20 seconds, stirring in between, until chocolate is melted and smooth. (Alternatively, melt chocolate in a double boiler.) Dip half of each meringue in chocolate. Place on wire rack to dry. Store in an airtight container.

▶ | COCOA POWDER

Cocoa powder, or just cocoa, is the brown component of chocolate. It's also the most concentrated source of chocolate antioxidants. Research has shown that adding cocoa powder to foods can provide the same health benefits as eating chocolate—for a fraction of the calories. The key is to use the right cocoa. Natural (unsweetened) cocoa powder contains the highest levels of healthful antioxidants. It's a better option than Dutch-processed (alkalinized) cocoa powder, which loses much of its antioxidant content during processing.

Cookin' With Cocoa

- **Add to Chili** Try a tablespoon of natural cocoa powder in your favorite chili recipe. If you're eating canned chili, a healthy pinch or two of cocoa can help spark up the flavor.
- **Swirl Into Yogurt** Add a teaspoon or two of natural cocoa powder to plain or Greek yogurt. Stir well and top with naturally sweet strawberries or raspberries.
- **Sprinkle on Oatmeal** Swirl a teaspoon of cocoa into hot cereal for breakfast.
- **Stir Up Chocolate Waffles** Add ¼ cup of cocoa powder (along with 1 tablespoon extra liquid such as water or milk) to your favorite pancake or waffle recipe.

DARK CHOCOLATE WINE SAUCE

Enjoy this antioxidant-rich sauce on ice cream or fresh berries:

1 cup Cabernet Sauvignon, Merlot, or other dry, full-bodied red wine
½ cup sugar
¼ teaspoon cinnamon
⅛ teaspoon allspice
A pinch cayenne pepper
½ cup natural cocoa powder
½ cup maple syrup
1 ounce (about 2 tablespoons) semisweet dark chocolate, chopped

Combine the wine, sugar, cinnamon, allspice, and cayenne pepper in a small saucepan. Simmer over low heat, stirring often, for five minutes until the sugar is completely dissolved. Whisk in the cocoa powder, and then add the syrup, stirring until smooth. Simmer on low, stirring constantly, for two more minutes. Remove from the heat. Add the chopped chocolate and continue stirring until the chocolate melts. Cool to room temperature before serving. Leftovers will keep in the refrigerator for up to one week.

good to know: ABOUT CHOCOLATE & COCOA POWDER

- Milk chocolate, which is chocolate made with milk or milk powder, has fewer antioxidants than dark chocolate and is usually higher in fat.
- White chocolate is not a healthful food. It is made from cocoa butter and sugar and contains none of the antioxidants found in dark chocolate.
- Buy good-quality dark chocolate made with a high percentage (look for around 70 percent) of cocoa solids.
- Store chocolate in a cool, dry place. Properly stored, chocolate should last for several months.
- Occasionally, a cloudy, whitish gray film will appear on dark chocolate. This "bloom" is the result of fat or sugar coming to the surface from being kept in too warm or too moist an environment. It doesn't look nice, but it doesn't affect the taste or healthful properties of the chocolate.
- Store cocoa in an airtight container in a cool, dark place—but not in the refrigerator, where high levels of humidity can cause it to spoil.

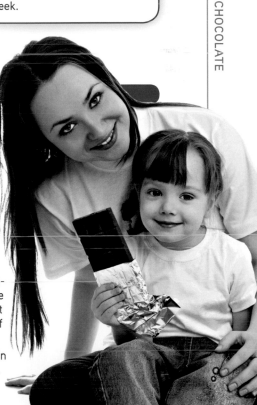

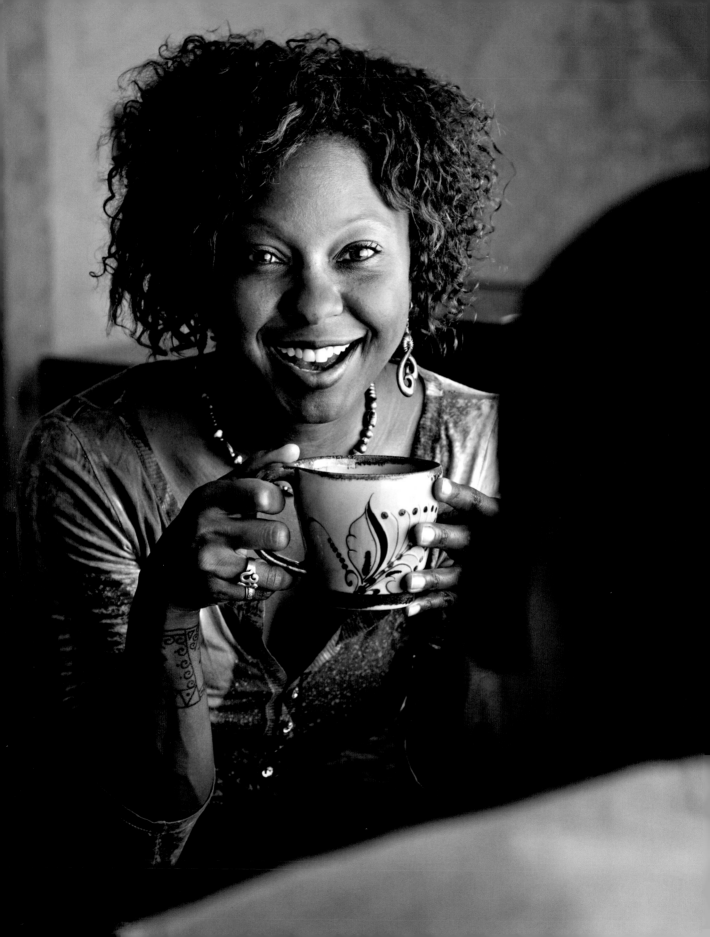

Coffee & Tea

9 CUES FOR HEALTH IN A CUP

Tea? Or coffee? From the standpoint of promoting good health, have either—or both. These two beverages are intimately associated with human culture, though tea has been with us much longer. According to legend, a Chinese emperor supposedly took the first sip of tea by chance in 2737 B.C. when dried leaves of the tea bush accidentally fell into a pot of boiling water. Whether or not that's true, by the fourth century A.D., Chinese texts were consistently mentioning tea, and just a few hundred years later, tea had soared in status to become China's national drink. Tea drinking spread to Japan and Europe, and from there to England and the colonies of the New World. Today, tea is second only to water as the world's most popular drink.

Coffee drinking is thought to have sprung up in Ethiopia and nearby parts of tropical Africa. By the mid-15th century, coffeehouses were serving coffee across the Middle East. After a slow start, coffee took Europe by storm during the 1700s. Capitalizing on the trend, the Dutch established coffee plantations in Java and quickly eclipsed the Arabs as the leading exporters of coffee. By the mid-1800s, coffee was being grown on plantations in many parts of the world, and coffee drinking had become an integral part of everyday life for millions of people.

Historically, tea and coffee were more than simple beverages to be sipped and shared. They were also used medicinally, primarily as stimulants and diuretics. In the late 1970s, several studies raised concerns about coffee's safety and linked it to an increased cancer risk. Recent investigations, using superior research methods and larger groups of people, have put those fears firmly to rest. Current studies show that coffee and tea are rich in antioxidants and other compounds. Used wisely, they help protect against heart disease, cancer, and much more.

good to know: ABOUT COFFEE & TEA

— Preheat the teapot before making tea by filling it with hot water and letting it sit for a few minutes. Warm the teacups in the same way. Pour out the warming water before making and serving tea.

— To keep tea fresh, store it in an opaque, airtight container in a cool, dry place. Avoid using glass jars, as this exposes the tea to light.

— The best cups of tea and coffee are only as good as the water used to make them. Use filtered or bottled springwater. Distilled water is not recommended, as it imparts a flat taste to the brew.

— Fresh water, with a high oxygen content, is also important to make a good cup of tea or coffee. Don't use hot tap water or water that has already been boiled once to brew tea or coffee. Also don't let water boil too long.

— Store freshly roasted coffee in an airtight container on the counter. There's no need to refrigerate or freeze it.

— A six-ounce cup of black coffee has just seven calories. But watch what you add to it. A splash of real cream or a liquid nondairy creamer will add about 50 calories and a teaspoon of sugar will add about 25 more.

▶ | TEA

Teas are made from the leaves of *Camellia sinensis,* including green, white, black, and oolong. Their differences are due to variations in processing the leaves. (Herbal teas are not tea in the same sense, but rather infusions of hot water and parts of medicinal herbs, including flowers, leaves, stems, and roots and rhizomes.) All types of tea made from *C. sinensis* contain a host of biologically active chemical compounds, including potent antioxidants, particularly substances called catechins. Studies show that green tea, for example, appears to help lower cholesterol levels, fight atherosclerosis (particularly in the coronary arteries in the heart), and help prevent certain types of cancer. It may also act to regulate blood sugar levels and therefore help control diabetes, protect against Alzheimer's and other forms of dementia, reduce inflammation in the digestive tract, protect against rheumatoid arthritis, and even help the body burn fat. Studies on black tea show that it can boost the immune system, help lower blood pressure, and possibly control diabetes by slowing the absorption of glucose by cells. Taken together, the evidence suggests that getting green or black tea into your diet may positively affect your health.

Turn to the Tea Leaves

■ *Brew Green Tea* To make the perfect cup of green tea, use 1½ heaping teaspoons of green tea leaves per cup of water. Bring water to a boil and then let it sit for three to five minutes (brewing green tea with just-boiled water can cause bitterness and an astringent taste). Pour the water into a teapot into which you've put the tea leaves, and let steep briefly, one to three minutes. (The smaller the leaves, the less time you should let the tea brew.)

■ *Try Black Tea* Brew black tea as you would green tea (see the previous paragraph), although it's fine to use just-boiled water. Allow to steep for three to five minutes. Pay attention to the taste, rather than the color. Let it steep until it tastes right to you.

■ *Cook With Tea* In many Asian cuisines, tea is added to foods to enhance color and flavor. To use green or black tea in cooking, steep tea leaves naturally using room-temperature water for 20 to 30 minutes. Here are a few ideas: Add a tablespoon of strong black tea to meat gravies and salad dressings. Add ¼ to ½ cup to soups, stews, and chili. Instead of water, use green tea to poach shrimp or cook rice.

GREEN TEA, KEFIR, & BLUEBERRY SORBET

Try this refreshing antioxidant-rich sorbet as a light dessert. Kefir is a fermented, yogurt-like drink that contains probiotics (see pages 179–180).

1 cup filtered water   2 tea bags organic green tea
½ teaspoon cinnamon   Pinch of cloves
¼ cup brown rice syrup, maple syrup, or honey
1 cup organic unsweetened 100% blueberry juice (not concentrate)
½ cup organic unsweetened 100% pomegranate or cranberry juice (not concentrate)
¼ cup organic raspberry kefir (with live probiotic cultures)

In a medium saucepan, bring the water to a boil. Remove from heat and let sit two minutes to cool. Add the tea bags, cinnamon, and cloves and steep three minutes. Remove the bags. Stir in the rice syrup (or maple syrup or honey) until well blended. Put in the refrigerator and chill 20 minutes. Add the fruit juices and kefir to the chilled tea mixture and stir well. Pour into a freezer-safe container, cover, and freeze for two hours. Remove and, using the tines of a fork, scrape and break up the frozen mixture. Refreeze for another hour and repeat the scraping. Repeat twice more, or until you have a well-frozen, granular slush. Serve in bowls garnished with fresh mint.

▶ | COFFEE

Many of us couldn't face the day without our morning cup of java. Evidence is mounting that this dark, robust beverage offers many health benefits. Research has shown that compared with non-coffee drinkers, people who drink coffee are less likely to have Parkinson's disease, type 2 diabetes, or dementia. They have fewer cases of stroke, abnormal heart rhythm (arrhythmia), and liver cancer, too. Despite these potential benefits, there are limits to how much coffee you should drink. Depending on how strong you drink it, coffee can contain a lot of caffeine, which in large quantities can bring on the jitters and interfere with good sleep. Too much coffee can also make heartburn worse. So do as the old adage advises: All things in moderation, including coffee.

The Joys of Java

- **Buy It Fresh** There are many ways to brew coffee. The way to ensure the best cup no matter what the brewing technique, though, is to use coffee as soon as possible after it has been roasted. Because fresh-roasted coffee is essential, purchase coffee in small amounts—just enough to last a week or two.

- **Grind Your Own** You'll also get the best tasting cup of coffee if you grind it just before you brew it. Use about 1 to 2 tablespoons of ground coffee for every 6 ounces of water (everyone's tastes are different, though, so adjust these amounts to suit yours).

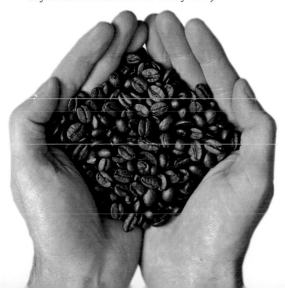

SELECTING COFFEES & TEAS

Remember when tea and coffee choices were limited to a brand or two of black teas or ground coffee sold in big, vacuum-packed, sealed cans? Today, consumers enjoy a bonanza of choices that even an emperor would envy—hundreds of offerings of bulk or tea-bagged green, black, oolong, and white teas. Green teas are dried tea leaf, retaining the green color. Black teas are fermented before drying. Oolong is partially fermented, and white tea is the carefully hand-plucked immature leaf buds. All provide a different flavor experience. Experiment and enjoy.

The same goes for coffee: An array of whole-bean or ground coffee choices is available from farmers from Africa, South and Central America, and Indonesia. Small boutique coffee roasters are as common as microbreweries. Whole freshly roasted coffee beans offer the richest flavor. Dark roasts have a more robust flavor than lighter roasts. Look for fair trade and certified organic offerings at natural food and grocery stores or gourmet shops. Ultimately, let your nose and taste buds be your shopping guides.

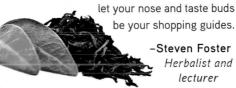

–Steven Foster
Herbalist and lecturer

- **Check the Heat** If you're brewing coffee manually—for example, using a cone filter or a French press—let the water come to a full boil, then turn the heat off and let the water rest a minute before pouring it over the grounds.

- **Drink Up** For the best taste, drink coffee right after it's made.

- **Add to Foods** Like tea, you can add coffee to sweet and savory dishes to get its benefits and add a wonderful depth of flavor as well. Try adding strong coffee or espresso to beef stews, black bean chili, and barbecue sauce. Use freshly ground coffee as an ingredient in spicy meat rubs. Replace some of the liquid in cake and cookie recipes with coffee, or use it in homemade pumpkin pie!

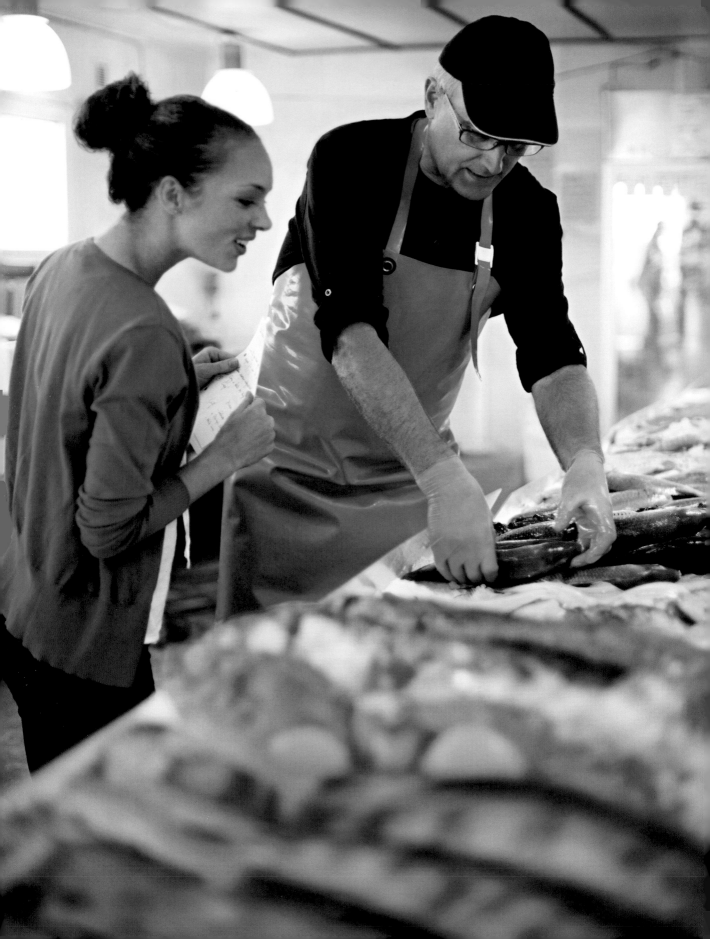

Fish & Flaxseed

13 WAYS TO GET GOOD FAT

All fats are not created equal. And scientific research is revealing that different kinds of fats have different effects on our bodies. Saturated fats are those that come mostly from animal sources such as meat and dairy products—think butter, bacon grease, cream, and cheese. When consumed in large quantities, some saturated fats appear to raise low-density lipoprotein (LDL, or "bad") cholesterol levels in the blood. So do synthetic "trans fats" such as partially hydrogenated oils found in margarine and many snack foods. A high level of LDL cholesterol in the bloodstream has been linked to an increased risk of cardiovascular disease.

Most nutrition experts recommend consuming very modest amounts of saturated fats. The American Heart Association, for example, recommends limiting saturated fat to 7 percent of a person's total daily calories. Nearly everyone agrees that we should avoid trans fats altogether.

Unsaturated fats are found primarily in plants and fish and they're usually liquid at room temperature. There are two basic types of unsaturated fats: monounsaturated and polyunsaturated. Olive oil and avocados (see page 171) are among the best sources of monounsaturated fats you can find. And—you guessed it—fish and flaxseed take the prize for being incredibly rich in polyunsaturated fats. Clinical studies have shown that when people replace saturated fats with unsaturated fats, LDL levels decrease along with the risk of cardiovascular disease. Unsaturated fats are also exceptional sources of a particular type of polyunsaturated fat that's making headlines these days: omega-3 fatty acids. Many studies have shown that omega-3 fatty acids can help decrease the risk of coronary artery disease, protect against irregular heartbeats, and help lower blood pressure. They also fight inflammation and may protect against cancer.

▶ | FISH

Evidence has been accumulating for decades that eating fish bestows impressive heart-healthy benefits. A number of studies have shown that adding fish to the menu on a regular basis can slash a person's risk of cardiac arrest in half. Other studies have found that eating fish provides similar protection against stroke. A diet that includes fish also helps prevent or delay dementia, reduces the chance of getting type 2 diabetes, guards against age-related macular degeneration, lowers the risk of certain types of cancer, and reduces inflammation linked to many other illnesses. All that, and fish are delicious, too! But before you fill your grocery cart with seafood, there are two things to keep in mind: Choose fish that contain the highest amounts of omega-3 fatty acids. And for the fishes' sake, choose species harvested sustainably, so they will be around for a long time to come.

Get Schooled on Fish

■ *Select Salmon, Carefully* Salmon is high in omega-3s, has a rich texture and unique flavor, and can be prepared in many different ways, starting with simply sautéing and drizzling with fresh-squeezed lemon. From both a flavor and sustainability standpoint, choose fresh or frozen wild-caught Alaskan salmon. Canned wild-caught salmon is also fine.

- **Reach for Farmed Arctic Char** Farmed sustainably in an ecologically responsible manner in cold Icelandic waters, Arctic char has a delicate flavor. Its light pink flesh is rich in omega-3s.
- **Go With Pacific Halibut** It has sweet white flesh that is tender and flaky when cooked. When buying halibut, make sure it's from Pacific, not Atlantic, waters. Atlantic halibut has been seriously over- fished, but the Pacific halibut fishing industry is sustainably managed.
- **Try Mackerel** Superbly heart healthy, mackerel can work in many recipes and is a treat both grilled and smoked. Choose smaller mackerel varieties such as Boston mackerel. Avoid king mackerel, a species that contains high levels of toxic compounds and represents a mercury-poisoning risk.
- **Consider Cod** Both Pacific and Atlantic cod are delicious. To buy sustainably, look for Atlantic cod from Iceland and New England caught by hook and line (avoid those caught by trawling) and Pacific cod from U.S. waters.
- **Opt for Pollack** Make it Alaska pollack or Atlantic pollack caught sustainably in Norwegian waters, though. Alaska pollack is the fish often sold as frozen fish sticks or fillets; it is also made into imitation crab.
- **Think Small** Pacific sardines and anchovies are packed with omega-3s, protein, and other good things. Because they are small and not at the top of any ocean food chain, they contain relatively low levels of toxins. Avoid sardines caught in the Mediterranean, because of overfishing; Atlantic herring (often sold as sardines) and Pacific sardines, however, are harvested from well-managed fisheries using ecologically friendly methods.
- **Choose Your Tuna** Many tuna species are critically endangered. Albacore is still somewhat abundant. Be aware, however, that although some albacore (and skipjack) tuna are certified sustainable, many of these fish are caught using methods that kill other ocean species, including sea turtles. And nearly all tuna carries the risk of high mercury levels. Canned wild-caught pink salmon is a perfect substitute.

RECIPE FOR HEALTH

SMOKED SARDINES WITH MIXED GREENS & FIG-OLIVE DRESSING

6 fresh figs, stemmed and quartered (If you can't get fresh figs, dried ones are fine, but be sure to soak them in hot water for a few hours or overnight to soften them up.)

¼ cup pitted green olives (my favorite is picholine), chopped

Juice of 1 lemon

2 tablespoons extra-virgin olive oil

2 roasted red peppers, store bought or homemade

¼ pound mixed greens (Try to find a greens mix with arugula in it, as its peppery notes pair perfectly with the other flavors in the salad.)

2 4-ounce cans smoked skinless sardine fillets

Salt

For the dressing, toss together the figs, olives, lemon juice, and olive oil in a small bowl. Season with salt and toss to combine.

   Cut the peppers into strips and divide between two serving plates. Divide the greens between the plates. Drain the sardines and separate the fillets. Place the sardines on top of the salad, then spoon vinaigrette dressing over the top. Serve immediately. Serves two as a main course.

–Barton Seaver

FLAXSEED

Look at flaxseeds and you may wonder how something so tiny can be so powerful in promoting good health. Yet the small, brown, slightly flattened seeds of flax plants are the richest known plant source of alpha-linolenic acid, an omega-3 similar to some of the fatty acids in fish oil. Flaxseed is also packed with phytochemicals—chemical compounds occurring naturally in plants—called lignans. In the digestive tract, bacteria convert lignans into estrogen-like molecules that circulate in the body and bind with estrogen receptors on cells. There's some indication that this may reduce the risk of certain hormone-related cancers, such as breast cancer, although more research is needed. High in soluble fiber, flaxseed is also good at lowering cholesterol and keeping constipation at bay. It's easy to get into your diet. Crush or grind the seeds before use, or buy flaxseed meal. Whole seeds will sail right through your body without much benefit.

⚠ **CAUTION:** Flaxseed may interact with some prescription medications, so check with your doctor before adding it to your diet. Women with breast cancer should not take any supplements without their doctor's approval.

Mix It Up With Flax

- ***Slip In a Spoonful*** You can add ground flaxseed to all sorts of foods. If you don't like the flavor as is, try adding a teaspoon of ground flaxseed to yogurt or cottage cheese. Add a similar amount to breakfast smoothies and power shakes. Or slip a spoonful into pancake and waffle batter. Just add a little extra water, because flaxseed tends to absorb moisture.

- ***Make Porridge*** Make a hot cereal by adding two parts boiling water to one part ground flaxseed in a bowl. Stir well and let thicken for a few minutes. Then add a pinch of salt and flavor with nut butter, cinnamon, berries, maple syrup, or chopped fruit. Or make a savory porridge by stirring in shredded cheese and chilies, garlic, or chives.

- ***Add to Treats*** Baking brownies, muffins, or cookies? Make them more healthful by adding a teaspoon of finely ground flaxseed into the batter.

- ***Use as a Laxative*** As an alternative to bulk laxatives, you can mix a teaspoon of ground flaxseed into water or juice. Because flaxseed absorbs water, be sure to drink plenty of fluids during the day.

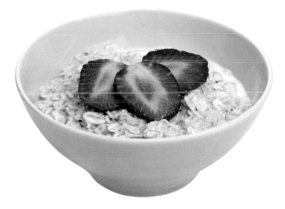

good to know: ABOUT FISH & FLAXSEED

— You don't need to eat huge slabs of fish. Small portions, just three to four ounces, deliver significant health benefits.

— For help in making healthful and environmentally friendly fish choices, use the "Seafood Decision Guide" and the "Seafood Watch" seafood guide made available online by National Geographic and the Monterey Bay Aquarium, respectively.

— Look for fish and fish products that bear the logo of the Marine Stewardship Council, which certifies sustainable fisheries and practices.

— Flaxseed supplements are available, but use caution. At high doses—and it's not clear how much is too much—lignans might turn into cancer promoters.

— Nutritionists suggest adding one to two tablespoons of ground flaxseed to your daily diet. Start with a smaller amount to avoid intestinal upsets and work up to the suggested amount.

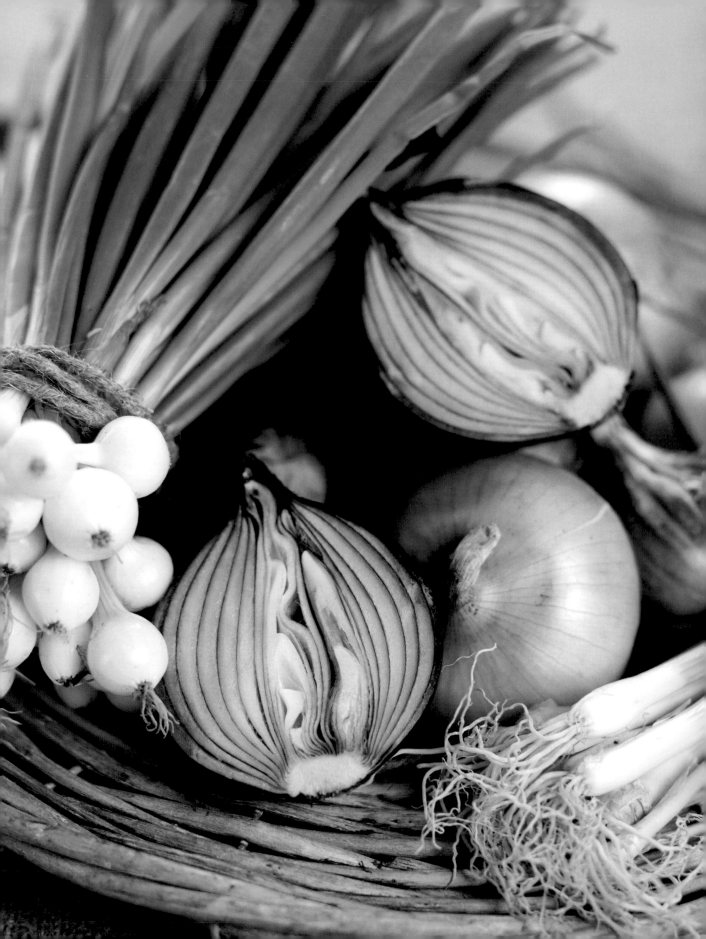

Garlic & Onions

11 SAVORY SUGGESTIONS

Garlic and onions have a lot in common. Both belong to the plant genus *Allium* and have the slender green leaves and plump bulbs wrapped in papery skin to prove it. Both have pungent, persistent aromas that linger in the kitchen long after you've cooked them—and on your breath long after you've eaten them. And they've both been a part of human cuisine and culture for thousands of years. Garlic and onions are among the oldest cultivated crops, first planted as many as 5,000 to 7,000 years ago. In ancient civilizations, however, they were more than simply foods. They were also associated with power and powerful beliefs. Olympic athletes in Greece ate garlic before competitions for strength and stamina, and the Egyptians reverently placed onions in tombs, believing their odor could help restore the dead to eternal life.

Over the centuries, garlic and onions were also valued greatly as medicinal plants. The first scientific proof of garlic's healing properties came in 1858, when French microbiologist Louis Pasteur demonstrated that garlic juice inhibits bacteria. More recent research confirms that garlic can fight a wide variety of infectious agents. Onions also fight infection. What's more, there is now a large and growing body of evidence that both onions and garlic may help prevent cardiovascular disease, boost the immune system, and even protect against certain types of cancer.

▶ | GARLIC

The medicinal benefits of garlic are tied to its sulfur-containing compounds, in particular a substance called allicin. When allicin and other compounds are released from cells making up a garlic clove—for instance, when you mince or crush it—they quickly break down to form a collection of infection- and disease-defying antioxidants. A number of studies have shown that garlic can help lower cholesterol to some degree, slow the development of atherosclerosis (hardening of the arteries), and slightly lower blood pressure—all actions that reduce the risk of heart disease and stroke. In addition to its antibacterial properties, garlic inhibits many types of viruses and fungi, and kills some parasites. Some laboratory studies suggest that garlic is able to inhibit the growth of cancer cells as well. Although clinical studies are needed to confirm this anticancer action in people, population studies have shown that people who consume quite a bit of garlic tend to have a lower incidence of certain types of cancer than people who eat very little. More research is needed before clear conclusions can be drawn about garlic's cancer-fighting powers, but in the meantime, take advantage of the bulb's known health benefits by adding it regularly to your diet.

Love Those Cloves

■ *Add Garlic to Salads* Fresh garlic contains the highest concentration of healthful compounds, but few people can stand to eat raw garlic straight. The solution is to add garlic to foods in the freshest form possible. When making a salad, cut a garlic clove or two in half and rub the inside of the salad bowl with the cut ends. Then chop or crush the halves and add to a tablespoon or so of olive oil, depending on how much dressing you need. Add a splash of lemon or a dash of balsamic vinegar, whisk together, and drizzle over the salad greens.

- **Make Garlic Butter** Heat a stick of butter in a saucepan, or gently in the microwave, until it liquefies. Add several crushed or minced garlic cloves and stir well. Pour the melted butter mix into a glass container with a tight-fitting lid and chill in the refrigerator. Use a little of this garlic butter to flavor breads, pasta, seafood, and other foods.
- **Heat It Gently** Heat does deactivate some of garlic's health-supporting compounds. However, garlic that is crushed and then only lightly cooked—either by sautéing or baking—still provides most of the health benefits

found in raw garlic. When a recipe calls for sautéed garlic, heat it only briefly before adding to other ingredients. When a recipe calls for sautéing onions and garlic, sauté the onions first until they are almost done. Then add crushed or minced garlic and heat for only an additional 15 to 30 seconds.

- **Mix It In** Mix crushed or minced garlic into dips, salsas, sauces, and salad dressings. Pureed vegetable dips such as baba ghanoush, hummus, and tzatziki are rich in garlic.
- **Add to Marinades** Add minced garlic to marinades for almost any type of meat. Rub the cut ends of garlic cloves on shrimp and other seafood before cooking.

⚠ **CAUTION:** Garlic is safe and well tolerated in the regular diet. Because garlic has blood-thinning properties and can alter the function of certain prescription medications, including anticoagulants and drugs to treat HIV, do not eat large quantities of garlic (more than four cloves daily) or take garlic supplements without first talking to your health care provider.

RECIPE FOR HEALTH

SIMPLE ROASTED GARLIC

Roasting garlic in the oven gives it a rich, nutty flavor and creamy consistency.

6 large garlic bulbs
Extra-virgin olive oil

Strip away the outermost layers of papery skin on the bulbs (leave the skins on the individual cloves intact). With a sharp knife, trim off the tops of the cloves (the pointy bits) to expose the flesh. Drizzle several teaspoons of olive oil over each trimmed bulb, coating well. Wrap each bulb tightly in aluminum foil. Place the wrapped bulbs on a baking sheet, in the cups of a muffin tin, or nested together in a casserole dish, with the trimmed ends up. Bake at 400°F for 30 to 35 minutes or until the bulbs are soft. Let cool for 10 to 20 minutes, and then unwrap. Press the soft roasted garlic out of each clove. Mash and spread on toasted bread, mix into cooked pasta, top baked potatoes or sautéed vegetables, spread onto pizza crust as a base beneath sauce . . . or just eat it warm all by itself.

▶ | ONIONS

Like garlic, onions are rich in sulfur-containing compounds. Onions also contain an antioxidant called quercetin that research has shown to halt the development of cancerous tumors, at least in animal studies. Quercetin helps fight something else, too: the development of *Helicobacter pylori*, a type of bacteria thought to be the cause of most stomach ulcers, and one that is sometimes linked to stomach cancers. Thanks to a high concentration of anti-inflammatory compounds, onions also help relieve inflammation and congestion.

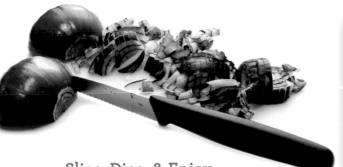

Slice, Dice, & Enjoy

- **Use Thin Slices** Raw onions, like raw garlic, contain the highest concentration of health-promoting compounds. For eating raw, choose sweet, mild onions. Add thin slices to burgers or sandwiches. Or toss them into salads (purple onion slices add wonderful color).

- **Sauté or Roast** Although heat does degrade some of the healthful sulfur compounds in onions, studies have shown that sautéing and roasting onions actually enhances their quercetin content. And sautéing and roasting makes onions taste sweeter too. Serve sautéed sliced or chopped onions as a side to grilled meats or stir them together with green beans or lightly steamed asparagus. Roast onion halves by slicing them along the onion's "equator" (slice into thirds if using large onions) and drizzling them with olive oil and balsamic vinegar, seasoning with salt

and pepper, and roasting in a 375°F oven for 30 to 45 minutes or until the onions are very soft and beginning to brown.

- **Add to Soups and Sauces** Add raw or sautéed onions to meat- and vegetable-based soups and almost any kind of savory sauce such as tomato sauce or sweet and sour sauce.

- **Prepare a Classic** French onion soup may be one of the best ways to enjoy the deep, sweet flavor of onions. Recipes—from the simplest to the most complex—abound!

PURPLE ONION TEA

The purple coloring in purple onions is due to the presence of antioxidants called anthocyanins (see page 184). Chopping the onions and letting them sit for a few minutes helps release infection- and disease-fighting compounds from onion cells. At the first sign of a cold or nasal stuffiness, try this tea:

¼ small red onion (about 2 tablespoons)
1 teaspoon honey
1 teaspoon freshly squeezed lemon juice

Chop the onion finely, put it in the bottom of a cup, and let sit for ten minutes. Add hot, but not boiling, water and let steep five minutes. Strain, and add honey and lemon juice. Sip slowly.

good to know: ABOUT GARLIC & ONIONS

— Research has shown that the best way to release garlic's healthful compounds is to mince or crush the cloves and then let stand for ten minutes before using.

— To make garlic paste, chop a clove with a knife, add a pinch of kosher salt, and mash the salt and garlic pieces together with a fork or the flat side of the knife.

— Choose garlic bulbs that are firm, plump, and undamaged. Store in an open container in a cool, well-ventilated place, but do not refrigerate.

— Always use fresh garlic. The pre-minced product packed in water is a culinary offense.

— Onions make you cry when you cut them because sulfur compounds released from the onion drift up and mix with moisture on the surface of your eyes to form sulfuric acid. The acid burns, stimulating profuse tearing to wash the irritant away. Try refrigerating onions before you cut them, or cut them under running water.

— Another way to avoid "onion tears" is to cut them on a cutting board placed near a gas burner. The flame sucks in the sulfur-laden air and burns off the offending particles.

— Lessen the bite of raw onions in salads and other foods by rinsing them briefly in water before using.

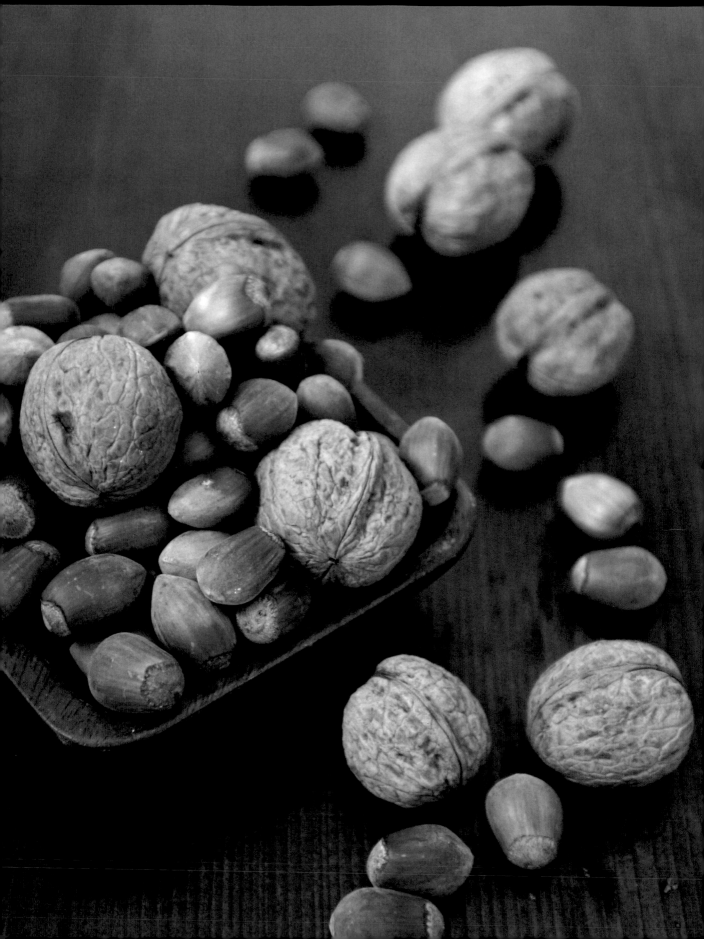

Nuts

12 WAYS TO GO NUTRITIOUSLY NUTTY

Nuts prove the old adage that good things come in small packages. They are loaded with protein, high in fiber, full of vitamins and minerals, and yes, rich sources of fat. It's because of their fat content that nuts used to be shunned. Yet research shows that people who eat nuts regularly have a lower incidence of heart attack than people who don't. Why? The fat in nuts packs a surprisingly healthful punch. Most nuts are high in unsaturated fat. When this "good" fat replaces saturated fat in the diet, it helps to naturally reduce the level of low-density lipoproteins, or LDLs (aka "bad" cholesterol), in the bloodstream. LDLs are known to increase the risk of cardiovascular disease.

Walnuts are among the best plant sources of alpha-linolenic acid, an omega-3 similar to some of the fatty acids in fish oil. Omega-3s help the heart by reducing inflammation and by preventing irregular heartbeat, which can lead to heart attack. Most nuts contain several other health-promoting substances, too, including antioxidants like vitamin E, cholesterol-lowering plant sterols, and the amino acid L-arginine, which keeps artery walls flexible and therefore less prone to developing blood clots.

The secret to taking advantage of the nutrients in nuts is simple: moderation. A small handful—about an ounce—can provide dramatic health benefits for less than 200 calories a day.

As a bonus, these tasty nuggets are also quite filling. Half a dozen nuts will satisfy hunger better than a whole stack of fat-free crackers. In fact, studies have shown that people who eat nuts regularly typically weigh less than those who avoid them!

▶ ALMONDS

Almonds are one of nature's best sources of vitamin E. A one-ounce serving (about 23 nuts) provides nearly 40 percent of the recommended daily intake of this vitamin. They're also a decent source of calcium, magnesium, potassium, and phosphorus. Almonds also contain

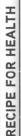

RECIPE FOR HEALTH

BROCCOLI SALAD

¼ cup balsamic vinegar

2 tablespoons spicy brown mustard

¼ teaspoon salt

4 tablespoons extra-virgin olive oil

1/3 cup blue cheese, crumbled

2 large heads broccoli, cut into bite-size pieces

½ cup lightly toasted almonds, coarsely chopped

2 tablespoons maple syrup

¼ teaspoon freshly ground black pepper

1 small red onion, sliced thin

½ cup dried tart cherries, preferably unsweetened

Steam broccoli pieces for three to four minutes, until just tender. Remove from heat and plunge into cold water to stop the cooking process. Drain. In a large bowl, stir together vinegar, mustard, maple syrup, salt, and pepper, and then whisk in the olive oil until the mixture emulsifies, about 30 seconds. Add drained broccoli, onion, almonds, and cherries to the bowl and toss with the oil and vinegar mixture. Serve with a small amount of blue cheese crumbles sprinkled on top.

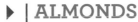

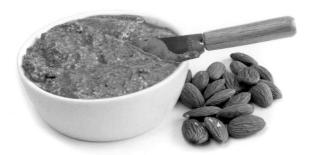

as many flavonoids—compounds that reduce inflammation and fight cell-damaging free radicals in the body—as a cup of green tea or a serving of broccoli. Research has shown that adding almonds to a healthy diet can prevent a spike in blood sugar following a high-carbohydrate meal, lower blood pressure, and lower cholesterol as much as some prescription drugs.

All-Good Almonds

- *Try Almonds to Go* Like all nuts, almonds are the perfectly portable snack. Carry some in your purse, backpack, or briefcase as a healthful food to nibble on. Almonds are ideal "carry-ons" for plane trips, where healthful food options are often limited.
- *Start the Day Right* Add whole or chopped almonds to breakfast cereal, granola, or oatmeal.
- *Move Over, Peanut Butter* If you've never had almond butter, you're in for a treat. Spread a teaspoon of freshly ground almond butter on toast or a bagel or onto a celery stick, or swirl into Greek yogurt.

▶ | PECANS

Pecans contain several different types of the antioxidant vitamin E and are particularly rich in one form of the vitamin called gamma-tocopherols. Recent research has shown that after eating pecans, gamma-tocopherol levels in study participants doubled and unhealthy oxidation of LDL cholesterol in the blood—which increases the risk of cardiovascular problems (specifically atherosclerosis)—decreased by as much as 33 percent. Pecans contain a wide variety of vitamins and minerals, including vitamin A, folate and other B vitamins, calcium, magnesium, phosphorus, and potassium. And vegetarians take note: Pecans also contain significant amounts of zinc, a mineral most often found in animal-based foods.

A Premium Nut

- *Upgrade Your Granola* Toasting pecans gives them a rich flavor. Drizzle honey over pecans, dried fruits, and regular (not instant) oats. Stir in a dash of cinnamon and a splash of almond or walnut oil, spread on a cookie sheet, and bake at 350°F until lightly browned.
- *Perk 'Em Up* Not fond of Brussels sprouts? Try with a dash of balsamic vinegar and a tablespoon of chopped toasted pecans. A combo of roasted asparagus spears, roasted red peppers, and toasted pecans is hard to beat.

good to know: ABOUT NUTS

— Freshly ground almond and other nut butters are far superior to what you find on grocery store shelves. You can often grind them on the spot in natural food stores. Or grind your own at home using a food processor.

— Toast almonds and other nuts to bring out their flavor. Spread shelled nuts on a rimmed baking sheet and pop into an oven that's been preheated to 300°F. Bake for seven to ten minutes, stirring once or twice. Alternatively, toast in a frying pan on the stove over medium heat, stirring constantly for about five minutes (be careful not to scorch them). Let cool completely.

— Buy almonds and other nuts whole rather than chopped, for freshness.

— When buying pecans in the shell, choose those that are a dull brown. Pecans with shiny, reddish shells have been artificially colored.

— Shelled pecans will keep about nine months in the fridge and a year in the freezer.

— When buying walnuts and other nuts in the shell, look for whole, clean shells without cracks, holes, or stains.

— Like other nuts with a high fat content, walnuts can become rancid. To preserve flavor and prevent spoiling, keep shelled walnuts refrigerated in an airtight container for up to six months or in the freezer for up to a year.

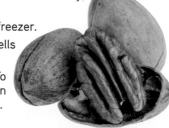

- **Gorgonzola Grapes** For a fantastic appetizer, beat together equal parts firm yogurt cheese (see page 180) and crumbled Gorgonzola cheese. Divide the mixture into roughly one tablespoon portions. Embed a red seedless grape into each lump of cheese, shaping it to completely enclose the fruit. Roll cheese-coated grapes in finely chopped, toasted pecans. Chill 15 minutes and serve.

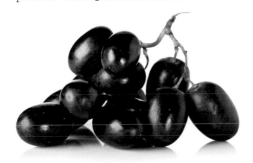

▶ | WALNUTS

They're bumpy and a bit weird looking, but walnuts may be the most healthful of all nuts and one of nature's most perfect ready-made foods. Walnuts are exceptionally high in antioxidants and omega-3 fatty acids. For this reason, they are very heart-healthy foods. The National Institutes of Health recommends that people consume at least 2 percent of their daily calories as omega-3 fats (some nutritionists suggest even more). For a person eating 2,000 calories a day, that equates to two grams of omega-3s. One serving of walnuts contains what amounts to 2.3 grams. As with all nuts, however, small amounts are sufficient—don't forget that these tasty nuggets are calorie-dense foods.

The Wonderful Walnut

- **Swap Oils** Substitute walnut oil for other oils in homemade salad dressings. Nut oils lack the fiber of whole nuts but are still an excellent source of omega-3 fatty acids and vitamin E.
- **Power Up a Smoothie** Add ¼ to ½ cup walnuts to a smoothie to boost nutrition and add fiber. A tablespoon of chopped walnuts is also a great topping for oatmeal, nonfat yogurt, sliced fruits, and salads.
- **Go Gourmet** A nut crust can turn a simple chicken breast or fish filet into an even tastier treat.
- **Rev Up Rice** Add chopped walnuts to cooked brown rice to add omega-3s and other nutrients and depth of flavor.

RECIPE FOR HEALTH

FETTUCCINE WITH ONIONS & WALNUTS

2 tablespoons extra-virgin olive oil
½ teaspoon kosher salt
¼ dry white wine (or low-salt chicken broth)
Additional salt and freshly ground pepper to taste
3 ounces (about ⅓ cup) shredded Comté
  cheese (alternatively, use Gruyère)

4 cups thinly sliced mild yellow onions
3 garlic cloves, minced
12 ounces fettuccine
½ cup toasted walnuts, chopped
¼ cup fresh basil, chopped

Heat olive oil in a large lidded skillet or Dutch oven over medium heat. Add onions and salt. Cook, stirring frequently, about 15 minutes until onions are cooked and translucent but not browned (if they start to brown, reduce heat slightly and stir more frequently). Reduce heat to low. Cover and cook an additional 20 to 25 minutes, stirring occasionally, until onions have turned a deep golden color and are very tender. Stir in garlic and wine (or broth); simmer about a minute, remove from heat, and cover. Cook pasta according to package directions. Drain pasta, reserving ¼ cup of pasta water. Add the hot pasta, pasta water, basil, and toasted walnuts to the onion mixture. Toss well to combine. Add salt and pepper to taste and serve immediately, with a scattering of shredded cheese on top. Serves four to six.

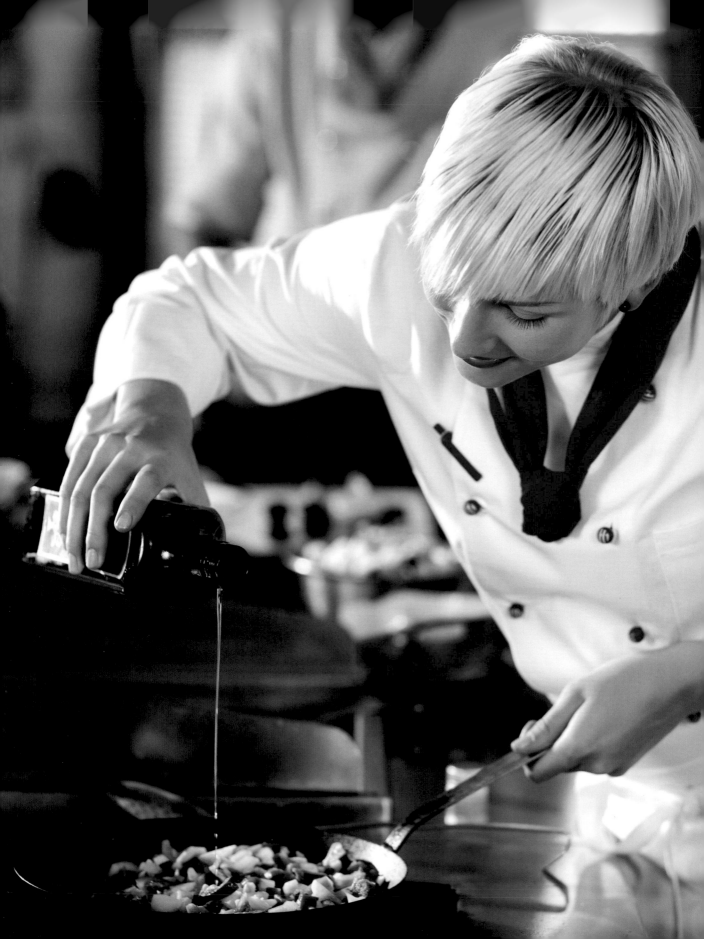

Olive Oil & Avocado

12 GOOD WAYS TO FAT-IFY YOUR DIET

Ask someone to list favorite fruits, and the list will very likely go something like this: strawberries, cherries, apples, peaches, plums, blueberries, pineapple, raspberries, mangoes, and so on. It's very unlikely that anyone's list—except perhaps a botanist's—would include olives and avocados. Yet olives and avocados are indeed fruits (as the botanist would tell you) that, like peaches, have a large, hard pit surrounded by a fleshy outer layer. Most people think "sweet" when they think of fruit, though, and olives and avocados are definitely not that (raw olives are incredibly bitter). But what these two fruits lack in sweetness, they make up for in wonderful, healthful fat.

Olives and avocados are two of the richest sources of monounsaturated fat in the human diet. Many research studies have shown that replacing saturated fat in the diet with unsaturated fat—monounsaturated fat as well as polyunsaturated fat (see page 159)—reduces the risk of cardiovascular disease. The replacement strategy is more effective, in fact, than simply reducing the total intake of fat.

People have been cultivating olives and avocados for thousands of years. Avocados hail originally from Central America. When Europeans arrived in the New World in the 15th century, these green, bumpy-skinned fruits were being grown by Native Americans from Mexico all the way down to Peru. Olives are indigenous to the Mediterranean region. Olives and olive oil have been part of civilizations in southern Europe, the Middle East, and North Africa since the early Bronze Age, some 5,000 years ago. Ancient peoples valued olives and avocados as foods with healing properties. We should today as well.

▶ | OLIVE OIL

Olive oil appears to be one of the world's most healthful fats. Researchers came to this conclusion back in the last century, after studying the health—and the diets—of Greeks living on the island of Crete. Greek men were found to have very low rates of coronary heart disease and a longer life expectancy than men from other European countries or North America. Although the classic "Mediterranean" diet these men were eating was high in fat, that fat was mostly olive oil. Subsequent studies have confirmed that olive oil lowers LDL ("bad") cholesterol—the type that contributes to cardiovascular disease—and raises HDL ("good") cholesterol, which helps guard against it. Olive oil is also rich in antioxidants that scavenge harmful free radicals and prevent them from damaging cells, as well as anti-inflammatory compounds that fight inflammation linked to heart disease, Alzheimer's, type 2 diabetes, and cancer. Olive oil is worth incorporating into your daily diet.

A Fat to Love

■ *Replace Saturated Fats* Use olive oil instead of saturated fats in cooking. For example, you can reduce the saturated fat in butter sauces by substituting beef or chicken stock thickened with olive oil. Instead of frying chicken,

MARINATED MUSHROOMS

2 pounds whole small button mushrooms, cleaned and stems trimmed

¼ cup fresh lemon juice

2 tablespoons minced fresh parsley

2 cloves garlic, crushed

1 teaspoon salt

¼ cup extra-virgin olive oil

½ cup white wine vinegar

Place the mushrooms in a large saucepan. Cover with water and add lemon juice. Bring to a boil and simmer for one minute. Remove from heat and drain. In a bowl, combine the remaining ingredients and whisk together well. Pour the mixture over the mushrooms, cover, and let marinate in the refrigerator overnight.

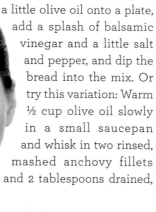

fish, or vegetables in butter or other solid shortening, sauté them in olive oil.

- **Try as a Dip** Make a dipping sauce for vegetables by combining olive oil, a dash of salt, and freshly ground pepper. Instead of smearing butter on bread, pour a little olive oil onto a plate, add a splash of balsamic vinegar and a little salt and pepper, and dip the bread into the mix. Or try this variation: Warm ½ cup olive oil slowly in a small saucepan and whisk in two rinsed, mashed anchovy fillets and 2 tablespoons drained,

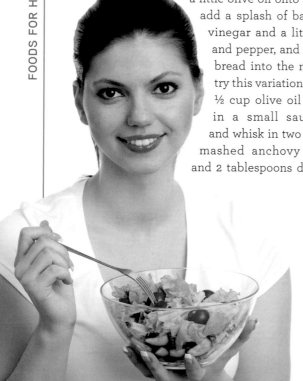

rinsed capers until the mixture is smooth and fluid. Use as a dip for crusty bread or drizzle over grilled fish or chicken breasts.

- **Stir Up Salad Dressing** One of the simplest and most healthful salad dressings is made by combining olive oil, balsamic vinegar, garlic, herbs, and salt and whisking together to emulsify. There are dozens of possible variations on this basic theme.

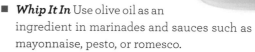

- **Whip It In** Use olive oil as an ingredient in marinades and sauces such as mayonnaise, pesto, or romesco.
- **Infuse It** Make your own flavored olive oil to use on salads by infusing the oil with fresh herbs. Add 2 to 3 sprigs each of fresh thyme, rosemary, and oregano, along with 3 or 4 basil leaves to a 12-ounce glass bottle. Fill with extra-virgin olive oil, cover tightly, and refrigerate. Because harmful bacteria can grow on fresh herbs, use this oil within two to three days.

▶ | AVOCADO

Avocados have the distinction of being the fattiest fruit on the planet. (They definitely live up to the nickname "butter pear.") They're an incredibly rich and concentrated source of healthful monounsaturated fat. Avocados are also a good source of fiber and protein (more than any other fruit) as well as potassium and folate, a water-soluble B vitamin that helps prevent changes to DNA that may lead to cancer. The oily fat in avocados is a healthful fat, but a medium-size avocado contains about 250 calories. In other words, small amounts—just a few slices—go a long way. Use avocados as a substitute for less healthful fats in your diet, not as a source of additional fat.

Avocado Adventures

- **Mash and Spread** Rather than putting butter on toast or a bagel, mash up a little avocado and spread it on instead. You'll save a surprising number of calories doing this: A tablespoon of avocado contains about 25 calories, whereas a tablespoon of butter has just over 100.

- **Replace Mayo and Sour Cream** Mayonnaise and sour cream are both high in saturated fat. Use a tablespoon of mashed avocado instead of mayonnaise as a sandwich spread. Top a baked potato with mashed avocado instead of sour cream or butter.
- **Fill the Middle** For a delicious, unusual appetizer, quarter an avocado, leaving the peeling on. Fill the "dip" in the middle with drained, rinsed capers, and enjoy.
- **Enhance Eggs** Adding about a tablespoon of diced avocado to an omelet gives it a unique texture and flavor. Add it to the egg mixture when you'd normally add vegetables during cooking.
- **Sprinkle Into Salad** Top a bed of greens with a few chunks of fresh avocado instead of croutons. And remember that avocado is a fruit, so it combines well with others—mix diced avocado with sliced apples, strawberries, blueberries, peaches, and grapes to make a healthful, colorful, and filling fruit salad.

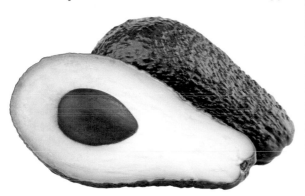

AVOCADO & MELON SMOOTHIE

Start your day with this creamy, nutritious drink—although you might need to eat it with a spoon:

1 ripe avocado
1 cup cantaloupe melon chunks
Juice from 1 lime (about 1 tablespoon)
1 cup almond or soy milk
1 cup fat-free, plain yogurt
½ cup orange juice

Cut the avocado in half, remove the pit, and scoop out the flesh. Place avocado and the rest of the ingredients in a blender and blend until smooth. Serve cold.

good to know: ABOUT OLIVE OIL & AVOCADO

- To get the most of what's good for you in olive oil, choose one labeled "extra-virgin" and "cold-pressed" to use in salad dressings or for dipping. Extra-virgin means the oil is made from the first pressing of the ripe olives, and cold-pressed indicates the oil has been extracted from olives by pressing alone, not chemically. Olive oil labeled "virgin" is fine for sautéing, as some of the flavor in extra-virgin oils is lost with heating.

- Store olive oil in the refrigerator to prevent it from becoming rancid. However, chilled olive oil solidifies and, depending on the size of the bottle, can take 10 to 30 minutes to liquefy again at room temperature. To ensure that you always have liquid oil conveniently at hand, keep about ½ cup handy on the counter in a dark bottle you can cork or cap. Replenish from a large bottle you keep in the fridge.

- Olive oil is a healthful oil, but don't forget that it's still a fat, with about 120 calories per tablespoon. Consume it in limited quantities as part of a balanced diet.

- Avocados are ripe when the flesh gives slightly under pressure. To encourage ripening, put slightly green avocados in a paper bag for a day or two. Or place them in a bowl with a banana, which naturally releases ethylene gas, a natural ripening agent.

- When the flesh of an avocado is exposed to air, it oxidizes and turns brown. To prevent this, coat the cut surface with a light film of olive oil, wrap in plastic wrap, and refrigerate.

- Darker, rough-skinned Hass avocados have a higher fat content than those with smoother, lighter green skins.

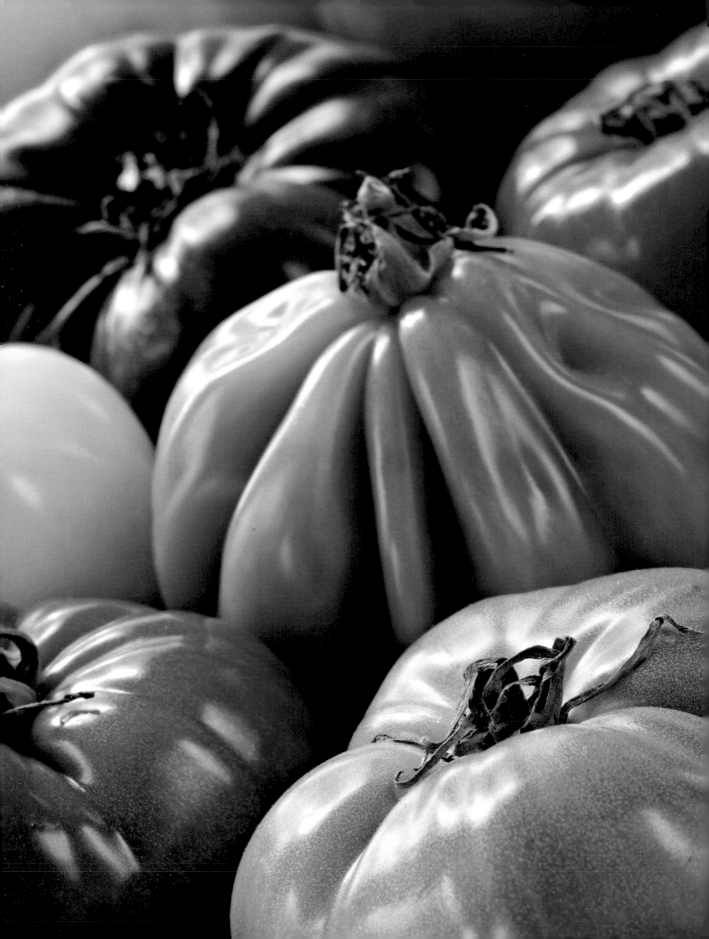

Pomegranate & Tomato

14 WAYS TO RELISH THESE REDHEADS

In 1544, the Italian herbalist Pier Andrea Mattioli puzzled over how to classify the strange, plump and juicy fruits that Spanish explorers had brought from the New World. He decided that tomatoes were kin to the herb mandrake, a known aphrodisiac. Soon nicknamed "love apples," tomatoes slipped comfortably into the cuisines of Spain, Italy, and other lands bordering the Mediterranean. But they got the cold shoulder in England, where John Gerard, an influential English herbalist, claimed tomatoes were "ranke and stinking." His pronouncement kept English and colonial American cookery free of the fruit until well into the 1700s.

Gradually, though, opinions changed and tomatoes entered American cuisine. Thomas Jefferson, an avid gardener, began planting several varieties of "tomatas" at Monticello in 1809. His son-in-law, Thomas Mann Randolph, mentioned that by 1824 everyone was eating them because they "kept one's blood pure in the heat of summer."

Pomegranates were slow to catch on in America too. Native to the Middle East, the orange-size fruits are linked to health, abundance, and rebirth in that part of the world, and have been since ancient times. Their delicate seeds, filled with tart ruby-red juice, are essential ingredients in a variety of Middle Eastern dishes. But for a long time, many Americans considered the pomegranate too unusual or perhaps too labor-intensive to eat, with its tough, leathery skin and fragile seeds encased in bitter, inedible membranes. A 2002 New York Times article cited a survey indicating that only 5 percent of Americans had ever tasted pomegranates. Attitudes changed, though, when science began showing that pomegranates are exceptionally healthful foods.

▶ POMEGRANATE

Pomegranate juice has a unique flavor, and contains a unique set of vitamins, minerals, and phytochemicals, including potent antioxidants. Research has shown that some of these antioxidants can help prevent cardiovascular disease by reining in "bad" cholesterol, reducing the risk of blood clot formation, and lowering blood pressure. There is growing evidence that pomegranate compounds have antibacterial properties and may help to prevent ulcer formation in the digestive tract. Pomegranate's anti-inflammatory nature makes it potentially helpful for arthritis pain, diabetes, and perhaps even Alzheimer's. But it's pomegranate's anticancer effects that are making headlines. Recent research has shown that pomegranate extracts inhibit the growth of breast, prostate, colon, and lung cancer cells in the lab. In animal studies, consumption of pomegranate extract inhibited growth of lung, skin, colon, and prostate tumors too. Clinical trials have shown that pomegranate juice can slow the progression of prostate cancer in some men with the disease.

POMEGRANATE & SPICED PEARS

3 ripe yellow or red pears, peeled, cored, and sliced into thin wedges
Seeds from 1 whole pomegranate
1 tablespoon freshly squeezed lemon juice (organic lemon)
1 teaspoon fresh lemon zest (organic lemon)
2 tablespoons maple syrup
½ teaspoon cinnamon
¼ teaspoon nutmeg
pinch kosher salt
3 tablespoons roasted, chopped pecans

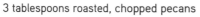

Place the sliced pears and pomegranate seeds into a large bowl. Add the lemon juice and lemon zest and mix gently. Combine the syrup and spices in a small bowl and add to the fruit. Blend gently to coat. Cover and refrigerate two hours. Serve, topped with chopped pecans.

⚠ **CAUTION:** Pomegranates and pomegranate juice are generally very safe. However, because the juice can interfere with how the blood thinner warfarin (Coumadin) and some other medications are metabolized in the body, check with your health care provider before drinking pomegranate juice.

Pomegranate Pleasures

- **Eat Fresh** Nothing beats the flavor of fresh, ripe pomegranate. Here's how to remove the delicious seeds. Use a sharp knife to cut the fruit in half along its equator. Place one half of the pomegranate in your palm with the cut side down. Holding it over a bowl, beat the skin with the handle of a knife or a wooden spoon. The seeds will begin to fall out of the membrane. Rotate the fruit as you continue beating to release all of the seeds. Once familiar with this method, you can get a whole fruit's worth of seeds in just a few seconds.
- **Add to Salad** Add jewel-like pomegranate seeds to green salads, fruits salads—even shrimp salad!
- **Eat With Olives** It may sound like an odd combination, but the tart yet sweet flavor of pomegranate seeds goes well with cured green or black olives. Serve the seeds alongside olives or sprinkle them over or into olive tapenade.
- **Make Chutney** Mix pomegranate seeds with citrus rind, citrus juice, honey, and a little salt and olive oil to make chutney to complement Indian and Asian curries.
- **Add to Drinks** Add festive color to sparkling wines by dropping a few pomegranate seeds into glasses just before serving to guests.
- **Build Into a Meal** Use pomegranate seeds as unusual ingredients in appetizers: Sprinkle them onto goat cheese spread on rounds of toast, or process a handful of seeds with roasted red peppers, walnuts, and olive oil to create a classic Middle Eastern spread. The seeds go well with roasted or grilled meats, in sauces or au naturel.
- **Use the Juice** To juice the seeds, place inside a potato ricer and squeeze over a bowl. Alternatively, put the seeds in a large, zip-top plastic bag. Push out the air, seal, and then flatten with a rolling pin to crush the seeds. Working over a bowl, snip one of the bag's lower corners and let the juice flow out while the seeds stay behind. If this sounds like too much work, 100 percent pomegranate juice is available at most grocery stores (look for unsweetened brands). Actually, there's a big plus to drinking the juice. Some of pomegranate's health-promoting antioxidants are found in the peel and the membranes around the seeds. Because commercial juicing involves squeezing the whole fruit, those compounds get into the juice.

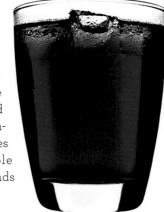

▶ | TOMATO

Despite their rocky beginning in American cuisine, tomatoes are now tops in popularity. We eat more tomatoes, both fresh off the vine and processed, than practically any other fruit or vegetable. Tomatoes are high in vitamins C and A,

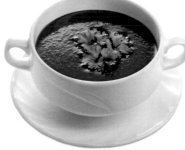

and the minerals potassium and iron. But they're absolutely packed with an antioxidant called lycopene that has anticancer properties. Studies have shown that lycopene seems to concentrate in the male prostate gland, where it appears to help fight prostate cancer or at least slow its growth. Other studies suggest that lycopene may also provide protection against breast, lung, and some other types of cancer. Interestingly, lycopene doesn't break down when exposed to heat, and more lycopene is released from a cooked tomato than a fresh one. What's more, it seems that lycopene is best absorbed through the intestine when eaten with a little fat, such as olive oil. So, if fresh tomatoes aren't your thing, know that tomato sauce, tomato paste, pizza sauce—even ketchup—packs an anticancer punch.

Savory, Saucy Side Dish

- **Eat Fresh** There is nothing that quite compares to the flavor of a vine-ripened, fresh tomato. Just eat out of hand, add to salad, or layer a slice or two in a sandwich.
- **Create a Caprese** This classic Italian salad has only a few ingredients. Slice fresh tomatoes and layer around a plate with fresh basil leaves and slices of mozzarella cheese. Combine olive oil and balsamic vinegar and drizzle over, adding a pinch of salt to taste.
- **Serve Up Salsa** Tomatoes are the backbone of most salsa recipes, usually a combination of chopped tomatoes, peppers, onions, lime, and cilantro. But there are as many versions of salsa as there are varieties of tomatoes.
- **Sauté, Stuff, and Stew** Sauté tomatoes for almost any kind of pasta sauce as well as sauces for chicken and fish. Scoop the seeds out and stuff large tomatoes with spicy combinations of meat and grains and bake until fragrant and steaming. Add tomatoes in any form to vegetable and meat stews and casseroles.
- **Don't Forget Soup** Tomato soup is an American classic. And homemade is infinitely better than canned (see the following recipe).

ROASTED HEIRLOOM TOMATO SOUP

Recipe from Bond, Breyer, and Gordon, *True Food*

5 pounds mixed, vine-ripened heirloom tomatoes, stemmed and halved

2 whole bulbs garlic, ends sliced off but still in skin

4 medium leeks, washed well, dark green parts removed, the rest chopped into chunks

3 red or yellow peppers, halved and seeded

6 tablespoons olive oil, divided

6 cups water

1 cup red wine

2 cups salt-free, 100% tomato juice

3 tablespoons pureed sun-dried tomatoes

1 tablespoon sweet paprika

1 cup basil leaves

4 cups low-fat milk (or soy milk)

Salt and pepper to taste

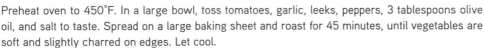

Preheat oven to 450°F. In a large bowl, toss tomatoes, garlic, leeks, peppers, 3 tablespoons olive oil, and salt to taste. Spread on a large baking sheet and roast for 45 minutes, until vegetables are soft and slightly charred on edges. Let cool.

Squeeze the roasted garlic out of the skins and add, along with the roasted vegetables, to a large pot along with the rest of the olive oil and all the remaining ingredients, except the milk. (Reserve a few basil leaves for garnish.) Bring to a boil, lower heat, and simmer 30 minutes. Add milk, then puree in a food processor or with an immersion blender until completely smooth. Season with salt and pepper to taste and garnish with reserved basil. Reheat briefly if necessary. Serves 12.

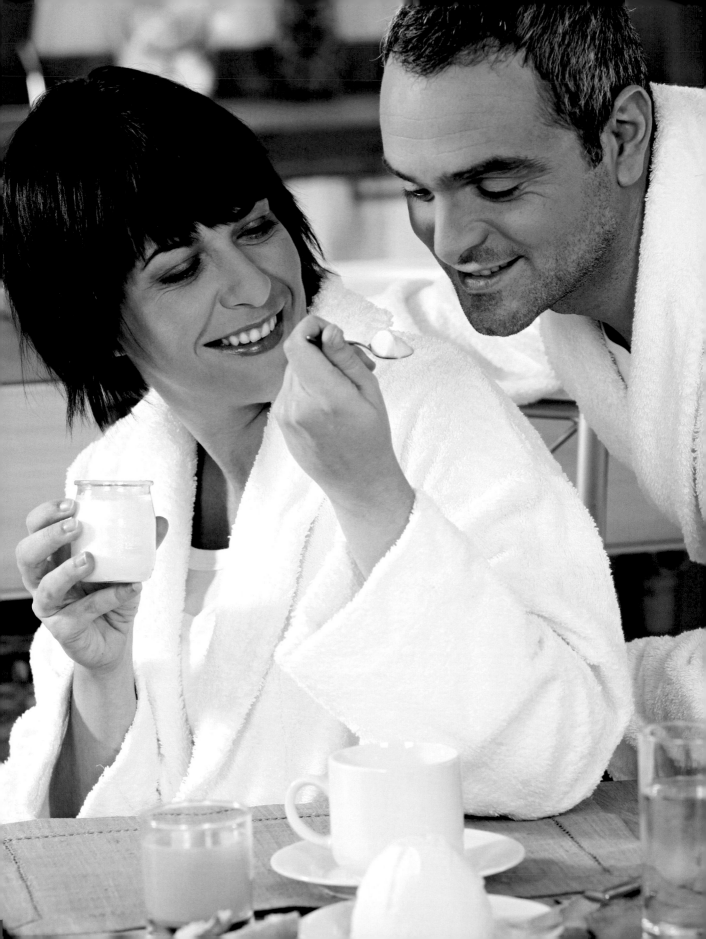

Probiotics

15 WAYS TO GO PRO

None of us is ever truly alone. That's because the average person is home to about 100 trillion microbes. Most of them are bacteria, and most of them live in the digestive tract. Before you panic at the thought of so many other organisms living inside you, know that you'd be in serious trouble without this internal menagerie. Beneficial bacteria in your small intestine and colon help to complete the digestion of many foods and add bulk to solid wastes. Equally important, they keep disease-causing microbes at bay by outnumbering them and entrenching themselves in places where these potential invaders would just love to take up residence.

Every once in a while, though, unfriendly microbes get their chance. An overseas trip might introduce a new strain of *E. coli* to your digestive tract. Eating tainted food might populate your intestines with something quite nasty. Stress or a poor diet might reduce the numbers of helpful bacteria. Or, in taking antibiotics for an infection, you might wipe out legions of the good guys, only to give bad bacteria the foothold they've been waiting for.

Probiotics are one way to fight back. Probiotic foods contain live cultures of bacteria that are very similar to the strains of healthful bacteria that normally inhabit our gastrointestinal tract. In addition to being generally good for you, probiotics can help prevent or treat certain types of intestinal upsets and disorders, including acute and antibiotic-associated diarrhea and irritable bowel syndrome. There is some evidence that probiotics may reduce the severity of certain allergic reactions, atopic eczema, childhood respiratory infections, tooth decay, and nasal pathogens, and may help ease the side effects associated with treatment for *Helicobacter pylori* infection, the cause of most stomach ulcers. Probiotic foods can be a delicious way to keep your intestinal inhabitants at peak performance and help fight many ailments too.

▶ | YOGURT, KEFIR, & BUTTERMILK

Thanks to high-profile advertising campaigns, yogurt is probably the best known probiotic food. Yogurt is made from milk that has been fermented using certain bacteria, including various strains of *Lactobacillus* bacteria. However, only yogurts that contain live bacteria ("active cultures") are truly probiotic foods. Read the nutritional label to make sure a product contains live bacteria. Kefir is a bit like liquid yogurt, although it contains different types of beneficial bacteria—often up to ten diverse strains. It's fermented using a mixture of bacteria and yeast together with milk proteins and complex sugars. Kefir can be made from cow's milk, goat's milk, or sheep's milk as well as coconut, soy, or rice milk. Modern commercial buttermilk is made by adding strains of lactic acid–producing bacteria to regular pasteurized milk.

Good for the Gut

- **Substitute Yogurt** Add probiotics to your diet by eating active culture yogurt and adding it to recipes and familiar dishes. For example, use yogurt in dressings and dips as a substitute for mayonnaise or cream.

- **Use Yogurt for Marinades** Yogurt adds distinctive flavor to marinades, and because it's acidic, it can help tenderize tough cuts of meat.
- **Use Yogurt Cheese** Yogurt cheese isn't really cheese; it's yogurt that's been drained of its liquid to form a product with a cream cheese–like consistency (see the following recipe). Use yogurt cheese in place of cream cheese or sour cream in dips, sauces, parfaits, dressings, on baked potatoes, and even in cheesecake.
- **Have a Kefir Breakfast** Kefir has a tart, refreshing taste. It's similar to yogurt, but in drinkable form. Start your day with a glass of kefir or use it as a base for a smoothie to which you add fresh or frozen fruit, spices, and fiber, such as ground flaxseed (see page 161).

FERMENTED FOODS

Our normal friendly "flora"—the bacteria living in and on us—form a key part of our defense against infection. Not only do these good bacteria outcompete "bad" microbes on our bodily surfaces, they also boost immune system function and aid digestion. No wonder antibiotics cause collateral damage, killing off the good with the bad. Scientists are learning that antibiotics may even produce enduring changes in our normal flora, thereby raising the risks of other infections and diseases.

What to do? Make fermented foods part of your diet. When you need antibiotics to combat an infection, take probiotics and continue for one to two weeks afterward.

–Linda B. White, M.D.
Educator and author

YOGURT CHEESE

Line a sieve or colander with six to eight layers of moistened cheesecloth. Fill the sieve with yogurt and set it over a bowl (make sure there's an inch or two of clearance between the bottom of the sieve and the bottom of the bowl). You should see a thin, clear liquid begin to drip out of the sieve and into the bowl. Cover lightly with a towel or plastic wrap and refrigerate. Let the yogurt drain for up to 12 hours; the longer it drains, the denser the cheese will be. Yogurt cheese will keep in the refrigerator for about a week.

- **Replace Milk With Buttermilk** You can drink buttermilk, although it's an acquired taste. Alternatively, get it into your diet by using it to replace cream or whole milk in your favorite recipes (think buttermilk ice cream). Or make a tangy smoothie by using half yogurt or kefir and half buttermilk.

▶ | ## MISO, TEMPEH, & NATTO

Another group of probiotic foods are those made from fermented soybeans. They include miso, tempeh, and natto. Miso is a staple in the traditional Japanese diet. It is made by fermenting soy, barley, wheat, or rice with a type of fungus that produces a red, white, or dark brown salty paste with a unique buttery texture. Tempeh is a food that originated in Indonesia at least 2,000 years ago. It is made by cooking soybeans, adding a fungus culture, and letting the beans ferment into a thick, meaty block with a nougat-like texture. In addition to promoting intestinal health, tempeh is high in protein and minerals. Natto is a probiotic food also made from fermented soybeans. A Japanese breakfast staple, natto has a strong, distinctive flavor and odor, and unique sticky texture—it's a food that most first-time eaters admit takes getting used to.

Soybean Surprises

- **Make Miso Soup** It's as easy as instant noodles. Heat some miso paste with water, stirring constantly over low heat. Enjoy as a salty broth, or add vegetables to make soup.
- **Whip Up Miso Dressing** Combine sesame oil, ginger, garlic, and a little miso to make an Asian-influenced salad dressing.

- **Move Over, Meat** Tempeh has a chewy, meatlike texture. Try substituting tempeh for ground beef in spaghetti sauce, chili, curries, and similar dishes.
- **Switch Out the Tofu** Use tempeh in any dish that calls for tofu—it's a more healthful option.

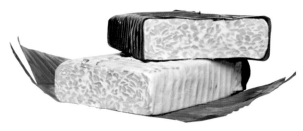

▶ KIMCHI & SAUERKRAUT

Probiotics can also come in pickled forms, such as the Korean food called kimchi and the eastern European favorite, sauerkraut. Kimchi is typically Chinese cabbage, eggplant, or another vegetable that has been allowed to ferment with red chili and other spices for at least a month—there are hundreds of variations. Kimchi is high in fiber, vitamins, iron, and several types of probiotic bacteria, including *Lactobacillus kimchii!* Sauerkraut, which means "sour cabbage" in German, is a dish made of finely shredded, salted, fermented cabbage and contains a variety of healthful bacteria as well.

Pickled Pickings
- **Try Solo or Combo** You can eat kimchi by itself or use it as an ingredient in many Korean recipes.
- **Boost Flavor** Use kimchi in a grilled cheese sandwich—it's the same principle as using sauerkraut in a Reuben.
- **Liven Up a Sandwich** Sauerkraut is the perfect complement to a ham and cheese sandwich, whether you layer it inside or eat it as a side dish.
- **Top a Potato** Mix yogurt cheese with sauerkraut and dill. Add a dollop on baked potatoes as a sour cream and butter substitute.

RECIPE FOR HEALTH

CRUNCHY SAUERKRAUT SALAD

1 large organic Braeburn apple, chopped
1½ cup natural sauerkraut (with active cultures), drained
1½ cups fresh fennel bulb, cut in thin slices
¼ cup lightly roasted pecans, chopped
3 tablespoons extra-virgin olive oil
2 tablespoons crumbled blue cheese

Toss all the ingredients except the cheese together in a bowl. Serve on a bed of lettuces, and top with a sprinkling of blue cheese crumbles.

good to know: ABOUT PROBIOTICS

— Kefir is a good choice as a probiotic dairy food if you are lactose intolerant, because most of the lactose it might originally have contained is broken down through fermentation.

— If you're taking antibiotics for something, be sure to compensate by eating probiotic foods, or by taking probiotic capsules (available at health food and some grocery stores). Follow package directions.

— Yogurt that contains a bacterium called *Lactobacillus reuteri* has been found to block the replication of certain illness-causing viruses. Not all brands carry that particular strain of beneficial bacteria, so look for a brand that does. When you feel a cold or the flu coming on, make a point to include this type of yogurt in your daily diet.

— Don't add yogurt, kefir, or buttermilk to foods that are boiling. Temperatures over 120°F destroy the beneficial bacteria these probiotic foods contain. Instead, add them off heat, after foods have begun to cool.

— To preserve the probiotic cultures in miso as much as possible, add it to hot foods off heat, at the end of cooking.

— Many commercial brands of sauerkraut do not contain live cultures. Look for fresh sauerkraut that does, and that has not been heated; heat kills the bacterial cultures.

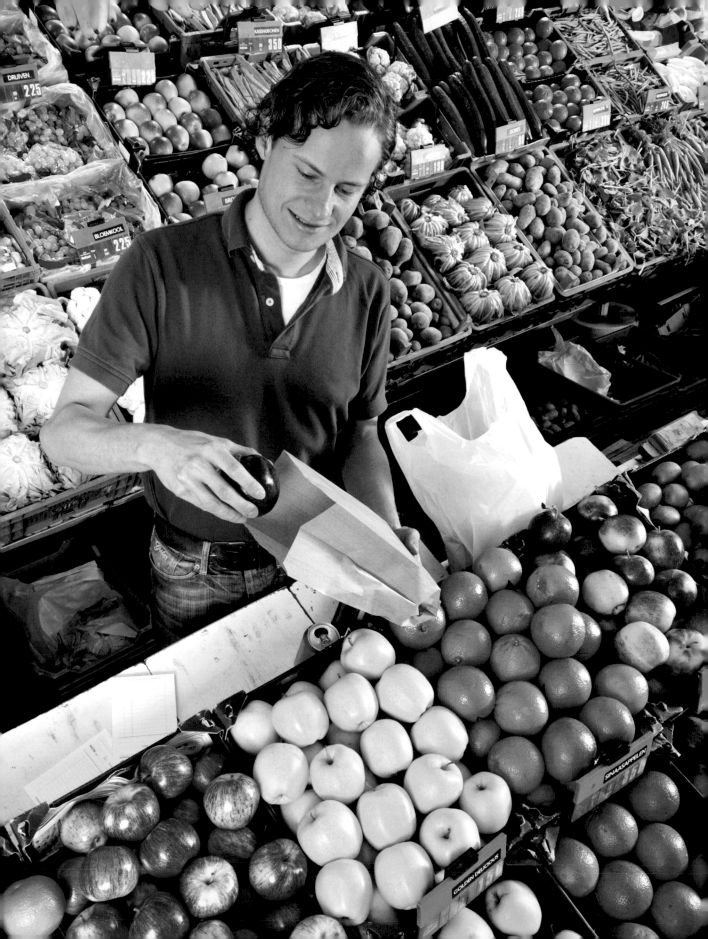

Rainbow Veggies

12 ROADS TO HEALTH AT THE END OF THE RAINBOW

Your mother may have told you to eat your greens. Turns out you need your reds, blues, oranges, purples, and yellows, too. Colorful vegetables and fruits are more than just eye candy. They provide a wide range of vitamins and minerals. They also contain an assortment of phytochemicals (*phyto-* is Greek for "plant"), including antioxidants that a growing body of research shows are both essential to health and our best defense against disease and age-related decline. Vegetables and fruits of particular colors contain different assortments of phytochemicals, so it's important to sample the entire color spectrum every day to get the best protection possible.

Studies have shown that, compared with people who consume only small amounts of vegetables and fruits, those who eat more of them and a wider variety as part of a healthy diet are less at risk from chronic diseases such as type 2 diabetes, some types of cancer, and particularly, cardiovascular disease. Fruit and veggie eaters also improve their chances of avoiding painful diverticulitis as well as cataracts and macular degeneration, two common causes of vision loss.

The average American, however, gets a mere three servings of vegetables and fruits a day. That's falling far short of what the latest dietary guidelines call for: 5 to 13 servings of these healthful foods daily, depending on a person's caloric intake.

▶ | ORANGE & YELLOW

There are two major groups of phytochemicals that act as antioxidants in our bodies: carotenoids and flavonoids. Orange and yellow vegetables and fruits tend to be especially rich in carotenoids. Of the more than 700 carotenoids scientists have identified, one of the most familiar is beta-carotene, which our cells convert into vitamin A. Sweet potatoes, pumpkin, and carrots are especially rich sources of beta-carotene.

Citrus fruits such as oranges and grapefruit aren't particularly high in beta-carotene, but are high in the antioxidant vitamin C.

Ode to Orange

- *Keep Fruit in Sight* If healthful fruits are hidden away in the refrigerator, you're less likely to reach for them as a snack or part of a meal. Keep fruits such as oranges, apricots, peaches, and mandarins in a bowl on the countertop.
- *Choose Orange* Potatoes, that is. White potatoes are considered more of a starch than a vegetable. Sweet potatoes are packed with healthful nutrients and they are easy to bake whole or sauté or roast in slices. Just don't negate their benefits by slathering them with butter, sugar, or marshmallows! Eat them au naturel, with a sprinkle of salt and a grind of black pepper. People who prefer a sweet rather than savory may find that a sprinkle of cinnamon does the trick.
- *Go Tropical* Try some orange fruits you might not know, such as papayas, mangoes, carambolas (star fruit), and guavas. They are just as nutrient packed as familiar oranges or yellow apples and will add variety to your daily choices for yellow and orange on the dietary color wheel.

▶ | RED

Red grapes and cherries. Rhubarb and tomatoes. Raspberries, strawberries, and pomegranates. And red apples, of course. Red fruits and vegetables are memorable for their rosy tints and ruby hues. A carotenoid known as lycopene is responsible for the red color in many of them (it's found in some orange fruits too). Research has shown that lycopene is a powerful antioxidant, and numerous studies link a diet high in lycopene-containing foods with a reduced incidence of cancer (including prostate cancer; see page 177), cardiovascular disease, and macular degeneration. Many deep red foods, such as pomegranates and cherries, also contain anthocyanins, thought to help reduce pain and inflammation and protect against the types of cell damage thought to lead to cancer, heart disease, and age-related memory loss. Red foods add an intense burst of rich color—and healthful nutrients—to any meal.

Recipes for Red

- **Mix Red With Green** Think red bell peppers sautéed with sliced green beans. Red grapes mixed with honeydew melon. Strawberries in a fresh spinach salad drizzled with a little balsamic vinegar.
- **Go for Tomatoes 'n' Eggs** It's been a classic English breakfast combination for generations. Dice fresh tomatoes and fold into an omelet. Or broil a half tomato (cut side up) for a minute or two and serve with soft-boiled eggs on toast. Research has shown that cooking tomatoes makes the lycopene they contain more readily absorbable by the body, boosting their health-promoting power.
- **Stuff Some Peppers** Red bell peppers can be transformed into the perfect edible containers for savory mixes of meat and rice, barley, or quinoa, or diced vegetables and

---

EAT LOWER ON THE FOOD CHAIN

Carnivorous predators are at the top of the food chain, and plants and bacteria and algae are at the bottom. The middle of the food chain includes herbivores, such as cows and deer. It is commonly agreed by scientists that the top of the food chain is the most toxic because many industrial chemicals such as polychlorinated biphenyls (PCBs) are stored in the fat of larger animals, and although such chemicals lodge in the plants low on the food chain, studies definitively show that the concentrations are many millions of times higher in predators. The takeaway? If you want to have the most chemical-free diet possible, you need to eat as low on the food chain as possible.

–Annie B. Bond
Author and eco-friendly living expert

---

bulgur. Roasted in the oven, stuffed peppers are a filling, hearty main dish or a good winter lunch.

▶ | BLUE & PURPLE

Anthocyanins are what give most blue and purple foods their colors. These natural antioxidant pigments are especially prevalent in berries (see page 143) such as blueberries, blackberries, cranberries, and raspberries. There are more blue and purple fruits than vegetables, although purple corn has been grown in South America for centuries, and has one of the deepest shades of purple found anywhere in the plant kingdom. You can spot purple cauliflower, purple string beans, and purple carrots at farmers markets and some grocery stores. The deep purplish red color of beets isn't due to anthocyanins but comes from another group of pigments—and strong antioxidants—called betalains.

Palate-Pleasing Purples

- **Top Your Cereal** Add ½ cup of mixed fresh berries, such as raspberries or blueberries, to hot oatmeal or granola.

- **Make Blackberry Syrup** Puree 2 cups of fresh blackberries in a food processor. Pour the pureed fruit into a fine sieve. Use the back of a spoon to help press out the juice; discard the pulp. Sweeten with a little honey if desired, and use as a topping for pancakes and ice cream or in salad dressings, marinades, and salsas.
- **Try Borscht** An eastern and central European soup made from beets, borscht can be served hot or cold. There are countless variations. Make a simple cold borscht by putting 1 heaping cup of cooked, sliced beets in a blender with a handful of chopped scallions and handful of peeled, sliced cucumbers. With the blender on low, add buttermilk until you reach the desired consistency. Salt to taste.

▶ | GREEN

You can probably name ten green foods in less than ten seconds: spinach, kiwi, broccoli, asparagus, green beans, peas—the list just goes on and on. Green fruits and vegetables are replete with many nutrients, but most are particularly rich in two carotenoids: lutein and zeaxanthin. Both are also found in the human eye, where they are thought to act as a sort of sunscreen for the retina. Studies have shown that people with high levels of these two carotenoids are much less likely to develop age-related macular degeneration, a cause of severe, irreversible vision loss, than people with lower levels. Leafy greens are naturals for salads and side dishes, and getting other green fruits and vegetables into your daily diet can be a snap.

Gourmet Green
- **Make Green Eggs, With or Without Ham** Add finely chopped fresh spinach to scrambled eggs, about 30 seconds before the eggs are completely set. The eggs don't actually turn green—they just look beautiful.
- **Move Beyond Iceberg** This lettuce has very little food value. Experiment with salads by trying different combinations of greens, including spinach, arugula, endive, Swiss chard, dandelion greens, escarole, and baby bok choy.

ORANGE-INFUSED RAW BEET SALAD

This refreshing and unusual salad may convince even people who say they don't like beets how tasty this purple-red vegetable can be:

1 pound young, fresh beets
¼ cup freshly squeezed orange juice
2 tablespoons red wine vinegar
2 tablespoons extra-virgin olive oil
2 tablespoons minced chives
Salt to taste
¼ pound fresh spinach

Peel the beets. Grate them using a food processor (use the shredding blade). Combine grated beets and chives in a large bowl. In a smaller bowl, whisk together the orange juice, vinegar, and olive oil. Pour over the shredded beets and toss to combine. Season to taste with salt. Mound some of the salad on a few spinach leaves and sprinkle with additional chopped chives. Serves four to six.

good to know: ABOUT PRODUCE

- Buy organic fruits and vegetables whenever possible. According to the Environmental Working Group's Guide to Pesticides in Produce, the 12 fruits and vegetables with the highest amounts of pesticide residues are apples, celery, strawberries, peaches, spinach, imported nectarines, imported grapes, sweet bell peppers, potatoes, domestic blueberries, lettuce, and kale and collard greens.
- For the freshest produce, visit your local farmers market. Make friends with the growers. They can be wonderful sources of information.
- Frozen vegetables are a good choice if fresh veggies are not available. Avoid canned vegetables; they are high in salt, and with the exception of tomatoes, many of their antioxidants and nutrients are damaged in heating and processing.

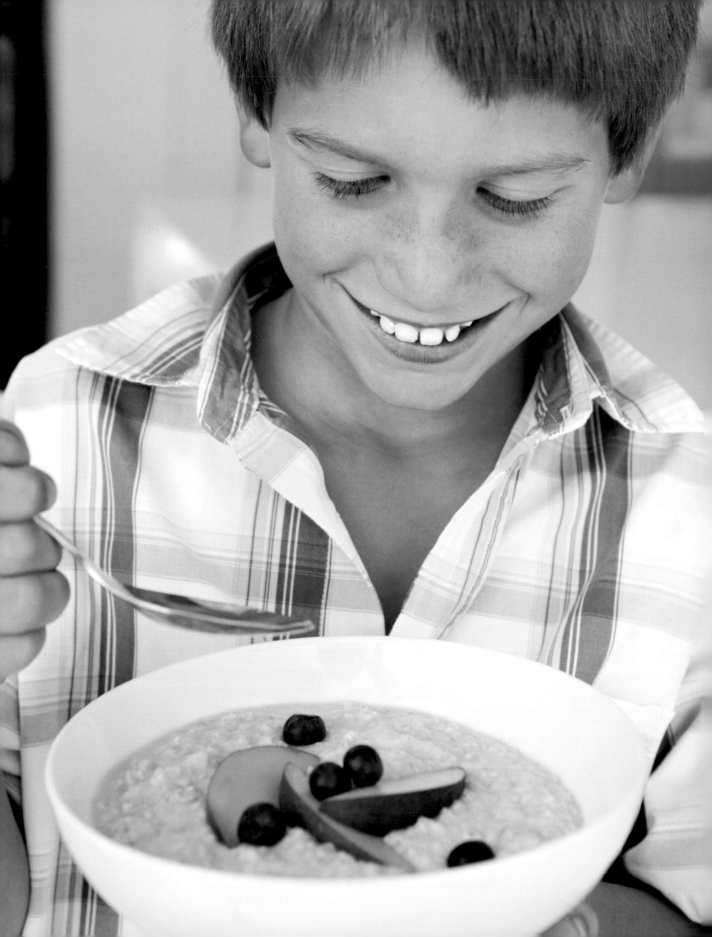

Whole Grains

15 REASONS TO GO WHOLE HOG ON WHOLE GRAINS

When our distant ancestors reached for grains—wheat, barley, oats, or rice—they took these edible seeds straight from the stalks of the cereal grasses that produce them. What they got in the bargain were carbohydrate-rich foods crammed with fiber, healthy fats, vitamins, minerals, and an astounding assortment of phytochemicals. The goodness packed into whole grains is rolled up into three basic parts. First, there's a tough, fibrous outer layer, called bran. Beneath this protective bran coat is the starchy endosperm, which acts as a source of stored energy for the seed's third part, the oil-rich germ. The germ is the seed's reproductive part, the embryo of a plant-to-be.

Our relationship to whole grains changed dramatically in the 1800s, when machines were invented to mill them. Milling strips away both bran and germ, leaving just the starchy endosperm. Milling makes grain (or what's left of it) easier to chew and digest. Milled grain often goes on to be refined, which turns it into fluffy flour that's great for making delicate pastries and airy breads, but largely devoid of its original nutrients.

In recent years, there's been a return to whole grains and all they offer. A growing body of research has shown that eating whole grains—and cutting back on refined ones—is a natural prescription for better health. Eating whole grains lowers cholesterol and inhibits the formation of blood clots, thus reducing the risk of cardiovascular disease.

▶ | BARLEY

For centuries, barley was the most important food grain in the ancient world. It was made into coarse, dense bread and, most famously, was and is the key ingredient in beer. Today, barley is often relegated to soups and little else. But this tasty little grain is loaded with cholesterol-lowering soluble fiber, vitamin E (in particularly potent antioxidant form), and selenium, a mineral that shows promising anticancer effects. When cooked, barley has a slightly chewy, pasta-like consistency. Look for hulled or lightly pearled barley; fully pearled barley has the least nutrients.

Barley Bits
- **Boil, Then Simmer** Barley is easy to prepare. Add 1 part rinsed barley to 3 to 3½ parts boiling water or broth. Let the liquid return to a

good to know: ABOUT WHOLE GRAINS

- When preparing any whole grain (except bulgur), rinse it thoroughly under running water and remove any dirt or debris.
- When cooking whole grains, use low-sodium vegetable or chicken broth instead of water for more complex flavor.
- Bulgur is sold by the size of the grains. Fine to medium grinds are commonly used for dishes like tabbouleh, whereas medium to coarse grinds are suitable for pilaf.
- Instant oatmeal is OK when you're in a rush, but flavored varieties are typically full of added sugar and artificial flavorings. Choose plain and add your own sweeteners, if desired, or fruit and nuts.

boil, then reduce heat to a simmer and cover. Simmer gently for 60 to 90 minutes.

- **Add to Salads** Add chilled, cooked barley to chopped vegetables and a favorite dressing to make a tasty cold salad.
- **Try It in Soups and Stews** Barley does go well in soup. Put it in soup and stews to add extra heartiness, fiber, and flavor.

▶ | WHOLE-GRAIN RICE

Rice is a staple food for roughly half the world's population. Most rice is milled to strip away the outer bran and the germ, resulting in far less nutritious, polished white grains. The carbohydrates in white rice break down relatively quickly during digestion, resulting in a sudden release of glucose (sugar) into the bloodstream—an effect known to foster diabetes over time. Whole-grain rice, like other whole grains with intact bran and germ, is digested much more slowly, meaning glucose is added to the bloodstream in a slow, healthy trickle. Research has shown that by swapping brown rice for white rice—even just some of the time—diabetes risk can be lowered, possibly by as much as 36 percent. Brown rice is the most popular and common whole-grain rice, but it also comes in other colors, including black, purple, and red.

Whole-Some Meals

- **Simmer Slowly** Rinse whole-grain rice and then add 1 part rice to between 2 and 2½ parts boiling water or broth. Turn the heat to low and simmer, covered, for 30 to 45 minutes.
- **Serve as a Side** Whole-grain rice makes a filling accompaniment to any main dish. Jazz it up by adding sautéed mushrooms or onions, chopped scallions, roasted pecans or other nuts, or sunflower seeds to hot, cooked rice just before serving.
- **Tuck It in a Pouch** For a substantial lunch, partially fill half a whole-grain pita with cooked whole-grain rice. Fill the remaining space with chopped vegetables and drizzle on a little of your favorite dressing.

▶ | BULGUR

A staple in the traditional Mediterranean diet for thousands of years, bulgur is a fast-cooking form of whole wheat. The whole grains have been cleaned, parboiled, dried, and then ground into smaller pieces. You can prepare this nutritious grain product with minimal cooking, usually in about 20 minutes. Many people just boil or

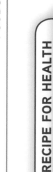

FOODS FOR HEALTH

RECIPE FOR HEALTH

ASIAN BLACK RICE PUDDING WITH MANGOES

Look for black rice, sometimes called forbidden rice, at Asian food stores and larger grocery stores.

1 cup black rice
3 cups water
¼ teaspoon salt + ⅛ teaspoon salt
½ cup organic palm sugar
1 15-ounce can organic unsweetened coconut milk, stirred
1 ripe mango, peeled, cut away from the seed, and chopped

Bring the rice, water, and ¼ teaspoon salt to a boil in a heavy saucepan. Reduce heat to low and simmer, covered with a tight-fitting lid, for about 45 minutes; rice will be tender but still wet. Stir in palm sugar, ⅛ teaspoon salt, and all but ¼ cup of the coconut milk. Bring the mixture to a boil, then reduce heat to low and simmer, uncovered, stirring occasionally, until mixture is thick and rice is tender but still slightly chewy, about 30 minutes. Remove from heat and let cool 30 minutes. Stir and spoon into bowls. Place about 2 tablespoons of chopped mango on top and drizzle with the reserved coconut milk. Makes six to eight servings.

CLASSIC TABBOULEH

1 cup fine bulgur
2 medium tomatoes
1 small English cucumber
5 scallions or 1 small onion
¼ teaspoon freshly ground pepper
3 tablespoons extra-virgin olive oil
1 cup fresh parsley, chopped fine
2 tablespoons fresh mint, chopped fine
Juice of 1 lemon
½ teaspoon kosher or sea salt

Place bulgur in a bowl and add 2 cups boiling water. Stir well and cover the bowl with a plate. Let sit for 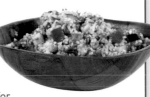 20 to 30 minutes or until soft. While the bulgur softens, remove the seeds from the tomatoes and cucumber. Chop them into roughly ¼-inch pieces. Cut the scallions into very thin slices (if using onion, chop into ¼-inch dice).

Strain the bulgur using a fine mesh sieve. Press out any excess water. Place in a large bowl and add the chopped vegetables, the parsley, and the mint. Combine the lemon juice, olive oil, salt, and pepper and add to the salad mixture, tossing well. Adjust seasonings, if necessary.

steam it and eat it like rice or couscous. It can also be added as an ingredient to other foods.

Obliging Bulgur

- **Try Tabbouleh** Bulgur may be best known to many as the main ingredient in tabbouleh (also spelled tabouli), a Middle Eastern salad traditionally made with bulgur, cucumber, and tomatoes, along with finely chopped parsley and mint (see the recipe above).
- **Use It Like Rice** In many Mediterranean countries, bulgur is used like rice. You can substitute it for rice in most recipes.
- **Combine With Meat and Veggies** Add fiber by adding bulgur to ground meat in main dishes or casseroles. Try beef and bulgur tacos!
- **Break Out of Your Breakfast Rut** Bulgur works well as a hot cereal and makes a nice

change from oatmeal. Just combine a cup bulgur and 1½ cups water in a saucepan. Cover and bring to a boil. Reduce heat and simmer gently for 10 to 12 minutes. Let stand five minutes before serving.

▶ | OATS

Oats are a premiere source of soluble fiber, which corrals dietary cholesterol within a sticky gel in the intestines and helps carry it out of the body—safely away from the blood. In addition to lowering cholesterol and therefore protecting against cardiovascular disease, the fiber in oats makes you feel full. Start your day with a bowl of rich, creamy oatmeal and you won't get hungry before lunch!

Opt for Oats

- **Go for Oatmeal** It's the classic day starter. All you need is 1 part regular rolled oats to 4 parts water. Mix the oats together with the cool water and a pinch of salt, then cover and cook at a simmer for 15 to 20 minutes, stirring occasionally. For creamier oatmeal, substitute low-fat or almond milk for half the water. Alternatively, try steel cut oats (also known as Irish oatmeal) instead of rolled oats, as steel cut oats are less processed.
- **Create Your Own "Instant" Breakfast** Not everyone likes cooked oatmeal. So try this instead: Mix together a handful of regular rolled oats, a big dollop of plain or Greek yogurt, and half an apple, grated. Cover and refrigerate overnight. In the morning, stir well and top with a dusting of cinnamon.
- **Use in Baking** Next time you make cookies, replace up to one-third of the flour with finely ground regular rolled oats (grind oats in a food processor for 15 to 20 seconds).

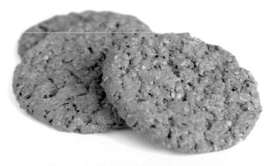

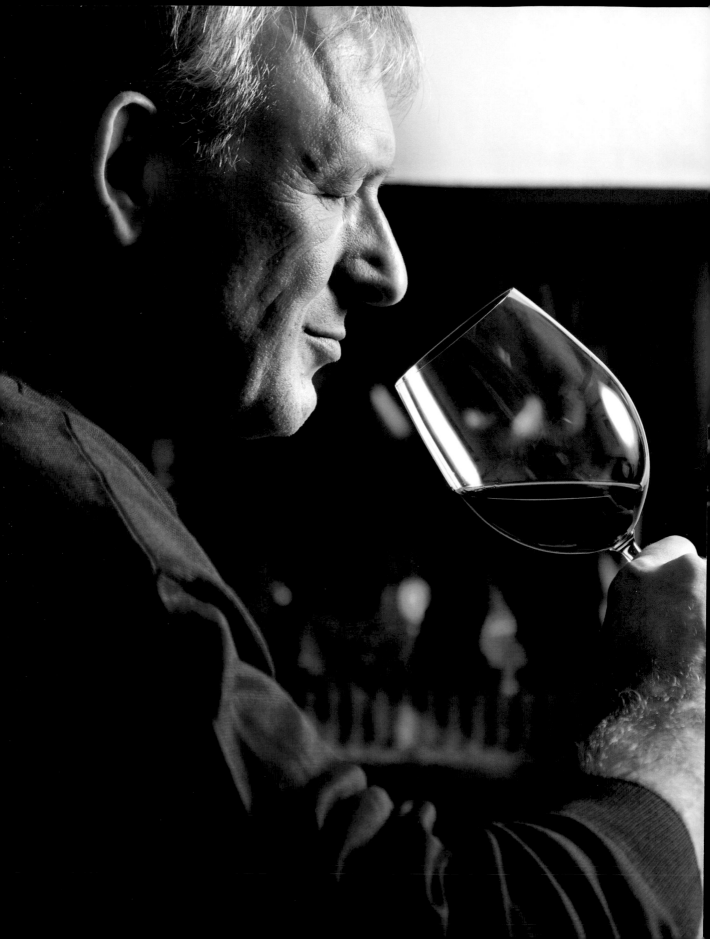

Wine & Grape Juice

15 WAYS TO REAP THE PLEASURES OF THE GRAPE

In 2003, scientists discovered the world's oldest wine—at least the dried remnants of it—in the bottom of clay jars unearthed at a site in Georgia, the former Soviet republic. Stone Age people had made it at least 8,000 years ago. Biochemical analyses found traces of tree resin in the dregs, evidence that these Neolithic vintners were deliberately trying to preserve their wine using resin's natural antibacterial properties. The archaeologists were only guessing, but they postulated that the ancient wine might have tasted something like retsina, a resin-preserved wine still popular in Greece today.

Wine is fermented grape juice. Yeasts are responsible for the fermentation process in wine—a process discovered by French chemist Louis Pasteur in 1857. Fueled by sugars in grape juice, yeasts grow and divide, producing ethanol (a form of alcohol) in the process. Yeasts do this until the alcohol concentration reaches about 10 to 15 percent, at which point it reaches a level toxic to the yeasts and fermentation stops.

Throughout recorded history, wine has been lauded as both food and medicine. Roman physician Pliny the Elder (A.D. 23–79) referred to "the healing powers of the vine." Current interest in the health-promoting aspects of drinking wine (and grape juice) can be traced to the early 1990s, when French researchers reported on what came to be known as the "French paradox": the fact that the French eat a diet high in saturated fat but have a low incidence of cardiovascular disease compared with those in many other countries. This finding sparked years of research on wine and its components. Studies have shown that wine does provide health benefits. Some benefits are derived from the alcohol in wine. Although alcohol in large amounts is toxic—and can have many harmful effects—moderate alcohol consumption appears to raise HDL ("good") cholesterol while lowering LDL ("bad") cholesterol, the type linked to increased risk of cardiovascular disease. One or two drinks of alcohol per day seems to reduce the risk of heart disease, death from heart disease, and premature death from any cause.

Red wine isn't just alcohol, though. Wine and the grapes from which it is made contain phytochemicals—chemical compounds occurring naturally in plants—that seem to have health-promoting properties of their own.

▶ RED WINE

Red wine is rich in antioxidants, substances that prevent free radicals from damaging cells throughout the body. One of these antioxidants, resveratrol, has been the focus of considerable research over the past few decades. Resveratrol seems to reduce inflammation, prevent damage to blood vessels, reduce LDL cholesterol, and prevent blood clots—all of which are associated with a reduced risk of cardiovascular disease. There is limited evidence that resveratrol may protect against some other diseases, including some types of cancer; in laboratory studies, for example, resveratrol seems to inhibit the growth of breast cancer cells.

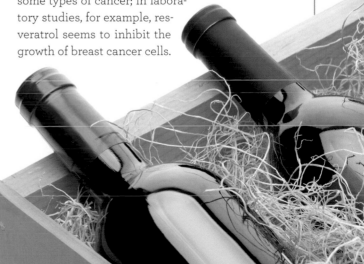

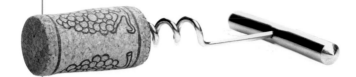

If you don't like wine, or don't drink, you can get resveratrol simply by eating red and purple grapes, or drinking grape juice.

> ⚠ **CAUTION:** If you don't drink, don't start just to prevent heart disease. If you do drink, drink in moderation. Moderate drinking is defined as an average of two drinks a day for men, and one drink for women. Drinking too much increases the risk of liver damage, certain types of cancer, and many other ailments. If you have a weak heart, avoid alcohol. Check with your doctor about drinking red wine, or any alcohol, if you take aspirin daily. Pregnant women should not drink alcohol.

Fruit of the Vine

- **Stick to the Limit** Experts recommend that women limit alcohol intake to one drink per day. Men should have no more than two. A serving of red wine is five ounces.
- **Serve Red With Chicken and Fish** If you want the benefits of resveratrol, red wine contains more than white wine. Don't worry about the rules that say "white wine with fish or foul." Light-bodied red wines, such as Pinot Noir, complement fish and poultry.

Save Cabernet Sauvignon, Malbec, and other full-bodied wines for heavier meats. But white wine drinkers can take heart. Some research studies have shown that white wines may offer heart benefits similar to those of red wines; whites contain little resveratrol, but they apparently contain other phytochemicals that offer cardiovascular benefits.

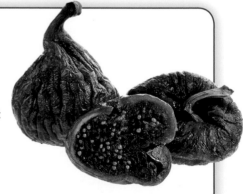

- **Make a Reduction** To make a rich sauce for meat, combine red wine and low-salt natural beef stock or broth in a 1:1 ratio. Pour them together into a saucepan, bring to a boil, and then reduce heat to a simmer and cook until the liquid is greatly reduced and the sauce is thick. (The alcohol in wine evaporates as it cooks.) Season with salt, pepper, and herbs, if desired, and drizzle over red meats.
- **Add Wine as an Ingredient** Recipes that call for red wine as an ingredient abound. Think pasta sauces, stews, and soups.
- **Create a Marinade** Add red wine to spicy meat marinades. It's a simple way to add flavor and moisture to meat.
- **Sauté Veggies** Add a splash of red wine at the end of the cooking and reduce it quickly to make a tangy glaze.

RECIPE FOR HEALTH

FIGS IN RED WINE SYRUP

3 long strips (about ½ inch wide) fresh organic lemon peel

1 cinnamon stick

5 black peppercorns

3 cloves

1½ cups dry, full-bodied red wine, such as Merlot or Cabernet

½ cup water

¼ cup organic palm sugar

1 cup dried Calimyrna figs, cut lengthwise into 3 slices

3 tablespoons freshly squeezed lemon juice

Place the first six ingredients in a heavy saucepan and bring to a simmer. Stir until the sugar is dissolved. Boil gently, uncovered, over medium heat for eight to ten minutes until the liquid is reduced to about 1½ cups; it will take on the consistency of syrup. Strain the mixture into a bowl, and return the strained liquid to the saucepan. Reduce heat, add the figs, and simmer, covered, about 30 minutes or until the fruit is plump and soft. Remove from heat and stir in lemon juice. Cool at least an hour before serving.

▶ | GRAPE JUICE

Red wine has received most of the press in terms of health benefits, but red and purple grapes and juice made from them offer the same good things. Many antioxidants, including resveratrol, are found primarily in the skins and seeds of grapes. These substances lower blood pressure, reduce the risk of blood clots, limit bad cholesterol, fight inflammation, and improve the flexibility of blood vessels. Some studies have shown that drinking grape juice can lower blood pressure and may also give the immune system a boost.

Grape Goodies

- ■ *Eat Whole Grapes* By eating whole grapes, you get the benefit of all their antioxidants, along with healthful dietary fiber.
- ■ *Color a Salad* Fresh grapes make a great addition to mixed green salads and fruit salads too. Consider using different varieties of red and purple grapes to add lots of color.
- ■ *Serve With Cheese* Fruit and cheese is a classic combination and a wonderful dessert. Grapes pair well with many different kinds of cheese, including feta and Gorgonzola. A little bit of cheese goes a long way; keep in mind that it is high in saturated fat.
- ■ *Cool a Curry* Sweet red grapes help balance the spicy heat of Asian and Indian curries. Slice a handful of grapes in half and offer them as a cooling condiment on the side.
- ■ *Yum Up Yogurt* Mmmmm … red grapes and Greek yogurt. Add sliced grapes to yogurt,

GRAPES & KIWI IN HONEY-LEMON SAUCE

1 cup organic seedless red grapes
1 kiwi, peeled and cut into ½-inch pieces
1 tablespoon honey
2 teaspoons fresh lemon juice
2 teaspoons fresh (organic) lemon zest

Place the grapes and kiwi pieces in a bowl. In a separate small dish, combine the honey, lemon juice, and lemon zest; stir to blend well. Pour over the fruit and stir gently to coat.

add a pinch of allspice, and enjoy. Or combine grapes with other fruits, such as bananas and berries, and add a dollop of yogurt on top.
- ■ *Perk Up Chicken Salad* Add sliced grapes and roasted pecans to your favorite chicken salad.
- ■ *Go Frozen* As a healthful summertime snack, try freezing red seedless grapes for a refreshing and quick treat.

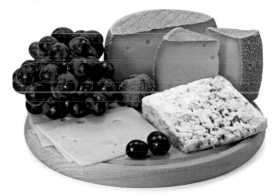

good to know: ABOUT WINE & GRAPE JUICE

— Other foods, including peanuts, blueberries, and cranberries, contain some resveratrol. However, it's not known how eating these foods might compare with drinking red wine or grape juice, or eating grapes.

— Wines made in cool climates appear to have the greatest amounts of resveratrol.

— Use only red wines in cooking that you would drink out of a glass. Cooking does not improve the taste of bad wine.

— Choose unsweetened 100 percent grape juice made from red and purple grapes. If it's too tart, add a little stevia powder to sweeten. Avoid products labeled as grape "drinks," which usually contain very little juice but a great deal of sugar.

— Always wash grapes before using them. Let them drip dry in a colander.

— Buy organic grapes to avoid harmful pesticide residues.

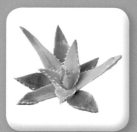
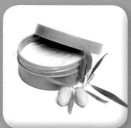
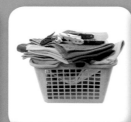
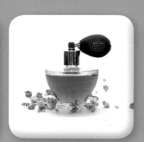
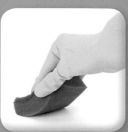

CHAPTER FOUR

clean, safe,

& beautiful

Clean & Natural

162 BEAUTY BASICS, INSIDE AND OUT

A trip down the personal care aisle in your local drugstore can be overwhelming. The number of facial cleansers, moisturizers, wrinkle creams, shampoos, conditioners, toothpastes, lip balms, deodorants, shave creams, hair styling aids, sunscreens, and cosmetics seems almost unlimited. Many announce that they are "natural" and "pure," but most are anything but.

Read the ingredient labels, and chances are you'll discover a list of scary substances including petrochemicals, synthetic compounds that disrupt hormones, known skin and eye irritants, and even carcinogens. What few consumers realize is that the U.S. government doesn't require health studies or premarket testing on cosmetics and personal care products. According to the watchdog Environmental Working Group, nearly 90 percent of the 10,500 ingredients used in personal care products have not been evaluated for safety by a publicly accountable institution.

House Beautiful?

Furthermore, the majority of commercial products we use in our homes to wash dishes and clothes, dust and polish furniture, clean rugs, scour sinks, kill mold and mildew, remove scum from showers, unplug drains, and "freshen" the air also contain harmful substances. Many are volatile organic compounds, or VOCs, often masquerading as "fragrances." There's a growing body of evidence that VOCs and other chemicals in cleaning products can cause asthma, allergies, headaches, eye irritation, dizziness, and nausea. Long-term

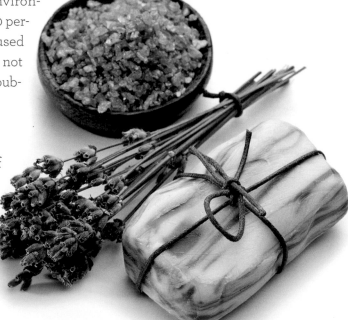

exposure has the potential to cause kidney and liver damage, nervous system disorders, and possibly cancer. The U.S. Environmental Protection Agency discovered that, thanks primarily to commercial cleaning products, the levels of roughly a dozen harmful organic pollutants are two to five times higher inside homes than out.

There Is Hope

There are simple, natural, healthy ways to look your best without applying a toxic soup of chemicals to your body. And there are safe strategies for cleaning your home that work in some cases better than conventional products and won't put your health (or the environment) at risk. But it's not easy to figure out how. Few experts besides our advisor, Annie B. Bond, have tackled the challenges of understanding the science behind hygiene and housekeeping products.

Building on Annie Bond's work, this chapter presents hundreds of simple solutions for healthy personal and home care, along with dozens of recipes ranging from moisturizers and body scrubs to DIY household cleaners and safe and effective insect repellents to keep bothersome bugs at bay. Nearly all are made with basic, relatively inexpensive ingredients you can find almost anywhere. Please note the cautions, however. Some recipes call for plant essential oils. These should never be taken internally and never applied in undiluted form to skin. And all cleaning agents, even natural ones, should always be kept safely out of the reach of curious children.

HOW TO GO GREEN

I once ran a survey on a large website asking questions about cleaning products. A full 94 percent wanted to switch to nontoxic and greener cleaners but only 40 percent did so. When the survey queried them further about their choices, their answer was that they were overwhelmed and didn't know what to choose. Plus, it became clear that three myths about green cleaning had affected their thinking: The first is that green cleaners didn't work as well, the second that they are too expensive, and the third that green cleaning takes more time.

I've actually been invited to EPA conferences to show how well simple household ingredients like baking soda work. And they do. As to cost, green cleaning products can be expensive, but a little goes a long way because most are concentrated. Swap out a few simple DIY recipes that cost pennies (see pages 233, 237, 240, 244, and 248), and you can save money in the end. Last, cleaning with less toxic ingredients doesn't take more time—you simply choose a different bottle. Or, if you are using DIY ingredients, most formulas work on their own while you are doing other things. For example, the best oven cleaner I use is applied before I go to bed: I sprinkle the oven with baking soda, spritz it with water, and when I wake up the next morning, the grime sponges out in a few minutes. No fumes, no elbow grease, and no extra time required.

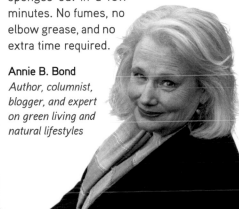

Annie B. Bond
Author, columnist, blogger, and expert on green living and natural lifestyles

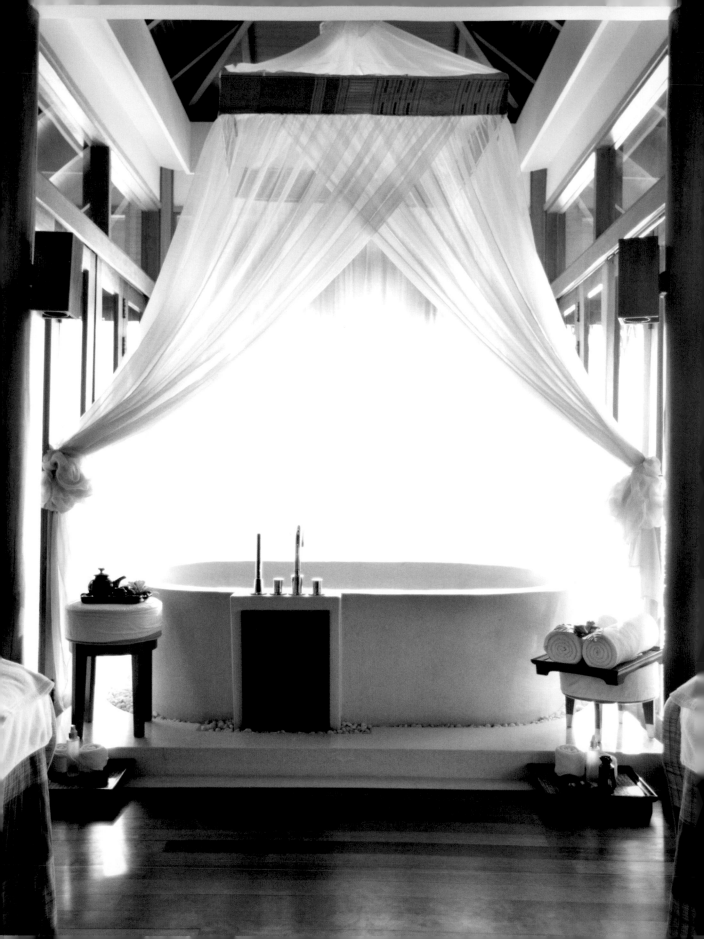

Body Scrubs & Healing Baths

9 WONDERFUL WAYS TO WASH

Try this little experiment: Lay a piece of Scotch tape across the back of your hand. Rub it gently to make sure it adheres, and then gently pull it off. Now hold it up to the light. The tape will be dotted with tiny flakes. Those are dead skin cells. Don't worry; it's perfectly natural. Everyone's skin is constantly shedding dead skin cells from the surface. As dead cells are lost, new cells move up from deeper skin layers to replace them. Removing dead skin cells on a regular basis is a very effective way to improve skin's appearance, stimulate circulation, and make it easier for natural oils and other skin-nurturing substances to penetrate the surface and be absorbed.

Facial scrubs and masks (see page 208) help exfoliate delicate facial skin very gently. Body scrubs are designed to exfoliate skin from the neck down. Commercial body scrubs abound. But keep in mind that because exfoliated skin more easily takes up what's applied to it, your skin is absorbing, to some degree, the petroleum-based chemicals, fragrances, preservatives, and artificial colors that most of these products contain. Fortunately, all-natural body scrubs, replete with wonderful ingredients that are good for your skin and your body, are among the easiest skin care products to make at home.

Body scrubs involve covering most of your skin with something that needs to be rinsed off, typically by showering or bathing (it's the easiest way). Bathing is a centuries-old ritual and one that has important therapeutic applications. Soaking in hot water—especially a tubful that's been enriched with herbs, natural plant oils, or salts—relaxes muscles, calms the mind, moisturizes and soothes skin, and stimulates circulation and the immune system. Showers are great for quickly getting clean, but they don't compare to a long soak in silky, herb-scented bathwater. Baths are a natural remedy for many ills and a habit worth adding to your life for their contributions to physical and spiritual wellness.

▶ BODY SCRUBS

Salt and sugar form the base for most natural body scrubs. But oatmeal, ground almond meal, ground rice, ground coffee, poppy seeds, and similar natural granular substances all make effective and mild exfoliating ingredients. Any one of these can be suspended in various liquids ranging from natural plant oil and herbal infusions to milk, honey, and yogurt. Making body scrubs is simple. Almost everything you need you'll find at grocery and natural food stores. There aren't many hard and fast rules, so use your imagination and feel free to experiment with different combinations of ingredients. Be careful not to use body scrubs too frequently, though. Once a week is usually sufficient.

Scrub-a-Dub-Dub

■ *Scrub Sweetly* Ordinary white sugar isn't something you want to include in your diet often, but as an exfoliant, the fine grains are very effective. Sugar is inexpensive and scent free and can easily be blended with a wide variety of oils and other ingredients. A basic sugar scrub can be created in minutes by combining ½ cup white sugar with enough almond oil to completely moisten the sugar, but not so much as to make the mixture runny with oil. Add a squeeze of fresh lemon and stir well to make sure the sugar is well saturated with the oil. Scoop up a little

with your fingers and massage onto an area of skin about the size of your outstretched hand, using small, circular motions. Continue until you've covered your entire body. Rinse and shower as usual. The following are variations on the basic scrub:

• Combine 1 cup of brown sugar with 3 drops rose geranium essential oil, 3 drops lavender essential oil, the contents of a vitamin E capsule, and ¼ cup to ½ cup almond oil (start with ¼ cup and add more oil, a tablespoon at a time, to reach desired consistency). Stir well to combine. This is a good scrub for dry skin.

• Mix ½ cup white sugar, ¼ cup Greek yogurt or organic sour cream, 1 tablespoon almond or jojoba oil, and a finely chopped fresh tomato. Natural acids in the tomato help chemically exfoliate skin, while the slightly abrasive action of the sugar exfoliates mechanically.

■ *Scrub With Salt* Salt exfoliates in much the same manner as sugar. Use sea salt or kosher salt rather than table salt. A basic salt scrub

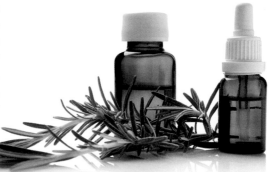

good to know: ABOUT BODY SCRUBS & HEALING BATHS

— Take a shower before using a body scrub. Your skin will be moist and soft, making it easier to exfoliate dead skin cells.

— Use your fingers to spread and massage a scrub gently over the skin in a circular motion. Avoid using a washcloth or loofah, as it's much easier to judge the correct pressure with just your fingertips.

— Gently rinse off the salt or sugar scrub and pat your skin dry.

— Use a scrub before shaving. The exfoliating action will result in a closer, smoother shave.

— Be aware—scrubs that contain oil can make a bathtub or shower floor very slippery.

— To make it easier to recline comfortably in a bathtub, place a full hot water bottle under your neck (and perhaps a second one under your lower back) for support and to relax against.

— If you have high or low blood pressure, avoid very hot baths.

— Some essential oils can cause skin sensitivity when dispersed in hot water. Avoid adding basil, oregano, thyme, nutmeg, clove, cinnamon, black pepper, and bay essential oils to homemade bath salts.

SOFT GLOW SALT SCRUB

1 cup sea salt (fine grain)
½ cup grapeseed or almond oil
¼ cup avocado or olive oil
Contents of 1 vitamin E capsule
10 to 15 drops essential oil (a blend is fine)

Mix the oils, vitamin E, and essential oils in a small bowl. Add the salt and mix well. Store in a container with an airtight lid.

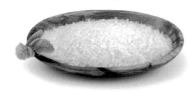

contains 1 cup of salt, about ½ cup light-textured oil such as almond or grapeseed, and 5 to 15 drops of a high-quality essential oil such as lavender, peppermint, rosemary, or lemon. Once it's mixed, the texture of the scrub should be moist enough to hold together, but not overly oily (adjust the amount of oil to achieve that texture).

- **Go Nuts** Ground almonds and oatmeal are also body scrub basics. To make a quick almond-and-oatmeal body scrub, put ⅔ cup coarsely chopped almonds, ⅓ cup regular (not quick) oatmeal, and ½ teaspoon dried sage or rosemary in a food processor. Pulse until the mixture resembles medium-coarse meal. Add enough plain yogurt, pure aloe vera gel, or almond oil to make a thick but spreadable paste.

▶ | HEALING BATHS

You may remember your parents or grand-parents talking about the soothing effects of soaking in a tub with Epsom salts. Bath salts, bath oils, and herbs can turn an ordinary bath into a heal-ing, calming experience. Mineral-rich bath salts help to soften skin, oils help to moisturize it, and herbs can be relaxing or energizing.

Tub Tonics

- **Soften With Salt** Bath salts range from vari-ous kinds of sea salt and Epsom salts to finely ground clay. The minerals in the salts make bathwater feel silky and leave skin both clean and soft. Making your own bath salts couldn't be easier. For the most basic, add 15 to 30 drops of your favorite essential oils to 2 cups of sea salt. That's it.

- **Combine Salts** Mix together 1 cup sea salt, 1 cup Epsom salts, 10 drops lavender essential oil, and 2 tablespoons dried lavender flowers in a jar. Add ¼ cup of this mixture to running water while the tub is filling. Swirl water well to distribute.

- **Soothe and Smooth** Using bath oil is especially good for moisturizing dry skin and fighting "winter itch." Add 1 or 2 tea-spoons of avocado, jojoba, or castor oil and a few drops of your favorite essential oil to the bathwater while the tub is filling, then settle in for a good soak. Be careful getting in and out of the tub, as the oil will make it slippery.

- **Experiment With Herbal Blends** You can add fresh or dried herbs directly to bathwater. But if you'd rather not contend with floating herbs and the resulting cleanup (and you'd rather not have the herbs go down the drain when you're done), enclose herbs in a muslin bag or a large handkerchief and tie this around the tub spigot. Turn on the hot water only and let it stream through the bag of herbs to create a strong herbal infusion. Then run enough cold water to bring the water temperature down to a comfort-able level. For a relax-ing herbal blend, put a handful each of dried cham-omile flowers, dried lav-ender, and dried rose buds or petals in the bag—or experiment with your own herb combinations.

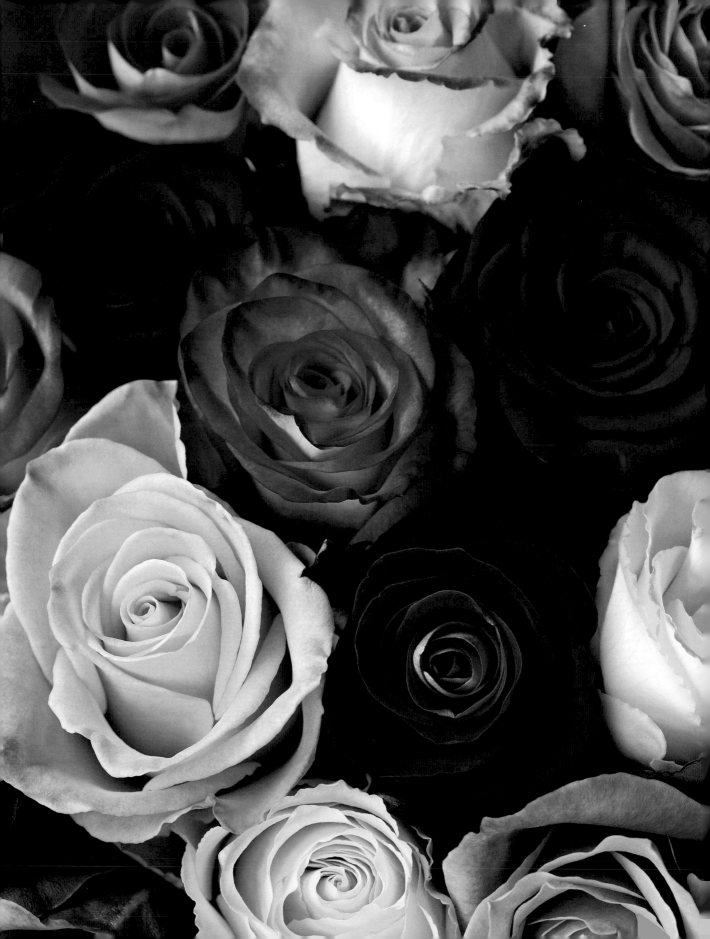

Fragrances
& Deodorants

13 SWEET SUGGESTIONS

In 2005, a team of Italian archaeologists working in Cyprus unearthed a 4,000-year-old perfumery. Scientists were able to reconstitute a dozen different perfumes from residues in clay jars found at the site. They extracted herbal essences from these residues, including cinnamon, myrtle, and laurel, all likely derived from local plants. Perfumery changed in the 19th century when it became possible to synthesize aromatic chemical compounds in the laboratory.

Many natural oils have been replaced with much less expensive synthetic substitutes. That floral fragrance reminiscent of lily of the valley or rose might not have any link to the real flowers but is instead the result of dimethyl-phenyl-ethyl-carbinol or 3,6-dimethyl-3-octanol.

In the past, people used perfumes not only to make themselves more alluring but also to mask unpleasant body odors. They also used natural deodorants. The Ebers Papyrus, written around 1530 B.C. and considered the most important medical texts to have survived from ancient Egypt, contains a recipe for a body deodorant. The first commercial deodorant was introduced in the West in the late 19th century, and a few decades later, antiperspirants—products that stop wetness as well as odor—appeared on the scene. Most modern commercial antiperspirants contain aluminum compounds that dissolve into skin at the first sign of sweat and cause pores in underarm skin to swell shut. Whether or not this pore-blocking effect is a health risk is still being investigated. What is known, though, is that synthetic chemicals aren't required for smelling nice.

▶ | FRAGRANCES

Natural perfumes are basically a blend of pure essential oils, alcohol, and water. The difference between a perfume and an eau de toilette or cologne is the ratio of essential oil to alcohol and water. Perfume has the highest essential oil content (between 15 and 30 percent), with the remaining liquid composed entirely of alcohol (or alcohol with a very small amount of water). Less potent fragrances, such as colognes, contain less essential oil and a higher percentage of alcohol and water. Making your own perfume or cologne involves experimenting with different essential oils to come up with blends that appeal to you. Use the purest essential oils you can find—unlike a drop of synthetic oil, a drop of pure plant essential oil placed on blotting paper will leave no residue behind as it evaporates; a synthetic oil will.

Essential Scents

■ *Start With a Known Combo* To make a natural perfume, you need an essential oil blend—the fragrance—together with a high-proof alcohol (vodka works well) and possibly a small amount of distilled water (it depends on the recipe). The first step is to choose (or create) an essential oil blend. Because there are dozens of essential oils and hundreds of potential combinations, take some of the guesswork out of crafting a fragrance by using established combinations known to be complementary. You can find entire books on perfumery that list such combinations; there are also similar resources online. In her book *Better Basics for the Home*, Annie B. Bond offers many combinations. The following are some she formulated:

- Rose, jasmine, rose geranium, and clove
- Lemon balm, thyme, nutmeg, and orrisroot
- Sandalwood, orange flower, sassafras, white thyme, cassia, and clove
- Basil, sage, dill, and sandalwood
- White rose, jasmine, orange flower, cassia, and myrrh
- Violet, cassia, rose, tuberose, orrisroot, and bitter almond
- Tuberose, jasmine, neroli, ylang-ylang, and clove

■ *Mix the Ingredients* Once you've determined your essential oil blend and the relative amounts of each oil to use in it, you can mix essential oils and alcohol to make a simple perfume. See the following recipe, also created by Annie Bond, for white lilac perfume as a guide.

WHITE LILAC PERFUME

The following perfume recipe is courtesy of Annie B. Bond, from *Better Basics for the Home*.

To make the essential oil blend, combine:

11 parts tuberose essential oil
6 parts orange flower essential oil
¼ part bitter almond essential oil

To create the perfume, combine:

3 parts pure essential oil blend
7 parts high-proof, good-quality vodka
20 drops (per ounce of perfume) orrisroot tincture (not essential oil; look for orrisroot tincture online)

Pour the mixture into a dark-colored glass bottle that has a tight-fitting cap with a glass eyedropper. Store away from light for one to two months before using, to allow the integration of the various scents. Apply to skin using the dropper, or put some into an atomizer and spritz on.

LIME ESSENCE COLOGNE

The following citrusy cologne with lavender and bay notes could work well as a men's cologne or aftershave:

1 cup high-proof, high-quality vodka
10 drops lime essential oil
8 drops lavender essential oil
5 drops bay essential oil
1 cup distilled water

Combine the essential oils and vodka in a dark-colored, pint-size glass bottle with a tight-fitting lid. Shake well. Allow to sit one month, sealed. Then add the distilled water, shake, and seal again. Let set one week, shaking once per day. At this point, the cologne is ready to use.

■ *Make It Oil-based* Oil-based perfumes are a mixture of essential oil blends and a light unscented oil such as jojoba. A basic "recipe" for an oil-based perfume is 1 ounce jojoba oil and 25 drops of an essential oil blend. Mix well and store in a dark-colored glass bottle that has a tight-fitting cap with a glass eyedropper (be aware that oil-based perfume can stain fabric).

■ *Go Solid* Solid perfumes are combinations of essential oil blends, a carrier oil, and beeswax to solidify the mixture. Solid perfumes are wonderfully portable—just keep them away from heat. The basic formula is 2 ounces beeswax, ⅛ ounce jojoba oil, and ¼ ounce essential oil blend. Heat the beeswax and oil in the top of a double boiler (or very gently on low power in the microwave, in ten-second intervals) until melted. Remove from heat and let cool slightly. Before the mixture begins to harden, add the ¼ ounce essential oil blend. Stir to combine, and pour into a dark-colored glass jar with a tight-fitting lid. Cap when cool.

■ *Create a Blend* If you're more daring, craft your own unique combination of essential oils. Place a drop of each essential oil you're considering

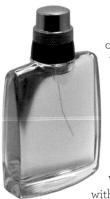

on the end of a strip of blotting paper. Wait a moment and then sniff each one (do not touch essential oils to your skin or nasal membranes). After you've selected several oils that you like, hold two or three or more different strips together and inhale the combination. Determine which oils work best together until you come up with a blend that's uniquely yours.

▶ | DEODORANTS

Body odor is most commonly caused by bacteria on the skin surface that are breaking down substances in sweat and producing odiferous compounds. There are no natural antiperspirants (substances that stop wetness), but you can find a selection of natural deodorants in natural food stores and some grocery stores and drugstores. Read the labels, though, to ensure the ingredients are truly natural—avoid parabens, polyethylene glycols, hormone-disrupting synthetic fragrances, petrochemicals, and antibacterial agents. Several simple substances, though, can be applied to prevent underarm odor (see the following).

Custom Combos

- **Dust On** Plain old baking soda can work as an effective deodorant by neutralizing body odors. Pour some in a dish, touch a powder puff to the surface, and dust your armpits with the powder.
- **Cool Off** Cooling, astringent witch hazel (look for real extract) makes deodorizing a snap. (Astringent tannins in the extract have an antibacterial effect.) Saturate a cotton ball in witch hazel and dab onto underarms. Let dry.
- **Go With Essentials** Add about 5 drops of lavender essential oil (which also has antibacterial properties) to 1 cup distilled water. Saturate a cotton ball and apply.
- **Mix It Up** Baking soda helps stop odor and cornstarch absorbs moisture. Use these two together as a natural deodorant by mixing a half cup each in a glass jar with a tight-fitting lid. You can add a couple drops of an essential oil, such as lavender, birch, bay, or cinnamon, to the jar to give it a little scent. Stir well and store in a tightly sealed jar. Use a powder puff to dab a bit of the powder under arms.
- **Make Your Own** Try the following recipe to create your own custom-scented naturally antibacterial underarm gel.

ONE-OF-A-KIND LIQUID DEODORANT

This recipe is adapted from Annie B. Bond's *Better Basics for the Home:*

¼ cup aloe vera gel
¼ cup real witch hazel extract
¼ cup bottled mineral water
1 tablespoon pure vegetable glycerin (less if the mixture feels too sticky)
10 drops antibacterial essential oils, such as lavender, thyme, bergamot, peppermint, or sandalwood

Combine all the ingredients in a spray bottle and shake well to blend.

RECIPE FOR HEALTH

---

good to know: ABOUT FRAGRANCES & DEODORANTS

- Essential oils are available from many online sources. Make sure what you are ordering is 100 percent pure, natural essential oil, not a synthetic.
- Essential oils derived from citrus plants, particularly bergamot, can increase the skin's sensitivity to sun.
- Do not use rubbing alcohol (isopropyl alcohol) or denatured alcohol to make natural perfumes or colognes. Rubbing alcohol is a toxic alcohol made from petroleum. Denatured alcohol is ethanol (the alcohol in wine and liquor) that has had bitter, poisonous substances added to it to prevent people from drinking it.
- When smelling and choosing essential oils for your own perfumes, colognes, or deodorants, work in a well-ventilated area away from kitchens and other rooms where there may be strong or lingering odors.

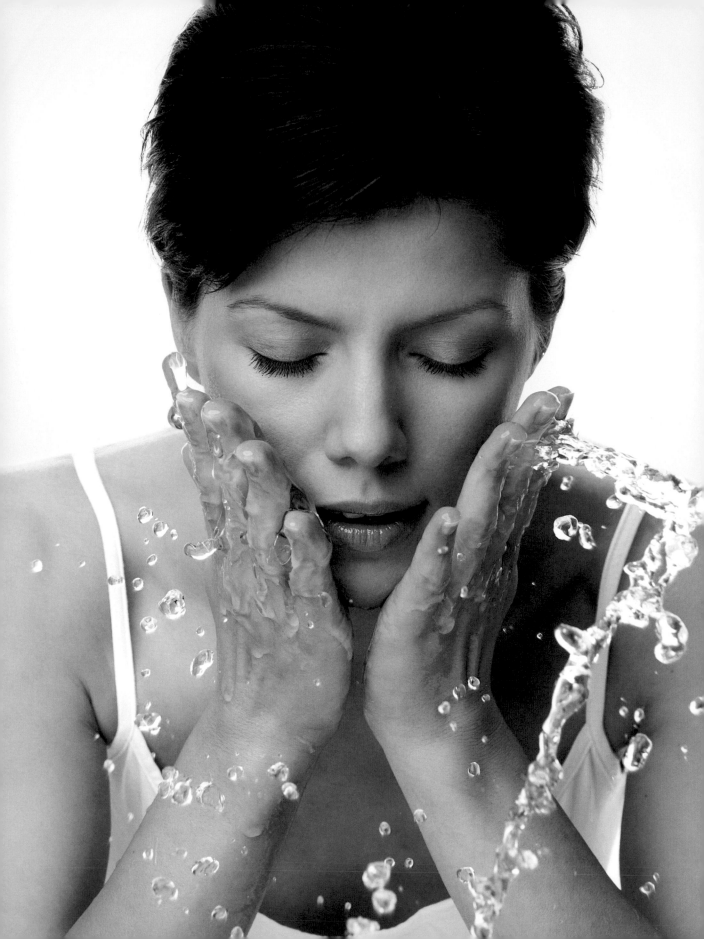

Fresh Face

14 BASICS, BRISK & BRACING

Clothing protects the skin on our bodies. But facial skin takes whatever the world dishes out head on. Dirt, dust, allergens, pollutants, and a host of other airborne contaminants settle on our faces every day, whether we work indoors or out. Add to that an accumulation of natural oils, dried sweat, dead cells, and proliferating bacteria, and it's no wonder our faces often look dull and dreary by the end of the day. The answer seems simple enough: If your face is dirty, wash it. But with what? Drugstore shelves are lined with a dizzying assortment of soaps, cleansers, and other skin care products. Yet reading their labels can be chilling.

Many of their ingredients—in addition to being unpronounceable—are hardly natural. Their safety, too, is questionable. Many personal care products contain hormone-disrupting phthalates (usually disguised under the catchall phrase "fragrance"), parabens (which have estrogenic effects), petroleum distillates (suspected carcinogens), formaldehyde (a known carcinogen), the pesticide triclosan, and other hazardous ingredients. More than 500 cosmetic and personal care products sold in the United States contain ingredients banned in similar products in Japan, Canada, or the European Union.

Yet a clean, fresh face is attainable, safely and naturally. Using simple ingredients you can find at your local health food or grocery store, you can make your own skin-cleansing and freshening products that work as well, or better, than most commercial brands.

▶ FACIAL CLEANSERS

Experts recommend a routine for achieving clear, clean, glowing skin. It begins with cleansing, usually morning and night—even if you have dry skin. Cleansing skin removes dirt, dead skin cells, oil buildup, and dissolves impurities that can block pores. It also improves circulation, protects against breakouts, and stimulates skin cell renewal. There are basically three types of natural facial cleansers: cleansing oils, milky lotions, and foaming gels.

Go for the Glow

- **Copy Cleopatra** One of the oldest and simplest ways to cleanse facial skin is to use what many ancient Egyptians did: pure olive oil. Simply smooth a little extra-virgin olive oil onto skin and massage it gently into the surface, avoiding the eye area. Rinse thoroughly with tepid water. Olive oil (or any natural plant oil) acts as a solvent to dissolve dirt and residues.

- **Choose a Cream-y Cleanser** Another ancient cleansing approach is to wash your

---

GENTLE SKIN CLEANSING OIL

Grapeseed oil tends to be easily absorbed into skin and doesn't feel greasy. Jojoba oil is also relatively light and easily absorbed. Lavender essential oil has antiseptic properties.

2 tablespoons grapeseed oil
1 tablespoon jojoba oil
1 tablespoon wheat germ oil
5 drops lavender essential oil

Combine the oils and pour into a dark glass bottle with a tight-fitting lid. Shake well to mix. Apply with fingertips and massage gently onto the face, avoiding the eyes. Rinse off with warm water.

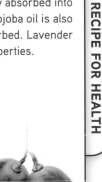

RECIPE FOR HEALTH

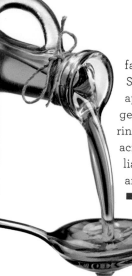

face in whole milk or cream. Simply use your fingertips to apply these dairy products in gentle circular motions, and then rinse. Yogurt, which contains an acid (lactic acid) that gently exfoliates dead skin cells, also makes an effective facial cleanser.

■ **Consider Castile** If you prefer a cleansing agent that lathers, try a castile soap, liquid or bar. Castile soap is made exclusively from plant oils rather than animal fat or synthetic substances. It tends to be far less drying than many commercial bar soaps, because it retains all of the natural skin-soothing glycerin that forms during the soapmaking process.

■ **Go for Natural Combinations** Slightly more complex natural facial cleansers can include herbal oils or tinctures, glycerin, fruit juices, and food products. Recipes for cleansers abound. The following is an example of a castile soap–based cleanser.

RECIPE FOR HEALTH

LAVENDER CLEANSING MILK

This recipe is courtesy of Annie B. Bond, from *Better Basics for the Home:*

1 cup lavender water (see the first paragraph of the recipe)

2 tablespoons unscented liquid castile soap

1 tablespoon vodka

1 teaspoon sweet almond oil

10 drops lavender essential oil

In a small saucepan, bring 1 cup water to a boil. Turn off heat and add a handful of dried lavender flowers. Let cool, cover, and steep in the refrigerator for 24 hours. Strain and reserve liquid.

Place the lavender water in a pint-size glass jar with a screw-top lid. Add the remaining ingredients, screw on the lid, and shake vigorously until well combined. Use a teaspoon or so of this soap to gently cleanse face morning and night. Rinse well with tepid water. Discard after one week.

NATURAL EXFOLIATORS

Exfoliating clean skin is a way to gently but thoroughly remove dead skin cells that are constantly forming on the skin's surface, a process that leaves skin soft, smooth, and vibrant. A plus: Exfoliating may help combat some of the visible signs of aging.

Shed Your Skin

■ **Try Almond Meal** Grind a small handful of almonds to a fine powder using a clean electric coffee grinder. Moisten about a teaspoon of the almond meal with enough purified water or plant oil (try avocado oil if you have dry skin or grapeseed oil for oily skin) to make a thin paste. Apply to skin using small circular motions. Rinse well.

■ **Be Fruitful** Fruit acids like those found in grapefruit, lemons, oranges, strawberries, grapes, and apples are natural exfoliants. Use about a teaspoon of fruit juice (freshly squeezed is best) per face cleaning. Dab on the juice, let it set for a few minutes, and then rinse off.

■ **Slice and Smooth** If you're in a hurry, simply slice a grape or strawberry in half and rub the cut surface over your skin.

■ **Go for Juicy Enzymes** Both pineapple and papaya contain natural enzymes that can effectively exfoliate skin. Cut a slice of either ripe pineapple or green papaya and rub the fruit over your face, avoiding your eyes. Leave on until the juice dries, then rinse thoroughly with lukewarm water.

TONERS

Using a toner on freshly cleansed, exfoliated skin helps close pores and can help improve skin tone. Most toners also work to restore skin's natural acidity. This "acid mantle," as it's sometimes called, naturally inhibits the growth of bacteria and fungi, thus promoting healthy,

RECIPE FOR HEALTH

SIMPLE & SWEET SUGAR SCRUB

This recipe is from Vermont Soapworks, cited in Annie B. Bond's *Home Enlightenment:*

2 tablespoons white cane sugar (not the most healthful sugar to eat, but wonderful for exfoliating)

2 tablespoons vegetable glycerin (available in health food stores)

½ teaspoon aloe vera gel

1 drop orange essential oil

1 drop lavender essential oil

Put the sugar and glycerin in a small bowl and blend. Add the aloe vera gel and the two essential oils and mix well. Put a dollop of the mix on your face and massage gently into skin. Leave on for three minutes (it will tighten as it dries). Rinse thoroughly with lukewarm water.

unblemished skin. All soaps—even the gentlest and most natural ones—are alkaline and disrupt the skin's acid balance to some degree. Toners counteract this effect.

Tonics for the Skin

- *Swish On Cider* One of the easiest toners is probably in your pantry already: apple cider vinegar. To prepare, combine equal parts vinegar (preferably organic) and bottled or filtered water. Use a cotton ball to apply to your face. Leave on five to ten minutes, and rinse with cool water. Another option is to mix equal parts of apple cider vinegar and cooled green tea and use in the same way.

- *Blend It* In a blender, puree a tablespoon of honey with a peeled, cored organic apple. Smooth this fragrant mixture on your skin, lie down so it doesn't drip off, and relax for 10 to 15 minutes. Rinse thoroughly with lukewarm water.

- *Make a Melon Mix* When watermelon is in season, mix 2 tablespoons watermelon juice (simply mash a piece of ripe watermelon to extract the juice) with 2 tablespoons filtered water and 1 tablespoon vodka or witch hazel (choose a brand made with real extract). Apply with a cotton ball. Wait a few minutes and then rinse.

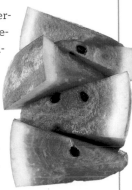

FOODS FOR HEALTH

A BETTER CHOICE

Many commercial beauty products are made from processed fish such as anchoveta and menhaden. Instead of buying these products—containing processed fish oils—eat fish rich in omega-3s and get the benefits from the inside out! Try canned sardines or anchovies over a salad for a delicious quick meal loaded with vitamins and minerals great for your skin and hair. Eating fish and staying away from products made from fish is better for you—and a boon for the anchoveta and menhaden populations that are currently being ravaged by reduction fisheries.

–Barton Seaver
Chef and sustainable food expert

good to know: ABOUT THE FRESH FACE

— Always treat facial skin gently.

— Make sure your hands are clean before you start cleaning your face.

— As a general rule, take three times as much time rinsing as you do cleansing to ensure that all traces of cleansers are removed.

— Never exfoliate the skin around your eyes. It is the most sensitive and delicate skin on your face and can easily be damaged.

— If you have acne, consult your dermatologist before using any type of exfoliant. Natural or commercial products that contain granules, no matter how small, can increase the risk of spreading pimples and infection.

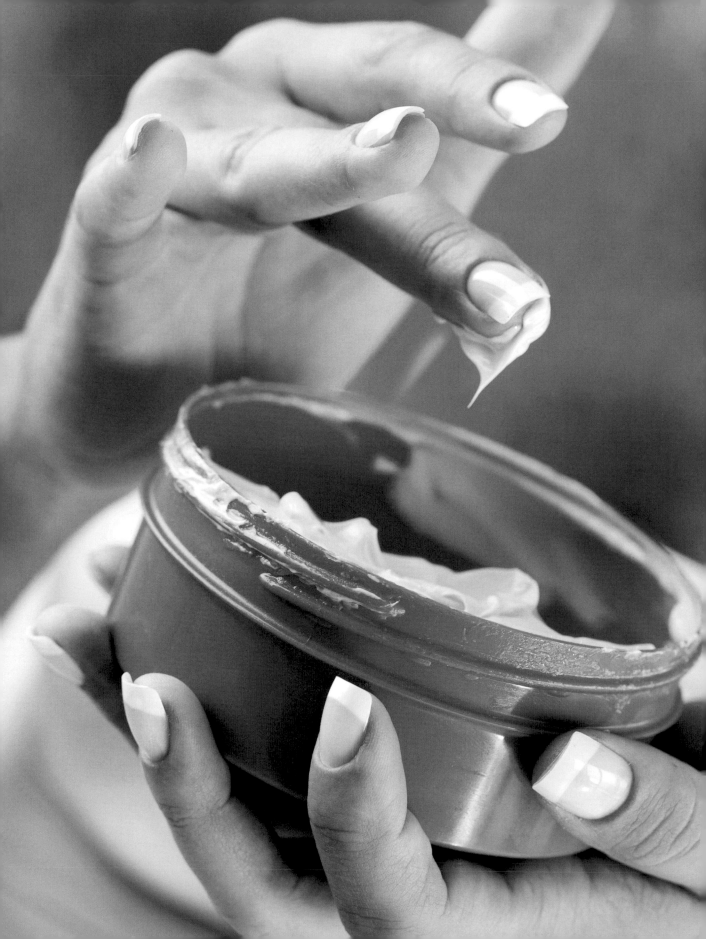

Hands & Nails

16 HELPFUL HANDFULS

On any given day, our hands take a beating. They're plunged repeatedly into water and exposed to dirt, detergents, grease, heat, cold, abrasive surfaces, sharp objects, and harsh chemicals. On bad days, we may cut, bruise, and even burn them. And although we're usually careful to dab sunscreen on faces and shoulders and knees, hands are often forgotten. It's not surprising that after all this wear and tear, our age, as well as our lifestyle, tends to show most on our hands. The solution usually seems to be to slather on hand lotion or splurge on a manicure.

But most commercial hand lotions and creams are much like those marketed for our faces. They're full of petroleum products and unpronounceable chemicals, some of which are hazardous to health. And nail polish? Just open a bottle and the odor of toxic solvents fills the air. Although you can find healthful hand lotions and creams if you look hard enough, you can also make your own quite easily. Transform hardworking hands into smooth, soft healthy ones by using natural remedies.

▶ BEAUTIFUL HANDS

Simple hand lotions and creams made out of all-natural ingredients can bring fast and effective relief to dry, chapped hands. Slightly more time-consuming treatments can help repair damage and promote healing. Scrubs, for instance, can gently exfoliate dead skin and rejuvenate the skin's surface. Soaks and masks help calm red, inflamed skin while restoring lost moisture.

Hand-Some Habits

- **Reach for EVOO** When it comes to skin care, extra-virgin olive oil is hard to beat. Wet your fingertips in a little oil and massage well into chapped hands and rough cuticles. If this feels greasy, dampen your hands slightly with a few drops of water and continue massaging; most of the greasiness will disappear.
- **Smooth On a Combo** For a simple oil-based hand lotion you can make in a few minutes, combine 4 teaspoons coconut oil, 2 teaspoons almond oil, and 2 teaspoons cocoa butter in a small microwave-safe bowl. Heat on low power in the microwave for just two or three seconds. Alternatively, warm ingredients in the top of

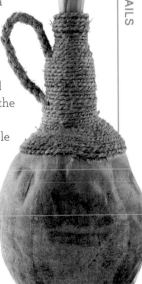

RECIPE FOR HEALTH

BUTTERY HAND CREAM

2 tablespoons shea butter

2 tablespoons mango butter

1 tablespoon cocoa butter

4 tablespoons sweet almond oil

1 tablespoon jojoba oil

20 drops lavender essential oil

15 drops lemon essential oil

10 drops geranium essential oil

In the top of a double boiler, gently heat the butters until completely melted. Add the almond and jojoba oil and stir until well blended. Pour the mixture into a small bowl and let cool about ten minutes, or until you see the first signs that it is beginning to solidify (get cloudy). Then using a whisk, beat the mixture until it turns into a cream with a light, fluffy consistency. Add the essential oils and whisk a minute or two more until completely blended. Store in a glass jar with an airtight lid. Keeps about six months.

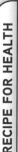
ANTI-AGING CARROT AND CRANBERRY SOAK

10 baby carrots
1 cup pure cranberry juice
   (unsweetened, no additives)
¼ cup avocado oil

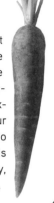

In a food processor, chop the carrot very fine. In a small saucepan, mix the chopped carrot and cranberry juice and let sit for an hour. Stir in the avocado oil and, on low heat, heat the mixture until it's warm, but not hot. Pour into a rimmed dish large enough to accommodate both hands. Soak hands for 10 to 15 minutes. Rinse well, dry, and apply a simple hand lotion or oil.

a double boiler until melted. Stir to combine and pour into a small glass jar, cool, and affix a tight-fitting lid. Massage a little of this rich, emollient mixture into hands as needed.

■ *Moisturize With Vegetable Glycerin* A humectant, glycerin is a substance that tends to absorb moisture from the air and "hold" it on the skin's surface. For a simple glycerin hand lotion, whisk together ¼ cup pure vegetable glycerin and ¾ cup rose water. Store in the refrigerator in a glass jar with a tight-fitting lid. Be sure you are buying real rose water, made from gentle steam distillation of rose petals. Look for it in natural food

stores, online, and in Greek delicatessens (read labels carefully).

■ *Go Dairy* To soften dry hands, soak for ten minutes in a bowl of lukewarm buttermilk. Rinse, dry, and massage in a natural oil or cream.

■ *Luxuriate in Lavender* Use a lavender "infusion" to relieve reddened, chapped skin on hands. In a saucepan, combine ¼ cup dried lavender flowers and ⅛ cup dried whole leaf sage, and add 1 cup water. Bring to a boil, and then reduce heat and simmer, covered, for 20 minutes. Cool, strain (discard the herbs), and add 5 drops lavender essential oil to the liquid. Shake well to emulsify. Saturate a cotton ball and apply the liquid all over hands.

■ *Exfoliate Gently* Removing dead skin cells can soften and brighten the skin on your hands. Fruit acids do this gently. Mash a handful of strawberries in a small bowl. Add a tablespoon of apricot kernel or grapeseed oil and a pinch of sea salt or kosher salt. Mix to make a paste and massage into hands, then leave on five minutes. Rinse and pat dry. If you don't have strawberries on hand, try this alternative: Mix a tablespoon of pineapple juice (fresh is best) with a teaspoon of Greek yogurt and the contents of a vitamin E capsule. Blend well and dab all over hands. Leave on ten minutes, then rinse.

■ *Delight in a Scrub* To exfoliate mechanically, you can mix almost any oil combined with

CHAMOMILE CHAPPED HANDS LOTION

2½ ounces apricot kernel oil
½ teaspoon essential oil of lemon, sweet orange, or bergamot
20 drops essential oil of German chamomile
1½ ounces shea butter
¼ ounce pure beeswax
4 ounces rose water
1 tablespoon pure vegetable glycerin

Combine the oils, shea butter, and beeswax in a double boiler over medium heat and warm until the wax is melted. Remove from heat and add the remaining ingredients. Blend with a whisk or electric mixer until creamy. Pour into a glass jar with a screw top and use promptly.

a slightly abrasive material such as ground oatmeal, ground nuts, salt, or sugar; adding a fruit acid will enhance exfoliation. Here's a simple hand scrub to try: Combine a small handful of brown sugar, about a tablespoon of apricot kernel oil, and the juice from a half lemon. Massage this mixture all over hands and around nails for a minute or two. Rinse well.

▶ | NICE NAILS

Well-groomed nails are beautiful without polish. Shape them with an emery board. Soak them in a natural nail "bath" that will moisturize dry, ragged cuticles and help remove stains. Then soothe them with fragrant combinations of natural plant and essential oils.

Nail File

- **Soften Cuticles With Fruit** Gentle fruit acids can help soften cuticles—no harsh chemicals needed. Soak nails for five or ten minutes in freshly squeezed orange juice, fresh pineapple juice, or apple cider vinegar. Rinse well.

- **Soak for Soothing** Combine ¼ cup honey, ¼ cup coconut oil, and 3 drops rosemary essential oil in a small bowl. Warm in the microwave to 15 to 20 seconds, or in the top of a double boiler. Soak nails for 10 to 15 minutes in the warm mixture. Rinse and pat dry.

- **Remove Ridges** Small ridges and grooves can be minimized by buffing nails with a gentle, slightly abrasive paste. Mix one part baking soda and two parts pulverized chalk (calcium carbonate) with enough pure vegetable glycerin to make a thick paste. Dab a little bit on a nail and use a small piece of flannel or other soft cloth to gently buff, working from side to side and up and down. Rinse well.

- **Coat to Protect** When cuticles get dry, they tend to become ragged. Keep them smooth and protected by applying wheat germ oil, twice a day. Dab a drop on each nail and massage it into the cuticle. Wipe off any excess. Alternatively, pierce a vitamin E capsule and use the oil in the same way.

- **Soothe While You Sleep** Blend 2 tablespoons almond or jojoba oil, the contents of a vitamin E capsule, and 3 drops each lavender and lemon essential oil in a small glass jar. Before bed, smooth a drop of this mixture onto each nail and the surrounding cuticle.

SALT & HONEY NAIL SCRUB

This scrub helps gently clean and moisturize cuticles and smooth nails:

1 tablespoon sea salt
1 tablespoon honey
1 tablespoon sweet almond oil
1 tablespoon real witch hazel extract

Combine all the ingredients in a small bowl. Working on one finger at a time, massage a little of the mixture all around the nail and cuticle area for one minute. Wipe off with a soft, clean cloth, then rinse briefly and dry.

good to know: ABOUT HANDS & NAILS

— If you're a gardener, protect your hands with gloves. Before you put them on, run your nails over a bar of soap to get some under your fingernails; it will act as a barrier to dirt. When you remove your gloves, use about a teaspoon of sugar and massage it over your hands while holding them under running water. The soap and sugar combination will help remove dirt and leave your hands smooth, clean, and unstained.

— Scrubs, masks, and soaks made with fruits or vegetables should be made fresh every time and discarded after use.

— After soaking cuticles to soften them, use the blunt end of an orangewood manicure stick to gently push the cuticles back from the nails. Avoid cutting cuticles, as this tends to toughen and thicken them and can foster infection.

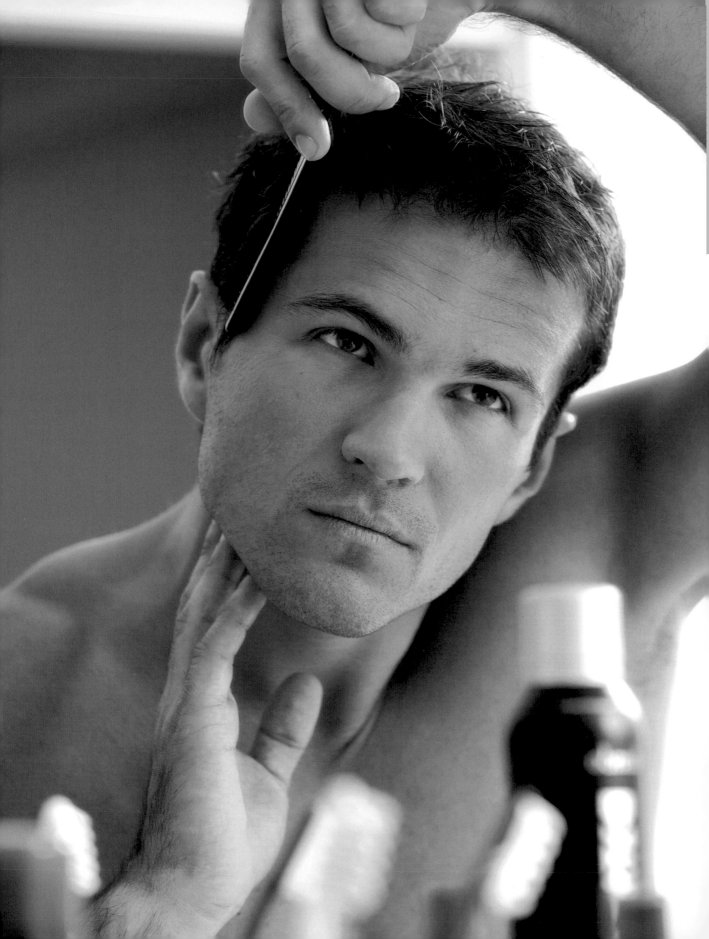

Healthy Hair

13 WAYS TO LUSHER LOCKS

Fair Rapunzel had magnificent hair, according to the story spun by the brothers Grimm. Rapunzel's hair wasn't just incredibly long. It was so healthy and strong it supported the prince's weight when he climbed to the top of her towering prison. A fairy tale? Of course. But so are the TV ads that try to convince us that the only way to get lustrous, bouncy, well-conditioned hair is to use brand-name shampoos and conditioners. Hair is made of the same protein found in fingernails. Each strand has a central shaft surrounded by an outer cuticle made up of cells that overlap like shingles on a roof. If the cuticle is damaged (think heat from blow dryers, chlorine, UV light, and certain chemicals), hair loses its moisture and natural oil to become lifeless, dry, and dull.

Conventional shampoos and conditioners can make hair look better, at least temporarily, but potentially at the risk of your health. For instance, most commercial shampoos contain sodium lauryl sulfate (SLS), a synthetic surfactant that creates wonderful lather but also dries out hair, irritates eyes, and triggers allergic reactions in many people. Very often sodium lauryl sulfate is accompanied by other undesirable ingredients. Natural hair care products are a healthy alternative. All you need are simple ingredients and a little time.

▶ | SHAMPOOS

Shampoos made of natural ingredients are a safe and easy approach to naturally clean hair. You can make a natural shampoo with just a few ingredients available at health food stores, some grocery stores, and many online retailers. And, you can tailor the ingredients to meet your needs.

Hair Dos (Without the Don'ts)
- **Use Castile** To make a basic natural shampoo with liquid castile soap, use the following recipe. It will not foam quite as luxuriously as commercial SLS-containing shampoos, but will leave your hair clean, shiny, and healthy.
- **Get Creative** Try different dried herb, natural oil, and essential oil combinations

to customize your homemade shampoo to suit your hair type. You can use these suggestions as guidelines, but don't be afraid to experiment to create your own unique recipes.
- *For normal hair:* Herbs include chamomile, lavender, rosemary, horsetail (mixtures

> **RECIPE FOR HEALTH**
>
> ### HOMEMADE BASIC HERBAL SHAMPOO
> 1¼ cups distilled water
> 2 tablespoons dried herbs (for example, chamomile, lavender)
> ¼ cup unscented liquid castile soap
> ¼ teaspoon almond or jojoba oil
> 20 to 30 drops of essential oil (for example, lavender, rose geranium, rosemary)
> 1 tablespoon aloe vera gel
>
> Bring the water to a boil in a small saucepan. Remove from the heat and add the dried herbs. Cover and steep 20 minutes. Strain the resulting herbal infusion and let it cool completely. Add the remaining ingredients, one at a time, to the herbal infusion, stirring well after each addition. Transfer the mixture to a plastic bottle with a flip-top lid for use in the shower or bath. Shake before using.

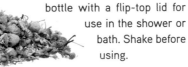

are fine); oils include almond, evening primrose, and borage seed oil; essential oils include lavender, rose geranium, chamomile, and rosemary.

- *For oily hair:* Herbs include lemon balm, basil, peppermint, yarrow; oils include almond, borage seed, grapeseed, and peach kernel oil; essential oils include lemon, eucalyptus, thyme, and cypress.

- *For dry hair:* Herbs include calendula, myrrh, burdock, parsley; oils include avocado, jojoba, and sunflower; essential oils include frankincense, patchouli, sandalwood, carrot seed, and jasmine.

■ *Experiment With Clay* For a truly unique shampooing experience, try Rhassoul clay, which comes from Morocco. It's a bit like putting mud on your hair, but the results explain why clay has been used on hair among North Africans for centuries. Rhassoul clay is available in some health food stores or online. You simply add enough water to a few teaspoons of the powdered clay until you have a mixture with the consistency of shampoo. Add a drop or two of essential oil to scent the mixture to suit your mood. Apply to hair, leave on about 15 minutes, rinse off, and wash hair normally with natural shampoo.

▶ HAIR RINSES

Natural soap shampoos are somewhat alkaline. Mildly acidic rinses and conditioners can help restore hair's slightly acidic pH. They also soften hair and help detangle it. Vinegar and herbal hair rinses have been used for centuries, for good reason: They're simple and effective.

Extra TLC

■ *Rinse With Vinegar* Organic apple cider vinegar makes a quick, inexpensive, and effective hair rinse that restores hair's natural pH, removes any soap residue, and even loosens and helps remove dead skin cells from the scalp. Mix equal parts vinegar and water and pour slowly through hair that's still damp from shampooing. Leave on for several minutes, then rinse.

■ *Rinse Away Dandruff* If dandruff is a problem, a clove and vinegar hair rinse may help. Combine 1 cup apple cider vinegar with ¼ cup rum and 10 drops clove essential oil. Shake to blend. Apply about ¼ cup of the mixture to hair that's been shampooed and toweled dry, working it well into the scalp. Wait five to ten minutes, and then rinse thoroughly with warm water.

■ *Try Glycerin* Glycerin forms a fine layer on hair, sealing the cuticle and attracting moisture. For a quick and easy glycerin conditioner to help tame dry, frizzy hair,

COCONUT-COCOA HAIR MASK

2 tablespoons natural cocoa
2 vitamin E capsules
1 tablespoon avocado oil
2 drops each rose geranium, lavender, bergamot, and orange essential oils

1 to 2 tablespoons warm milk
2 tablespoons coconut oil, warmed
1 tablespoon jojoba oil

Place the cocoa in a small bowl. Add enough warm milk—slowly, while whisking with a fork—to make a smooth, creamy paste. Pierce the vitamin E capsules and add their contents to the paste. Add the oils and essential oils and whisk until smooth and well combined. Apply to dry hair, massaging in from roots to ends. Pile hair on head and put on a plastic shower cap, and then wrap a large towel around your head. Relax for an hour. Rinse off in the shower, and then shampoo as normal.

mix 1 tablespoon pure orange blossom water (available at health food stores) with ½ cup distilled water and 1 to 2 drops of vegetable glycerin in a small spray bottle. Shake well to combine. Spritz a little on shampooed hair after towel-drying.

- **Add Honey and Lemon** Vinegar, honey, lemon, and herbs can combine for a gentle hair rinse that can add natural highlights, especially to blond hair. Make a cup of chamomile tea (see page 84). Stir in a tablespoon of honey, a tablespoon of freshly squeezed lemon juice, and ¼ cup apple cider vinegar. Mix well and slowly pour over damp hair. Work through to the scalp and let sit for five to ten minutes. Rinse well with lukewarm water.

⚠ **CAUTION:** Avoid chamomile if you are allergic to ragweed or other plants in the aster family.

▶ | TREATMENTS

Sometimes, shampooing and conditioning just isn't enough. A homemade hair mask can be an inexpensive and easy approach to nourishing and revitalizing hair without exposing it to harmful chemicals or causing further damage. And most of the ingredients for most natural hair treatments are as close as the grocery store.

Hair Repair

- **Get Help From Honey** Honey is a natural humectant. To deeply condition dry, damaged hair, mix ½ cup honey with 1 teaspoon olive oil and massage into clean, damp hair. Let sit for 20 to 30 minutes, and then rinse well with warm water. Wash hair with a natural shampoo and let air-dry.
- **Add Body With Beer** For limp, flat tresses, mix ½ cup flat beer with 1 teaspoon grapeseed oil and 1 raw egg. Whisk together well and apply to clean, damp hair. Wait 15 minutes, and then rinse with cool water. When hair is well rinsed, wash with a natural shampoo and let dry naturally.

⚠ **CAUTION:** Raw eggs may be contaminated with potentially harmful bacteria. Be sure to rinse hair well after using this mixture, wash hands thoroughly after handling the raw egg mixture, and avoid getting it in your mouth while using it on your hair.

- **Apply Avocado** One of the best natural hair-repair foods is avocado. Rich in monounsaturated fat (see pages 172–173), avocado adds gloss and manageability. Mash the flesh of 1 small avocado with 1 tablespoon of Greek yogurt, 1 teaspoon of almond oil, and a small squeeze of fresh lime juice. Massage into clean, damp hair and leave on 15 minutes before rinsing away with warm water. Wash hair with a natural shampoo and let air-dry.
- **Infuse With Essential Oils** The simplest way to tame frizzies and add shine to hair? Add 1 drop of rosemary and 1 drop of lavender essential oil to 1 teaspoon of avocado or olive oil. Rub a tiny bit of this mixture onto the palms of your hands, and then run your hands through your hair. Brush and go.

good to know: ABOUT HEALTHY HAIR

- Wet hair thoroughly before applying shampoo; it will distribute more easily (so you can use less).
- Apply shampoo mostly to the hair near your scalp. As you rinse it out, it will clean hair all the way to the ends.
- Wash and rinse your hair in warm water, rather than hot water, which tends to strip natural oils.
- Avoid washing your hair every day. Try every other day to allow hair to retain more of its natural oils.
- Heat from blow-dryers and curling irons is very drying and leads to dull, brittle hair. Let your hair dry naturally whenever possible.

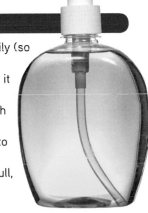

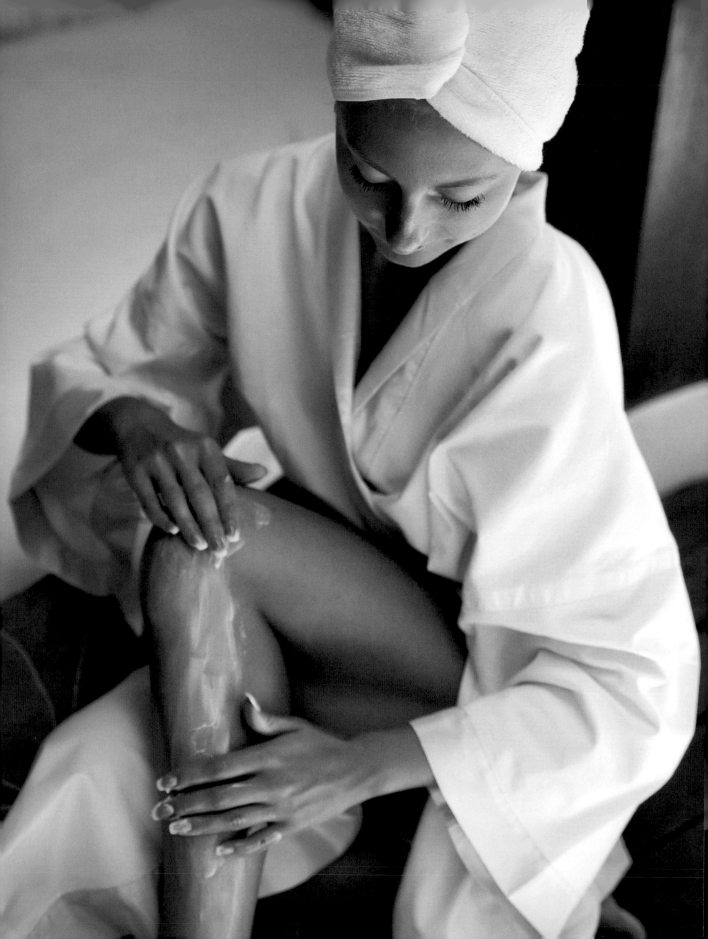

Moisturizers & Masks

11 SUGGESTIONS FOR SMOOTHER SKIN

There's nothing quite like a baby's dewy skin. It's soft, supple, and moist, replete with natural oils. Moist skin is healthy skin, but keeping it that way is a challenge. No matter what kind of skin we were born with, wind and dry air can steal its moisture away. So can washing it with harsh, oil-stripping soaps and exposing it to chemicals, solvents, and fragrances. Swim in a pool or sit in a hot tub at the gym, and you literally bathe your skin in moisture-stripping chlorine. Inevitably, skin also becomes drier as we age.

Keeping our bodies hydrated by drinking plenty of fluids is part of maintaining good health. But hydrating alone won't keep skin moist. That's where moisturizers come in. These are oils, lotions, and creams that help restore skin's lost moisture and oil, and protect it from losing even more. Moisturizers can also help soothe minor irritations, like those caused by shaving. Masks can be moisturizing, too. Some masks help restore moisture whereas others enhance skin's ability to absorb moisturizers more effectively.

Yet take a look at the ingredients of many commercial moisturizers, shave creams, and masks and you'll discover they're nothing short of a chemical soup: petroleum-based compounds, alcohols, synthetic fragrances, and a horde of preservatives. Some of these substances can actually increase skin's dryness. Others can trigger allergic reactions. A few are known carcinogens.

That's disturbing, especially because we tend to leave some of these products, particularly moisturizers, on our skin for long periods, and reapply them frequently. Fortunately, there are safer—and better—natural ways to moisturize and protect your skin.

▶ MOISTURIZERS

Moisturizing is an essential step in taking care of your skin. First cleanse and tone (see pages 207–209), and then moisturize. Not everyone's skin is the same, of course, so it's important to choose or create a moisturizer that is suited to your particular skin type, whether it's dry, oily, or something in between. Hands, legs, and feet probably need a heavier, richer moisturizer than what you'd use on your face. The fundamental ingredients in most natural moisturizing lotions and creams are plants oils; in addition to water, they are the simplest and most effective moisturizers known.

---

good to know: ABOUT MOISTURIZERS & MASKS

— Moisturize immediately after bathing, showering, or washing your hands while skin is still damp.

— Shower, bathe, and wash your hands in lukewarm, never hot, water. Keep showers short.

— Use a humidifier, especially during the winter months. Sleep with a humidifier in your bedroom (close doors to keep the moist air in). Try to keep the humidity level between 30 to 40 percent in your immediate environment.

— Eat foods high in monounsaturated and polyunsaturated fat (see page 331).

— Make a mineral water spritzer by combining 10 drops of your favorite essential oil with 1 cup of mineral water in a spray bottle. Mist your face and hands throughout the day.

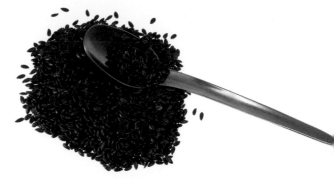

Lotion Potions

- **Look for Natural Oils** Choose lotions or creams that are rich in real plant oils such as shea butter, cocoa butter, almond oil, jojoba oil, and avocado oil. Truly natural products will likely contain other plant compounds, such as essential oils (lavender oil, rosemary oil) or essences (rose water), along with vegetable glycerin, a natural humectant (a substance that soaks up moisture from the surrounding air). Choose "paraben-free" and "phthalate-free" products. If ingredients such as 1,4-dioxane, octyl-demthyl, polyethylene glycols (PEGs), or anything else you can't pronounce are on the label, keep looking.

- **Go Basic** Simple, pure extra-virgin olive oil not only cleans skin effectively (see page 207) but also works well as a moisturizer. When your skin is still quite moist after cleansing, smooth several drops of olive oil over your face as well as knees, elbows, and any other rough skin areas. Olive oil is high in mono-unsaturated fats, which hydrates skin without leaving a greasy residue. Alternatively, try wheat germ oil (rich in vitamin E), almond oil, jojoba oil, or grapeseed oil as equally simple moisturizers.

- **Make a Gel** When flaxseed (see page 161) is combined with water, it creates a mucilaginous gel that can work as a natural moisturizer. Stir 1 teaspoon flaxseed into ½ cup cool water in a saucepan. Bring to a boil, reduce to low heat, and simmer until the mixture becomes thick and gelatinous. Cool and pour through a sieve to strain out the seeds. Dab the strained gel onto your skin and massage in. Keep refrigerated and discard after two to three days.

▶ SHAVING CREAM

Shaving every day is a bit like scraping sandpaper over your face or legs. Shaving can rob skin of its protective outermost layer of skin cells and strip away natural oils, exposing sensitive "new" skin every time. Many conventional shaving creams and gels are made from petroleum-derived chemicals, including isopentane (a degreaser that breaks down natural skin oils and smells like gasoline), and other compounds that are known irritants, hormone disruptors, and potential carcinogens. For a safer, more natural shave, try these simple approaches.

Smooth & Soothe

- **Use Oil** Pure plant oils, such as olive, almond, or grapeseed oil, act as natural lubricants and so help a razor glide easily over skin. You

ALL-NATURAL MOISTURIZING LOTION

Use different oils to produce a lotion suited to your moisturizing needs. Jojoba oil (actually a plant wax) is more stable than most plant oils, and rancidity is rarely a concern. Grapeseed oil is very light and easily absorbed. Apricot kernel oil is slightly richer. Avocado oil is richer still, and good for more mature skin.

2 tablespoons pure aloe vera gel
2 teaspoons vegetable glycerin

½ teaspoon jojoba, grapeseed, apricot kernel, or avocado oil
1 teaspoon pure beeswax

In a bowl, combine the aloe vera gel, glycerin, and oil. Melt the beeswax in the top of a double boiler. Add the melted wax to the ingredients in the bowl, whisking rapidly until blended, and then more slowly until the beeswax cools and the mixture thickens, about five to seven minutes. Scoop the lotion into a glass jar with a tight-fitting lid. Keeps two to four weeks.

WITCH HAZEL EXTRACT & GLYCERIN AFTERSHAVE LOTION

Courtesy of Annie B. Bond, *Better Basics for the Home:*

1 cup real witch hazel extract
½ cup high-proof vodka, rum, or brandy
1 to 2 tablespoons vegetable glycerin
10 to 20 drops each peppermint and
   eucalyptus essential oil (alternatively,
   use thyme and rosemary essential oil)

Combine the ingredients in a glass jar with a tight-fitting lid. Shake well to blend. To use, pat a little of the mixture onto just-shaved skin. The lotion keeps indefinitely.

don't need to use much. Simply pour a little oil into a dish, dip your fingertips in it, rub the oil into your hands, and then rub your hands over the area you need to shave. When done, rinse the shaved area and pat dry. Because the oil is a natural moisturizer, it will leave skin smooth, supple, and protected.

- **Try Infused Oil** Create a skin-soothing oil for shaving by adding 1 or 2 drops of chamomile or lavender essential oil to ½ cup plant oil. Or make a refreshing oil by adding a few drops of peppermint or eucalyptus essential oil to the same amount of oil. Use as previously advised.

⚠ **CAUTION:** Don't use chamomile if you are allergic to ragweed or other plants in the aster family.

- **Lather Up** If you'd rather lather up to shave, try using all-natural castile soap in liquid or bar form. It produces a rich, creamy lather naturally. Follow with a skin-softening natural aftershave lotion (see recipe above).

▶ | MASKS

Masks can be applied to the face and neck about once a week to help remove excess oil, open pores, exfoliate dead skin, draw out impurities, and help moisturizers absorb more deeply into skin. You can make simple, soothing, spa-quality masks using foods as close as the nearest grocery store. Although these natural ingredients are very mild, it's a good idea to do a patch test before trying something new. Simply apply of bit of the mask to the inside of your arm and wait a few hours to see if any reaction develops.

A Skin-Deep Solution

- **Apply Avocado** Oil-rich avocado pulp is particularly good for moisturizing dry, mature skin. Puree the pulp from ½ ripe avocado. (Optional: Add ¼ cup honey to the avocado and mix well.) Apply liberally and leave on for ten minutes. Rinse off using cool water.
- **Mash a Peach** For a peaches and cream complexion, combine two very ripe peeled and mashed organic peaches with ¼ cup almond or jojoba oil and 1 tablespoon organic heavy cream in a bowl. Whisk together to blend. Dab onto skin, leave on about five minutes, and rinse with warm water.

HONEY: SWEET FOR YOUR SKIN

Women have long enjoyed the benefits of honey on their skin. Now modern research has shown that honey is a potent antiseptic, helping to fight off the bacteria that cause acne and other skin problems. Honey also works as an anti-inflammatory, reducing irritation and redness of the skin. Considered a humectant, a substance that seals in moisture, honey improves skin hydration and decreases the appearance of fine lines. You can make your own honey mask at home for a fraction of the cost of store-bought products:

4 ounces plain yogurt
2 teaspoons raw honey
¼ teaspoon olive or almond oil

Mix all the ingredients together in small bowl. Apply to face, leaving on for 15 minutes. Rinse. Repeat one to two times per week.

–Tieraona Low Dog, M.D.
Author and integrative medicine expert

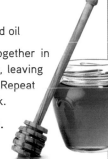

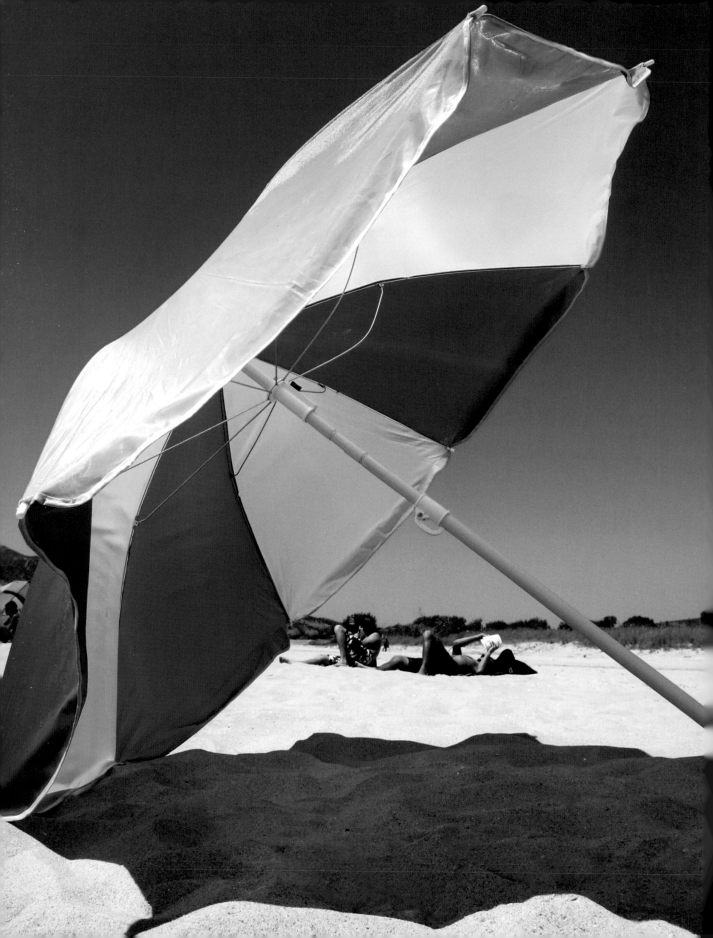

Natural Sun Safety

9 IDEAS TO ENSURE FUN IN THE SUN

Sunlight is something we all need in small doses. When sunlight strikes our skin, ultraviolet (UV) rays trigger the synthesis of vitamin D in our bodies, a vitamin essential to healthy bones and teeth and general health. About 30 minutes a day out in the sun is all it takes. Getting too much sun, though, isn't healthy. Overexposure to the sun's ultraviolet (UV) rays is what causes most of the skin changes that we associate with aging. The effects are cumulative. Over time, those invisible UV rays damage fibers in skin, causing them to break down. The result is sagging, stretching, and thinning that leads to lines and wrinkles as well as unattractive spots.

Besides these cosmetic changes, exposure to UV rays from the sun—and from tanning beds—is the number one cause of skin cancer, the most prevalent form of cancer in the United States. UV radiation damages the DNA in skin cells, triggering genetic disruptions that can lead to uncontrolled cell division and growth, and the development of tumors that can be benign or malignant. Malignant skin cancer, also called malignant melanoma because it involves abnormal skin pigment cells called melanocytes, accounts for 75 percent of all skin cancer deaths. It can develop and spread quickly, and if not caught early and successfully treated, can spread to other organs and is difficult to control.

Nothing can undo sun damage that's occurred earlier in life, but it's never too late to do a better job protecting skin from the sun's harmful rays. For years we've been told to protect ourselves by wearing sunscreens. Most of the chemical sunscreens that line grocery store and drugstore shelves work by employing synthetic chemicals that absorb the sun's rays, thus preventing them from damaging skin for a certain amount of time. However, some of these UV-absorbing chemicals present problems of their own. Several have been shown to mimic the hormone estrogen. In laboratory tests, estrogen-sensitive breast cancer cells in test tubes multiplied when they were exposed to some of these substances. Although their precise effects in the human body are still unclear, these research results are cause for concern

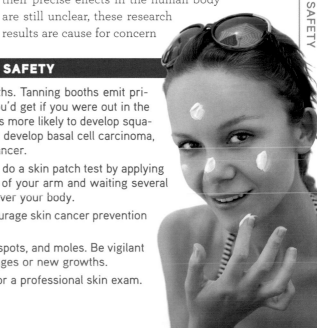

good to know: ABOUT NATURAL SUN SAFETY

- Avoid tanning in the sun, and avoid tanning booths. Tanning booths emit primarily UVA—as much as 12 times the amount you'd get if you were out in the sun. People who use tanning salons are 2.5 times more likely to develop squamous cell carcinoma and 1.5 times more likely to develop basal cell carcinoma, the two common types of non-melanoma skin cancer.

- When using sunscreen or any new skin product, do a skin patch test by applying a small amount of the product on the inner side of your arm and waiting several hours to see what happens before putting it all over your body.

- If you're a parent, be a good role model and encourage skin cancer prevention habits in your children.

- Get to know your skin and all its normal bumps, spots, and moles. Be vigilant (every month) about looking for suspicious changes or new growths.

- See your doctor or a dermatologist every year for a professional skin exam.

because chemical sunscreens are readily absorbed through the skin. Researchers at the Centers for Disease Control and Prevention found that nearly 97 percent of Americans have one of the most common chemical sunscreens, benzophenone-3, in their blood.

Furthermore, until recently, most sunscreens manufactured in the United States protected only against UVB, which is the type of radiation responsible for causing sunburn. Older chemical sunscreens did little to protect against UVA, which penetrates skin more deeply than UVB and has now been shown to damage cells in the basal (bottom) layer of the skin, where most skin cancers occur. Sunscreen manufacturers responded by creating "broad spectrum" sunscreens, products supposedly designed to block both UVB and UVA. The problem is that one of the most common UVA-protecting chemical sunscreens, avobenzone, may not offer all that much protection. Unless it has been chemically stabilized, it has a tendency to break down when exposed to sunlight, rendering it fairly useless. So . . . what to do?

▶ | SAFER SUNSCREENS

Zinc oxide is a mineral that can protect the skin from the sun's damaging rays quite effectively. Unlike chemical sunscreens, zinc oxide is what's called a physical sunscreen; it scatters light. When you apply a zinc oxide sunscreen, the mineral particles sit on the outermost layer of your skin and physically deflect UV rays away from

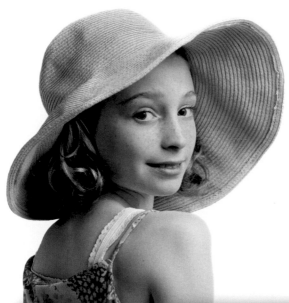

RECIPE FOR HEALTH

NATURAL ZINC OXIDE SUNSCREEN
Adapted from Annie B. Bond, *Better Basics for the Home:*

2½ ounces jojoba oil
½ ounce beeswax
1 tablespoon wheat germ oil
2 tablespoons uncoated pharmaceutical grade zinc oxide powder ("non-nano" or "nonmicronized")

1½ ounces coconut oil or cocoa butter
4 ounces distilled water
10 to 20 drops antiseptic essential oil, such as lavender

Melt the oils and beeswax in a double boiler over medium heat. Remove from heat and add the water. Mix with an electric handheld mixer until thick and creamy. Carefully measure out 2 tablespoons zinc oxide. Avoid stirring the powder and creating or breathing zinc oxide dust. Add the powder gently to the melted oils and stir it in slowly with a spoon to combine. When the zinc oxide is completely mixed into the oils (no visible dry powder), add the wheat germ oil and essential oils and return to using the electric mixer. Beat until the mixture reaches a smooth, creamy consistency. Store in a glass container with a tight-fitting lid for up to six months. ⚠ **CAUTION:** Zinc oxide, like most dustlike powders, may be a health risk if inhaled. When working with zinc oxide, wear a surgical mask to cover your mouth and nose. Do not stir the powder vigorously, dump it into the melted ingredients, beat with an electric mixer, or do anything else that might cause dust. Once the powder is completely mixed into the oils and other ingredients, it is no longer an inhalant risk.

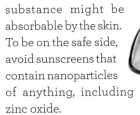

VITAL VITAMIN D

Among the sun-shy public worldwide, lack of vitamin D is now a serious problem. Few foods contain vitamin D. Further, insufficient amounts of vitamin D raise the risk of autoimmune diseases, allergies, asthma, bone loss, diabetes, cardiovascular disease, depression, and even some cancers.

To get enough vitamin D, consider this: During spring and summer, you can expose your skin (not your face) to about 15 minutes of sun a day. Or you can take supplements: 600 international units (IU) a day of vitamin D_3, 800 IU for those over 70. Some health care providers now recommend at least 1,000 IU—not to exceed 2,000 IU daily. Higher doses are needed to correct deficiencies. Ask your doctor about checking your levels with a blood test.

–Linda B. White, M.D.
Educator and author

the skin's surface, protecting the skin below. Zinc oxide is unique among sunscreen ingredients in that it is truly a broad-spectrum blocker that protects skin from all forms of damaging UV radiation.

Ban the Rays

- **Look for Zinc** As concerns about chemical sunscreens increased, a number of manufacturers responded by creating zinc oxide–based sunscreens. They are more expensive than chemical sunscreens, but they do offer proven protection.
- **Avoid Nano** Nanoparticles are particles so small they are measured in nanometers (one-billionth of a meter). That makes them still bigger than molecules, but there is some concern (although still not a lot of concrete evidence) that nanoparticles of any

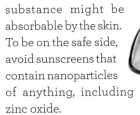

substance might be absorbable by the skin. To be on the safe side, avoid sunscreens that contain nanoparticles of anything, including zinc oxide.

- **Wear It** A sunscreen is effective only if you actually put it on your skin! Use a zinc oxide sunscreen with a sun protection factor (SPF) of at least 15 and reapply it according to directions. SPF doesn't refer to the amount of protection, but rather how long protection will last. For instance, if your skin would normally burn after 10 minutes in the sun, using a sunscreen with an SPF of 15 means you could stay out in the sun without burning for 10 × 15, or 150 minutes. But keep in mind this is a rough estimate. The actual protection depends on many things, including sun intensity and the sensitivity of your skin.
- **Watch the Clock** As a general rule, apply about two tablespoons of zinc oxide sunscreen to your entire body before going outside and reapply that amount often, and immediately after you've been sweating a lot, have been swimming, or after towel drying. Be sure to read the directions on the package of sunscreen you are using, however, as they may differ.

▶ SUN STRATEGIES

- **Wear a Hat** No matter what sunscreen you use, some UV radiation is going to reach your skin. So it's important to use other sun strategies along with sunscreen to give your skin the full protection it deserves. One of the simplest? Wear a hat and a long-sleeved shirt. It may not be the coolest option (in every sense of the word) but it's definitely effective.
- **Seek the Shade** The sun's UVB rays are most intense between 10 a.m. and 4 p.m. (UVA rays are pretty much the same during all daylight hours throughout the year). Avoid the most intense UVB period by staying out of the sun during the midday hours.
- **Wear Sunglasses** UV rays also damage eyes and can lead to the development of cataracts.

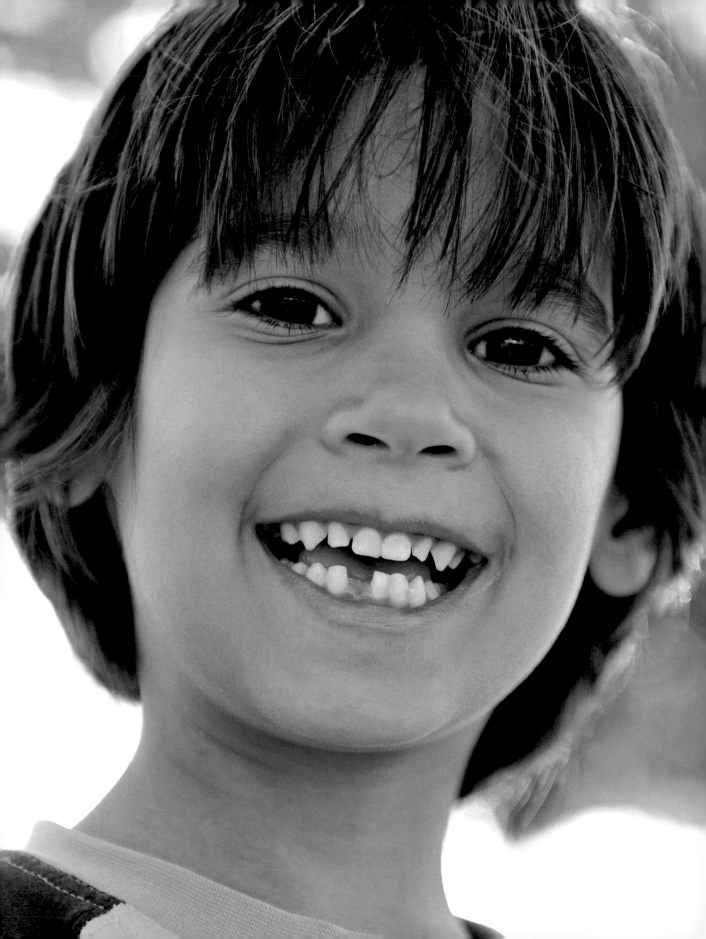

Tooth & Mouth Care

13 STEPS TO A SWEETER SMILE

Smiles reveal a great deal about personality, self-confidence … and dental hygiene. Clean teeth and fresh breath are signs of well-cared-for mouth. But stroll down the dental care aisle of any drugstore, and you'd easily conclude that the only way to achieve a healthy smile is by using tubes of sweet, glossy toothpaste and mouthwashes tinted in alarming shades of blue, green, and red. Read the labels on these products, though, and you might not want to put them in your mouth. Fluoride is added to most commercial brands of toothpaste to reduce the incidence of dental caries (cavities).

But some critics believe we're exposed to too much fluoride on many fronts, and fluorine-based chemicals have been linked to kidney damage and other health problems. Also hidden in that ribbon of toothpaste on your brush are petroleum-based detergents, potentially damaging bleaches, artificial colors, and in some brands, a controversial broad-spectrum antibacterial agent called triclosan that's been linked to a variety of health and environmental concerns. The good news is that for centuries, people have been getting clean teeth and fresh breath naturally, and you can too.

> ▶ ## TOOTHPASTES & POWDERS

Traditional cultures all over the world use herbs and plant oils and essences to clean teeth, stimulate gum tissue, and inhibit oral bacteria. Many familiar herbs, including rosemary, myrrh, tea tree, sage, thyme, anise, and fennel, fight germs that cause plaque to form on teeth, which in turn can lead to dental caries and periodontal disease. There are natural toothpastes and powders on the market that contain extracts of these and other herbs. But read labels carefully. Even some products marketed as "all natural"

RECIPE FOR HEALTH

ALL-NATURAL MINT TOOTHPASTE

Courtesy of Annie B. Bond, *Better Basics for the Home*:

4 ounces calcium carbonate (chalk)
2 ounces baking soda
$1/8$ teaspoon stevia powder
10 drops essential or peppermint oil
Food-grade glycerin (enough to make a paste)

Combine the first four ingredients in a small dish and blend well. Add enough glycerin to make a paste similar to toothpaste. Store in a glass jar with a tight-fitting lid. To use, place about ½ teaspoon of the mixture on your brush.

---

may contain some of the same ingredients you're trying to avoid in conventional toothpaste. Making your own toothpaste or powder is an alternative. It's the only way to control exactly what you are—and aren't—putting into your mouth.

A Better Brush

- ***Use a Natural Toothbrush*** For thousands of years, many traditional cultures have chewed the bark or twigs of certain plants to help clean teeth. These chewing sticks or twig toothbrushes—essentially the precursors of the modern toothbrush—are still used today in parts of Africa, South America, India, Asia, and the Middle East. In the

CLEANER TEETH MAY LEAD TO LONGER LIFE

It turns out that brushing your teeth is more than your mom's good advice. It was once thought that bacteria were the factor that linked gum disease to other infections in the body. However, more recent research demonstrates that inflammation from gum disease can be a sign of other chronic inflammatory conditions, such as diabetes, cardiovascular disease, and Alzheimer's. According to the American Academy of Periodontology, some 75 percent of adults suffer from some form of periodontal disease. Treating inflammation may not only help manage gum disease but other chronic inflammatory conditions as well.

To reduce inflammation, eat green, leafy vegetables; add more omega-3s to your diet; reduce simple carbohydrates like bread and pasta; exercise; get plenty of sleep—and *brush your teeth.*

–Dan Buettner
Author and lecturer on longevity

Middle East, the most common source of twig toothbrushes is a shrubby tree, *Salvadora persica*. A recent scientific study showed that an extract of *S. persica* worked as well as chlorhexidine gluconate—one of the best proven antiplaque agents. Look for natural twig toothbrushes (sometimes called miswak) in natural food stores or online; follow package instructions. Consult your dentist before using a twig toothbrush as a regular replacement.

- **Massage Gums** Some Ayurvedic practitioners recommend massaging gums as a way to promote healthy teeth and gums. Take a small mouthful of warm sesame oil and swish it around in your mouth for two minutes. Spit it out and then gently massage your gums with your index finger for about a minute. Rinse well.
- **Brush With Baking Soda** Plain old baking soda (sodium bicarbonate), applied to a damp toothbrush, is one of the simplest traditional approaches to naturally cleaning teeth (and it's probably right there in your pantry). It's been used for decades as a tooth cleaner. If the taste is unpleasant, mix several tablespoons of soda with a packet of stevia powder and add a pinch of cinnamon or cloves to create a palatable blend. To use, just dip damp toothbrush bristles.
- **Make a Paste** Myrrh is strongly antibacterial; it's an ingredient in some natural toothpastes available in health food stores. Mix ½ teaspoon powdered myrrh (available from natural food stores and online) with an equal amount powdered sage and about a teaspoon of honey or food-grade glycerin to make a thick paste. Use like toothpaste, rinsing well.
- **Clean With Salt** Bacteria-inhibiting salt is useful for treating minor infections such as canker sores (see page 45) and sore throat (see page 25). It will also effectively inhibit bacteria that cause plaque formation on teeth. Put it to work by combining equal parts popcorn

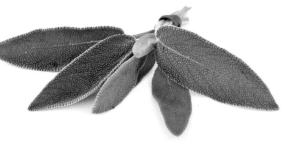

---

good to know: ABOUT TOOTH & MOUTH CARE

- Don't risk damaging the enamel that forms a tooth's outer surface. Use the softest bristle toothbrush you can find and avoid "scrubbing" teeth with hard pressure.
- Try an Ayurvedic exercise said to stimulate the energy meridians in teeth. *Gently* tap your teeth (top and bottom) together a half dozen times in succession.
- Avoid lip balms that contain camphor, which can sap moisture from already dry lips.
- Natural lip balms can do double duty as healing treatments for dry, ragged cuticles and to help combat brittle nails.

salt (because of its fine grain) and baking soda. To make it taste a little better, add a drop of your favorite "minty-fresh" essential oil, such as or peppermint.

- **Get Fancy** Use the recipe on page 227 to make a refreshing, basic toothpaste that works so well and tastes so good you'll never miss the commercial brands.
- **Floss With Flavor** You can turn ordinary dental floss into a bacteria-fighting tool by soaking floss (you'll have to unwind it from the spool) in a mixture of ¼ cup water and 40 drops of an antibacterial essential oil, such as thyme or tea tree. Steep in the liquid for four or five hours, then remove and let dry.

▶ | MOUTHWASHES

It's a common misconception that breath mints and minty mouthwashes will give you fresh breath. What'll they give you is minty-smelling breath that quickly reverts to whatever you started with. Or worse, because many breath mints contain sugar, which gives odor-causing oral bacteria even more raw material to work with. Most commercial mouthwashes contain alcohol, which can promote a dry mouth (another bad breath culprit). If you often have bad breath, see your dentist. Chronic bad breath can be a sign of periodontal disease. For ordinary, occasional bad breath, try a natural mouthwash that will help fight bacteria while at the same time driving away halitosis.

Swish & Spit
- **Make It Minty** You can make a simple minty mouthwash in less than 15 seconds. Add ¼ teaspoon baking soda or salt and 1 drop peppermint essential oil to about 4 ounces of filtered water. Stir, sip, swish, and spit.
- **Go Herbal** Place 1 teaspoon each dried peppermint leaves, dried rosemary leaves, and fennel seeds in a saucepan with about 2 cups water. Bring to a boil, turn off the heat, and let the herbs steep for 20 to 30 minutes. Cool and strain. The resulting mouthwash keeps in the refrigerator for several days.

▶ | LIP BALMS

When cold winds blow, furnaces run, or you're out in the sun or on the water, your lips can really suffer. Chapped lips have been drained of their moisture and need a protective, soothing boost. Commercial lip balms often disappoint. They feel good when first applied, but when they wear off, your lips are no better. That's because most of them contain a stew of chemicals and a high concentration of synthetic, petroleum-derived wax. All-natural lip balms are available. Look for those rich in plant oils, such as shea butter, which deeply moisturizes lips. Alternatively, make your own.

Lippity-Do-Da
- **Smooth On Oil** In a pinch, soothe chapped lips with a thin coating of any rich plant oil, such as olive or avocado.
- **Squeeze On Vitamin E** Keep a few vitamin E capsules handy as first aid for chapped lips. Pierce the capsule, squeeze some out, and smooth on.
- **Make Your Own** Making lip balm is easier than you might think. Double the recipe above and share some with friends.

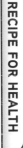

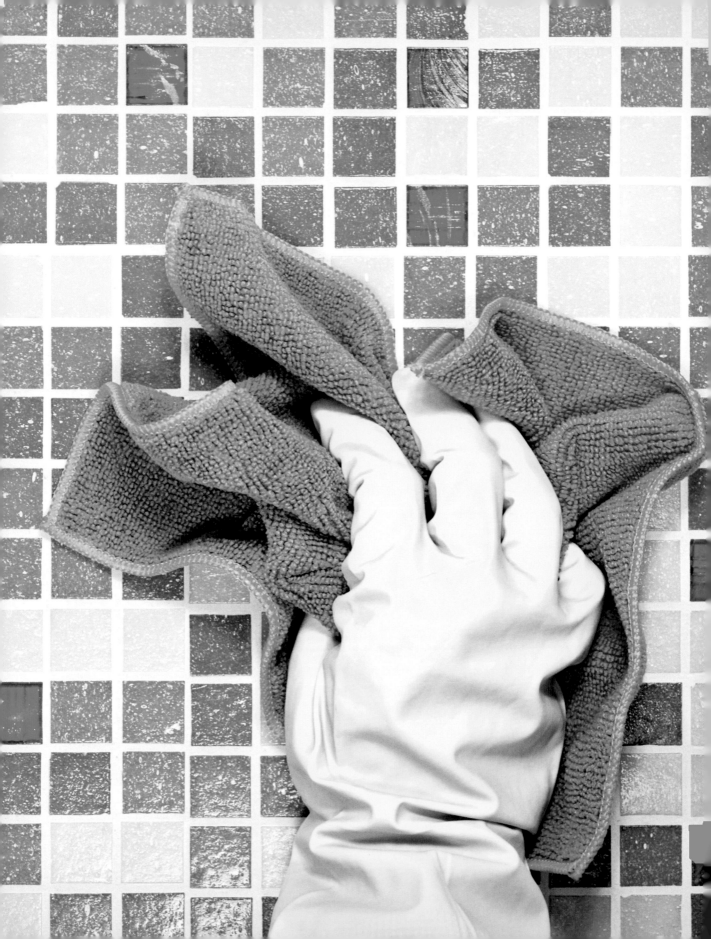

Disinfecting & Deodorizing

12 WAYS TO A SPOTLESS SHINE

Comic book heroes often have special high-powered senses that allow them to see what normal folks cannot. It sounds like a wonderful gift—until you realize there are things you might not want to see—like the billions of bacteria that lurk in your home. You'd guess the bathroom would be the most germ-infested place, right? Not by a long shot. Studies have shown that the average kitchen harbors more bacteria than any other room in the house. Often, 500,000-plus bacteria *per square inch* live in the drain of the kitchen sink alone. And germs don't just sit around idly; they multiply.

Given ideal conditions, a single bacterium can become more than eight million bacteria in less than 24 hours! For those ideal conditions, you don't need to look much farther than the kitchen sponge. The fact that it's moist and warm much of the time makes it an ideal breeding ground. A sponge that's been used no more than two or three days harbors millions and millions of bacteria. Every time you use it to wipe up a spill or wipe down a surface, you're spreading scores of bacteria around—and contaminating your hands, too.

Grocery and hardware store shelves are lined with disinfectants designed to kill bacteria. However, some contain antibacterial compounds—such as triclosan—that help foster antibiotic-resistant strains of these microbes. Other ingredients in common disinfectants are toxic. Read their labels carefully and you'll see all sorts of warnings and cautions: Don't inhale the fumes. Contact with skin can cause irritation. Poisonous if swallowed. Standing side by side with disinfectants on store shelves are dozens of home deodorizers: air fresheners, scented sprays, and cones of "odor-eating" gels. Yet the ingredients in deodorizers are frightening, too. They include formaldehyde (a carcinogen), petroleum distillates, and 1,4-dichlorobenzene, which causes skin, throat, and eye irritation—and possible nervous system damage. As if that weren't bad enough, a University of Washington study of top-selling air fresheners (and laundry products) found that all of them emitted at least one chemical regulated as toxic or hazardous under federal law—yet none of those chemicals was listed on the product labels. There are safe, natural alternatives to commercial disinfectants and deodorizers, and most of them can be made in minutes.

▶ DISINFECTANTS

Vinegar, baking soda, and hydrogen peroxide are safe, reasonably effective, eco-friendly germ fighters. True, none of them packs the true disinfectant, microbe-destroying punch of chlorine bleach, which kills most germs on contact, including *E. coli* and other microbes that can cause foodborne illnesses. Using bleach has many drawbacks, however. Topping the list is that combining bleach with other substances can be quite dangerous. When vinegar and bleach mix, for instance, toxic chlorine gas is formed; when ammonia (a very alkaline cleaner) and bleach combine, toxic chloramine gas is released. For this reason, bleach is considered one of the most hazardous of all household cleaning products. So, although natural antibacterials aren't perfect, they can go a long way toward banishing bacteria without the risks of bleach.

Safer Scrubbers

- *Clean the Cutting Board* Several studies have shown that vinegar, usually in combination with salt or hydrogen peroxide, can inhibit bacteria on cutting boards, including some strains of *E. coli.* You can sanitize

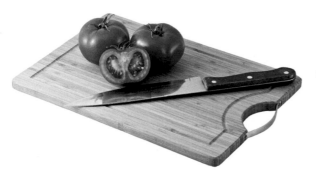

these surfaces—to some extent—by spraying with undiluted white distilled vinegar. Let sit for ten minutes or so. Rinse well and then apply a 3 percent solution of hydrogen peroxide. Let this solution saturate the board for ten minutes, then rinse. Finally, wash the cutting board thoroughly in hot, soapy water. Alternatively, clean the cutting board with hot, soapy water first, then spritz with vinegar and leave it to dry overnight.

- *Clean Produce* A study carried out at Virginia Tech found that the numbers of bacteria on fruits and vegetables could be greatly reduced (although not completely eliminated) by spraying first with undiluted vinegar, and then with hydrogen peroxide. Rinse produce thoroughly with water before eating.

- *Use Lemon* The juice of a lemon is quite acidic and, like vinegar, can act as a sanitizer on surfaces. Slice a lemon in half and rub the cut side over the surface of a cutting board, chopping block, or inside of a sink. Another option is to dip the cut side of the lemon in

good to know: ABOUT DISINFECTING & DEODORIZING

— Sponges can harbor millions of bacteria, and it is very difficult to get them really clean. One approach to sanitizing a sponge is to wet it thoroughly and then microwave on high power for two minutes. (Caution: The sponge will be very hot.) Use cellulose sponges rather than synthetic ones, which may be infused with harmful chemicals and may release harmful chemicals when heated.

— A better alternative to sponges is to buy a large supply of inexpensive cotton dishcloths. Use one for a day and then launder.

— In the kitchen, designate a cutting board specifically for meat. Use different boards for cutting vegetables, fruits, and so on. Research comparing plastic with wooden cutting boards has shown that wooden boards, especially those made of maple and other tightly grained hardwoods, harbor fewer bacteria than plastic. No matter what type of cutting board you use, don't give bacteria a chance to multiply. Sanitize and wash cutting boards thoroughly as soon after using them as possible.

— Scrub the sink—and the drain strainer or plug—before washing produce in it.

— Ventilate bath and laundry rooms to discourage mold and mildew.

— In kitchens and bathrooms, either run an exhaust fan frequently or open windows periodically to let in fresh air.

— Invest in a good dehumidifier to keep basements dry, especially during humid summers.

— Many houseplants are natural indoor air fresheners.

kosher salt (salt also inhibits bacteria) and scrub briskly with the salt-lemon juice mix. Rinse and let air-dry.

- **Sanitize the Toilet Bowl** Vinegar, a solution of acetic acid, has notable antimicrobial properties. Use it to sanitize surfaces, including the toilet bowl. Pour 2 to 3 cups of white distilled vinegar all around the bowl and under the rim. Let stand 30 minutes. Alternatively, follow vinegar with baking soda (see page 241).

- **Inhibit Mold** Spray mold with undiluted white distilled vinegar—it will inhibit but not necessarily banish it. Alternatively, spray with a solution of tea tree oil (about 1 teaspoon oil to 1 cup water) or hydrogen peroxide (¼ to ½ cup hydrogen peroxide to about 1 cup of water). Here again, give lemon a try. Spray undiluted lemon juice on mold. Let sit for ten minutes and then scrub with a handful of kosher salt. Let sit another few minutes and rinse well.

- **Freshen Drains** Add enough water to several tablespoons of baking soda to make a thick paste. Scoop up some of this paste with an old toothbrush and use it to scrub the metal rim of sink drains, where bacteria can collect. To freshen the drain itself, combine 1 cup fine table salt (or popcorn salt), 1 cup baking soda, and ¼ cup cream of tartar and store in a glass jar with a tight lid. Every week, pour ¼ cup of this mixture down each drain in your house. Let it sit for 10 to 15 minutes, then flush with hot water.

▶ | DEODORIZING

If you've ever hung clothes out to dry on a clothesline (a great energy-saving alternative to using the dryer), you know what "clean" smells like: intensely fresh and naturally deodorized, thanks to the power of air and sunshine. If only our homes could smell like that all the time! But odors often inhabit our indoor spaces. Sometimes the solution is simply to open the windows and let a cleansing breeze blow through. When that's not practical, skip the commercial air freshening sprays and solids. They only

BATHROOM-FRESHENING SPRAY

Keep a small spray bottle of this mixture in the bathroom to help banish unpleasant odors:

½ cup white distilled vinegar
1½ cups water
10 to 15 drops of lavender, cinnamon, lemon, or any other pure essential oil (a mixture is fine too)

Mix all the ingredients in a glass jar with a tight-fitting lid. Put about half of the mix in a small, attractive spray bottle or atomizer to keep in the bathroom (label it "air freshener" so guests will know what it is).

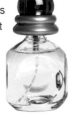

mask odors and add many harmful chemicals to the air. Instead, reach for these safe, natural solutions.

Odor Eaters

- **Reduce Carpet Odor** Sprinkle baking soda liberally onto carpets that smell less than fresh. Leave on for 30 minutes, and then vacuum thoroughly to remove the powder (empty vacuum canister or bags frequently).

- **Soak Up Odors** Place an open box of baking soda in the refrigerator to absorb odors. Replace every three months. To clean and deodorize refrigerator shelves and drawers, mix up a 1:1 solution of white distilled vinegar and water in a spray bottle. Spray liberally and wipe dry.

- **Zap Smells** Place an open bowl of vinegar in a room to banish odors quickly.

- **Use Coffee Grounds** To deodorize a freezer, fill an old stocking or a muslin bag with dry, used coffee grounds and place inside for several days. Use this to deodorize closets too.

- **Deodorize With Vodka** Vodka can work as an effective natural air freshener. Put some in a spray bottle and spritz lightly in the vicinity of odors. You can add a few drops of your favorite essential oil, such as lavender, if you want to actually add a scent.

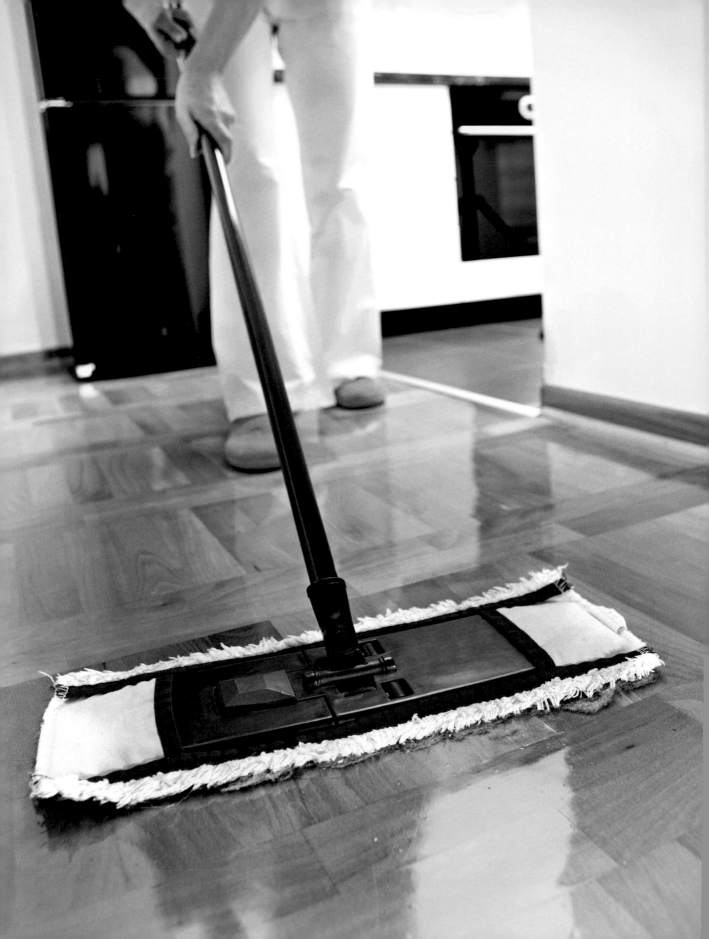

Floors & Furniture

12 MEASURES FOR BETTER MOPPING

Cleaning floors—whether stone, tile, wood, or carpeted—has to be one of the most tedious of all housecleaning tasks. So it's not surprising that new floor-cleaning products are constantly hitting the market, promising "easier," "faster," and "sparkling clean." Yet, like promises associated with other commercial cleaning products, all this hype comes with a catch. Most conventional floor and carpet cleaners are a stew of potentially toxic chemicals. Their "fresh" synthetic scents mask the true and nasty nature of what we're spritzing, swabbing, and sprinkling across the open expanses of our houses where babies crawl, children sprawl, and pets roll and scamper.

Traditional furniture dusting and polishing has given way in many homes to running a chemically saturated, disposable cloth over every surface where dust collects. You expose yourself and members of your household to toxic compounds (many labels don't even reveal what the ingredients are), and the cloths aren't reusable and end up in landfills. Many furniture polishes and dusting sprays contain nerve-damaging petroleum distillates. Some also contain formaldehyde, a known carcinogen. Because many of these products come as aerosol sprays, it's almost impossible to use them without inhaling some of those unhealthy substances.

▶ FLOORS & CARPETS

What do you require to safely clean floors and carpets? Despite what manufacturers might say about needing all sorts of special cleaners for the job, the fact is that a handful of natural safe cleaning agents will do. Start with a good broom or dust mop and a high-quality vacuum cleaner. A first step to making floor cleaning easier is to avoid letting floors get really dirty in the first place. Position a doormat at every entrance and don't be embarrassed to ask visitors to remove their shoes—it's your house, after all! Sweep, dust-mop, and vacuum on a regular basis—do it every few days if you or family members have pets—or allergies. When more thorough cleaning is needed, reach for the following "green" cleaners made with simple, inexpensive ingredients.

good to know: ABOUT FLOORS & FURNITURE

- Don't use oil soaps, wax cleaners, or products that promise they will leave a shine on any floor. They coat the floor, leaving a residue that builds up over time.
- Never use anything abrasive—steel wool, coarse scrubbie pads, or scouring powders—to clean any type of flooring (even ceramic tile), as it may permanently scratch the surface.
- To remove scuff marks on most types of floors, sprinkle on a little baking soda and use a damp cloth to gently rub away the marks.
- Old T-shirts (cut up to remove hems and seams) or old diapers make wonderful dusting cloths.
- Use a lot of cloths as you dust. To keep from simply spreading dirt around, reach for a clean one as soon as the one you're using shows an accumulation of dirt.
- Avoid feather dusters, no matter how pretty they are. They stir up dust rather than collect it, and some have quills that can scratch wood.

Floor Lore

- *Use Gentle Soap on Sealed Wood* If your wood floor has a surface finish (polyurethane is probably most common, but some wood floors are also sealed with varnish, epoxy, and acrylic coatings), use a damp mop and a gentle dishwashing detergent solution—about ¼

cup liquid detergent to a gallon of warm water. (Look for natural dishwashing liquids usually available at health food stores, rather than buying petroleum-derived detergents.) Too much water will cause wood to swell and warp, so be sure to use a mop that is barely wet. When finished, buff the floor dry with a towel by wrapping a towel around the head of the mop and securing with rubber bands.

- *Use the Same Technique for Tile* Use a damp mop on ceramic tile floors with the same gentle mixture of mild detergent and water noted previously. Mop a second time with water only and then towel-dry the floor.
- *Use Citrus for Oiled Wood* If your wood floor has been sealed with a penetrating oil, such as tung or linseed oil, clean with a natural citrus solvent made from citrus (orange) peel oil and a small amount of water. Look for this product online; it may also be sold at some paint stores as a natural alternative to mineral spirits. Read labels carefully.

- *Use Vinegar for Vinyl* For vinyl floors as well as cork and real linoleum, first use a damp mop with the mild detergent and water solution (provided previously). Follow this by using a damp mop with a dilute white vinegar solution—½ cup white distilled vinegar to 1 gallon warm water—to rinse and add a little shine.

- *Uncork the Club Soda* As a quick alternative for cleaning vinyl and linoleum floors, try club soda. The cleaning action is due to the slightly alkaline mineral salts in the liquid. Simply pour some into a spray bottle, spritz onto the floor, and damp-mop. Club soda can help remove stains from vinyl floors as well. Pour some over the stain, let sit a moment, and rub gently with a soft cloth.

- *Clean Carpets With Steam* Wall-to-wall carpeting is ubiquitous in many modern homes, and has the great advantage, compared to hard-surfaced floors, of being quiet. But it also traps dirt and animal dander, and provides a perfect home for dust mites. Synthetic carpeting and carpet pads are a source of toxic chemicals; even all-wool carpeting is typically treated with pesticides to kill moths. Ridding the house of carpeting is rarely practical, however. The best option to clean installed carpeting is to use steam. If you hire a commercial cleaner, insist that they steam-clean using a detergent that is without fragrance and that doesn't contain antibacterial substances of any kind. Or rent a steam cleaner and do it yourself using a small amount of natural, fragrance-free liquid detergent (available in natural food stores or online).

▶ | FURNITURE

Have you ever arrived at a party where you were greeted by the hosts at the door—along with the unmistakable and lingering smell of furniture

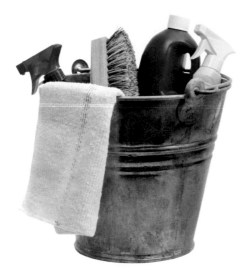

Dust Busters

- **Remove Dust** Naturally clean wood furniture begins with removing dust from the surface. Enhance the dust-attracting power of your dust cloths (pure wool or soft, 100 percent cotton work best) with this simple recipe: Mix 2 tablespoons lemon juice, 10 drops real lemon essential oil, and 2 to 3 drops of pure jojoba oil in a small spray bottle. Shake the ingredients until well mixed. Mist a cloth lightly (one squirt) and dust exposed wood surfaces. Make a fresh batch every time you dust, as this solution does not keep well.

- **Make a Simple Polish** An effective furniture polish can be made by mixing ¼ cup white distilled vinegar with a few drops jojoba oil. To tone down the strong vinegar smell (don't worry, it will disappear), add 2 to 3 drops of your favorite essential oil, such as lavender or lemon. Mix well in a spray bottle and spray onto a soft cloth. Apply to wood surfaces, work in well, and buff to a shine with a second clean cloth.

- **Shine With Wax** If you really want to make furniture glow, natural wax helps provide a lustrous natural sheen. Use the recipe below.

polish? It's a familiar odor that's been described as "lemon with a touch of engine oil." Most commercial brands of furniture polish are replete with petroleum distillates and solvents that are not only flammable but also toxic to animal nervous systems (think you and your pets). Say goodbye to those products and replace them with simple, natural alternatives. If you like, you can still have a lemony fragrance, but it will come from natural essential oils.

good to know: ABOUT CLEANING PRODUCTS

- Jojoba oil (actually a liquid wax) has the advantage when used in cleaning products of never going rancid. If jojoba isn't an option, replace with olive oil—but choose a lower grade as you don't need to use extra virgin olive on your furniture.
- Don't throw commercial cleaning products you've decided to stop using into the trash. Take them to a recycling center that handles petrochemicals and similarly toxic compounds.

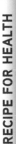

RECIPE FOR HEALTH

FURNITURE-POLISHING WAX

Courtesy of Annie B. Bond, *Better Basics for the Home:*

2½ ounces jojoba or olive oil

1½ ounces coconut oil

1 ounce pure beeswax

1 ounce carnauba wax

4 ounces distilled water

10 drops lemon essential oil

Warm the oils and waxes in a double boiler over medium to low heat until completely melted. Alternatively, warm in a microwave-safe bowl, heating for 10 to 15 seconds and then stirring; repeat in this fashion until waxes are melted. When waxes and oil are melted and warm, slowly add the water. Beat the mixture with an electric hand mixer until the ingredients emulsify and turn thick and creamy. Add the essential oil and blend well. Store in the refrigerator in a glass jar with a tight-fitting lid. To use, put a dab of the cream on a soft cloth and rub into the wood surface, using circular motions until the oils have been absorbed. Buff to a lustrous gloss with a second soft cloth.

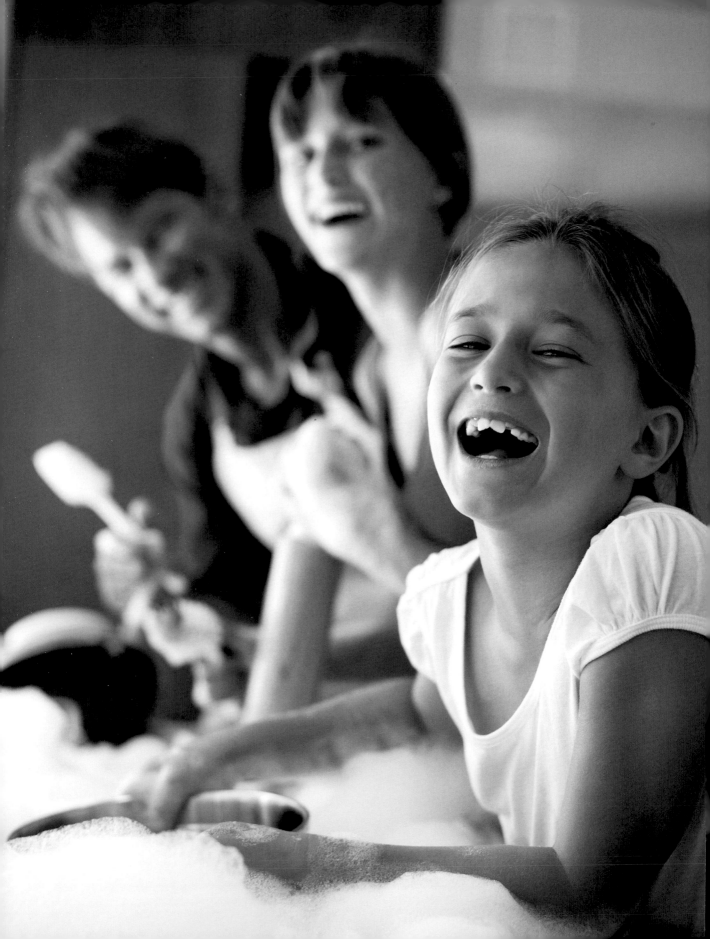

Healthy Household Cleaners

12 BREATHABLE CLEANING SOLUTIONS

Take a look at the cleaning products you've got stuffed under the kitchen or bathroom sink. Do you have a different spray or scrub or squirtable cleaner for each surface, from countertops and tile to mirrors and shower doors? If you believe the smiling models in television ads, you might think you need all those aids to degrease, shine, scour, scrub, and otherwise rid your home of grime. But reading the labels on these products might give you pause. Many contain petroleum-derived solvents and chemicals linked to a host of illnesses. In using them, you may be getting rid of dirt, but at the risk of contaminating the environment and maybe even harming your health.

Several generations ago, houses were most likely as clean as houses are today. But the average homeowner's arsenal of cleaning supplies probably consisted of just a half dozen natural dirt-defying agents, including baking soda, washing soda, simple soaps, vinegar, and borax. Alone or in combination, straight or diluted, this handful of natural cleaners was enough to handle almost any dirty job. They still are. You can use these time-tested standbys to make effective homemade cleaners. They are environmentally friendlier than most commercially formulated products, and in most cases, quite a bit cheaper, too.

▶ CLEANING SURFACES

Dirty windows. Greasy countertops. Scum-fogged shower doors. Imagine cleaning all these things and more with simple pantry staples. One of the best—and safest—household cleaning agents for many jobs is vinegar (a solution of acetic acid). White distilled vinegar removes grime, inhibits bacteria and mildew, helps banish odors, and can make windows sparkle. Almost as versatile is baking soda, aka sodium bicarbonate, the same alkaline white powder that makes biscuits rise. Baking soda can be

put to work shining faucets and fixtures, cleaning porcelain and tile, removing scum, helping dissolve away baked-on foods, and absorbing odors. When baking soda and vinegar combine, a foaming chemical reaction occurs, one that can be harnessed to clean toilet bowls and stinky drains.

On the Surface

- ***Wipe It Down*** Thanks to its acidic nature, vinegar dissolves grimy dirt, soap scum, and hard-water deposits. For a simple all-purpose cleaner, combine equal parts white distilled vinegar and water in a quart spray bottle (use less vinegar and more water for a milder solution). Use vinegar and water to clean countertops (except marble), stove tops and backsplashes, ceramic tile, and porcelain. (Vinegar has a sharp odor, but the odor dissipates very quickly as it dries.)

⚠ **CAUTION:** Do not use vinegar on marble, as it will permanently etch (dull) the surface.

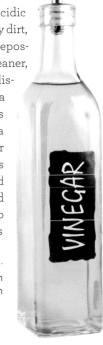

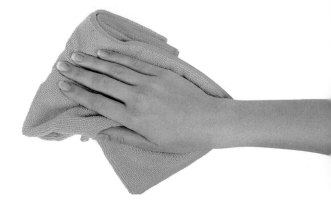

- **Make It Shine** A mixture of equal parts vinegar and water is also an effective window cleaner, one that cleans without streaking. To help cut through greasy dirt on glass (more likely to be found on the inside of windows due to a buildup of airborne grease from cooking), mix in one drop of a simple, natural liquid detergent into the vinegar and water mix. Shake well, spray on windows, and wipe clean with soft cotton or linen rags.

- **Dissolve Deposits** Dissolve hard-water deposits with undiluted vinegar. Soak a cleaning rag in vinegar, wring it out, and wrap around the base of a faucet, where such deposits typically form. Remove after a few minutes and the deposits should easily scrub away. For hard-water deposits that threaten to clog the holes in showerheads, pour ¼ to ½ cup vinegar in a plastic bag, wrap around the showerhead so the showerhead holes are submerged, and attach securely with rubber bands. Leave on for an hour or two. Remove and scrub the showerhead with a stiff bristle brush. Be sure to protect your eyes from spatters while scrubbing.

- **Beat Oven Grime** If your oven isn't self-cleaning, sprinkle a thick layer of baking soda on the bottom to clean baked-on spills and splatters. Spray with water until the powder is saturated. Fill a bowl with very hot water, set it on an oven rack, and close the oven door. Replace the hot water every hour and re-dampen the baking soda by spraying with water. After eight to ten hours, wipe out the baking soda—along with the oven grime. Rinse well to remove all the soda.

- **Combine Vinegar and Baking Soda** When acidic vinegar meets alkaline soda, a chemical reaction takes place in which the two substances neutralize each other; as they do, bubbles of carbon dioxide are released. In short, you get foam! Try this trick for cleaning the toilet bowl: Pour a bucket of water into the toilet to force water out of the bowl and expose most of the interior. Drizzle undiluted white vinegar all around the bowl and under the rim (use 2 to 3 cups). Let sit for a few minutes. Then sprinkle in about 1 cup of baking soda. The mixture will foam vigorously. Use a toilet brush to scrub the interior with the foam, and then rinse away.

RECIPE FOR HEALTH

TOUGH JOB CLEANER

Courtesy of Annie B. Bond, from *Better Basics for the Home,* this recipe for cleaner will remove most types of common dirt and grime. Washing soda (sodium carbonate) is a stronger cousin of baking soda. Borax (sodium borate decahydrate) also forms a strong alkaline solution when mixed with water. ⚠ **CAUTION:** Washing soda and borax can irritate skin, eyes, and—if inhaled—lungs. Wear rubber gloves when using this cleaner, and protect your eyes from splashes. Keep out of the reach of children.

½ teaspoon washing soda
2 teaspoons borax
½ teaspoon castile soap
2 cups hot water

Put the first three ingredients into a spray bottle. Add the hot water, screw on the top, and shake until well mixed. Test in an inconspicuous place before spraying over a large surface area. Do NOT use this cleaner on fiberglass or aluminum. Spray and wipe off with a soft cloth.

- **Clean a Drain** Put the vinegar and soda reaction to work to clean sink drains. Pour about ¼ cup baking soda into the drain, and then slowly drizzle in about the same amount of vinegar to create foam. After the bubbling has subsided, flush with hot water.
- **Use Ashes** The glass front on wood-burning stoves can turn dark from creosote and soot. Don't use commercial oven cleaner to remove this, as some stove manufacturers might suggest. Instead, when the stove is cold, don a pair of rubber gloves and grab a few paper towels. Dampen a paper towel in water and dip it into some of the fine ash in the stove. Smear the wet ash onto the glass and rub gently. Repeat with more ash until the glass is clear. (When ashes mix with water, an alkaline substance called lye is formed.) When the glass is clean, spritz it with vinegar and water solution to neutralize, and wipe dry.

▶ | SINKS & TUBS

Many commercial scouring powders (and other products) contain chlorine bleach. Bleach whitens effectively and also kills bacteria, but combining it with other cleaners can be dangerous. When vinegar and bleach combine, for instance, toxic chlorine gas is formed; when ammonia (a very alkaline cleaner) and bleach combine, toxic chloramine gas is released. Replace chlorine bleach–containing cleansers with natural versions you can make at home.

Homemade Helpers

- **Scrub With Soda** Baking soda is mildly abrasive. Use it like cleanser; just sprinkle it on a damp rag to clean tubs and sinks.
- **Mix Soda and Soap** Enhance a basic baking soda scrub by adding a natural soap to help cut greasy residues. Add enough liquid castile soap or scent-free natural liquid detergent to a cup of baking soda to make a thick paste (about the consistency of frosting). Store in a glass jar with a tight-fitting lid. Scoop out enough for an area and scrub gently with a soft cloth.
- **Go With Borax** Borax has a more powerful cleaning action than baking soda, with the advantage that it cleans mildew. Sprinkle borax onto shower stalls, sinks, and bathtubs, and rub with a damp rag. (Always wear rubber gloves when using borax.)
- **Try Feldspar** If you need a cleanser with a little more grit than baking soda can provide, look for a natural, commercial brand made of finely ground feldspar (a natural mineral), baking soda (sodium bicarbonate), and washing soda (sodium carbonate).

---

good to know: ABOUT HOUSEHOLD CLEANERS

- If you run out of vinegar, you can wash windows with club soda. Put some in a spray bottle, spritz, and wipe. The alkaline mineral salts in the soda help loosen dirt.
- To banish cooking smells in a room, place a bowl of vinegar on the counter or a table for several hours. Or saturate a dish towel in vinegar, wring out hard, and whirl the towel through the air for a few minutes. Great for removing the smell of burned toast!
- Place a dish or open box of baking soda inside the refrigerator to absorb odors. Replace every month or two.
- Pure cellulose sponges are a better choice than those made from polyurethane foam. Cellulose sponges are made from wood pulp, a by-product of the logging industry; they are biodegradable. Synthetic polyurethane foam sponges are made using petrochemicals and can emit formaldehyde (a known carcinogen). Avoid any sponge labeled as "antibacterial"—it probably contains the environmentally harmful antimicrobial triclosan.
- Keep all cleaning solutions and cleansers out of the reach of children, on a high shelf or in a locked cabinet.

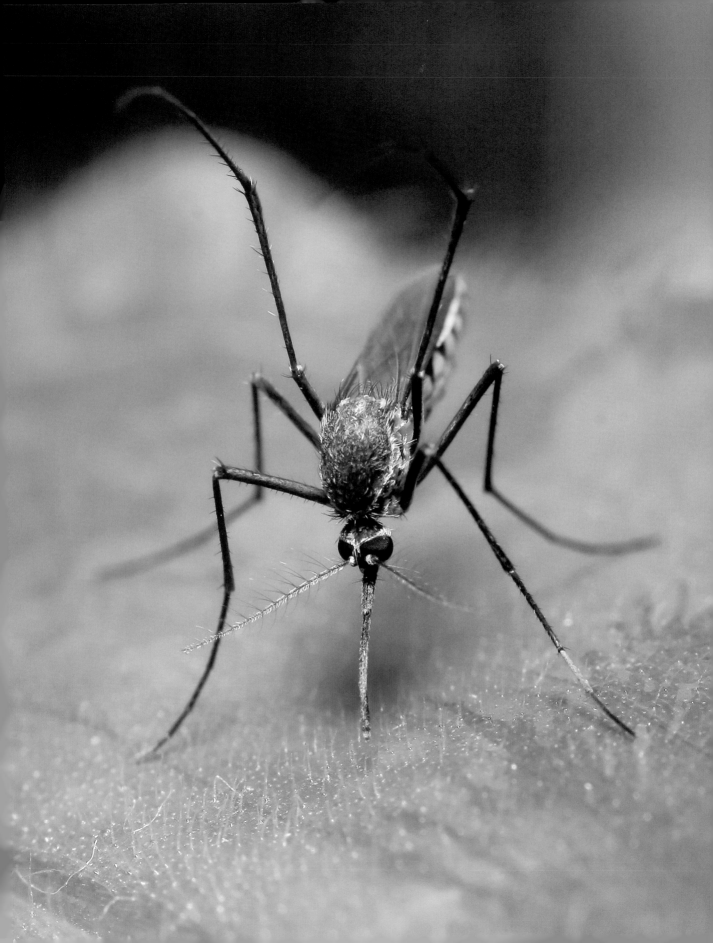

Insect Control
14 PEST CONTROL POINTERS

Take a lazy summer day, add a welcoming hammock and an irresistible book, and you've got the makings of a perfect afternoon—until a high-pitched whine announces the mosquitoes have arrived. Earth is home to anywhere from four million to six million different kinds of insects. Most of them are remarkably beneficial, but some are mighty pesky pests. Mosquitoes, gnats, and biting flies can make time spent outdoors unpleasant. Moths and silverfish can gnaw holes in clothes, whereas ants and roaches can invade the pantry. And out in the garden, small armies of grasshoppers, aphids, bugs, and beetles can munch through beautiful blooms or an entire crop of vegetables in no time at all.

When insect pests invade our personal spaces, a first impulse may be to reach for chemical repellents to keep them at bay or powerful insecticides to kill them. The problem is, most conventional insect repellents come with serious risks, and some insecticides are almost as poisonous to people as they are to pests. What's more, many insecticides aren't very selective. You may get rid of a pest by using an insecticide, but you'll likely kill helpful species at the same time. Why spray or scatter toxins in your home and garden—or apply them to your skin—when there are natural, safe solutions to control annoying and damaging insect pests?

▶ | INSECT REPELLENTS

Biting, swarming, and buzzing insects can be more than an annoyance in some places. In parts of North America, for instance, mosquitoes transmit West Nile virus and the rare but often fatal eastern equine encephalitis. Most conventional insect repellents contain a substance called N,N-diethyl-m-toluamide, or DEET for short. DEET repels insects, especially mosquitoes, very effectively. But it can irritate eyes and skin, and there's some evidence DEET may cause neurological problems, including seizures. DEET-containing insect repellents have their place (see page 244). But where disease transmission isn't a threat, natural repellents may be all you need.

Shoo Fly Shoo

- ***Wash and Go*** Many natural plant essential oils make reasonably good insect repellents. You can make a simple insect-repelling hand and body wash by adding 10 to 15 drops of lemon balm, rose geranium, or lavender essential oil to roughly 2 tablespoons of liquid castile soap. Wash exposed areas of skin with some of this soap mixture (rinse off and dry) before heading outdoors.

⚠ **CAUTION:** Never apply undiluted essential oils directly to skin, as they can burn and irritate.

- ***Make a Rub*** In a small jar, thoroughly mix together about 20 drops of an essential oil such as lavender, thyme, lemongrass, or peppermint, 2 tablespoons almond oil, and 2 to 3 teaspoons aloe vera gel. Wet your fingertips with some of this mixture and apply lightly to exposed skin or to cuffs, collars, and other areas of clothing adjacent to bare skin where biting insects might be tempted to land.

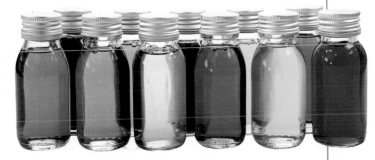

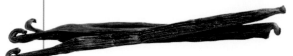

- *Back Off, Blackflies!* If blackflies are a problem, mix 10 to 15 drops cinnamon essential oil with ½ cup grapeseed oil and ¾ cup filtered water in a plastic spray bottle. Mix well. Mist this mixture lightly onto clothing (avoid face and eyes) or squirt a little into your hand and then dab onto exposed skin.

- *Shoo and Soothe* Natural witch hazel mixed with a few drops of a plant essential oil can make a repellent that both keeps insects away and soothes insect bites. Try mixing about 10 to 15 drops of essential oil (thyme oil is quite effective for repelling mosquitoes) with about 2 tablespoons real witch hazel extract. Dab onto clothing or exposed skin.

- *Try Vanilla for Gnats* An old folk remedy for keeping biting gnats at bay is to dab pure vanilla extract onto skin.

▶ | IN YOUR HOME

Insects find their way into our homes no matter how tidy we try to be. They squeeze in around window frames and slip through cracks in foundations. They follow us inside when we open doors and hitch rides on clothing and shoes. And once inside, there are lots of places to hide. Many household insects are fairly easily controlled with simple concoctions made from ingredients you can find at grocery and natural food stores.

Pest Patrol

- *Drive Away Moths* Clothes moths produce caterpillar-like larvae with a taste for wool. For generations, the go-to moth repellent was mothballs. They contain naphthalene, a possible carcinogen known to harm blood cells and cause liver and neurological damage. If you see signs of clothes moths, hang items

MOTH-AWAY SACHETS

There are a number of herbs that clothes moths appear to dislike. Try this combination to make small sachets that you can hang in closets and slip into drawers:

¼ cup dried mint leaf
¼ cup dried rosemary
2 tablespoons dried thyme
2 tablespoons dried lavender
1 cup whole cloves

In a small bowl, mix all the ingredients until well blended. Divide the mixture into ten roughly equal portions. Place each portion in a small muslin tea or sachet bag (available at natural food and some craft stores) and tie securely shut. Place where needed. Replace every three months with fresh dried herbs.

good to know: ABOUT NATURAL PEST CONTROL

— Wear long pants and long-sleeved shirts to minimize the amount of skin exposed to biting or stinging insects.

— In areas where disease-carrying mosquitoes or other insects are a threat, you must weigh the risk of using DEET repellents versus potentially being bitten. If you do choose to use DEET, opt for the lowest concentration you can find. Use as little repellent as possible, and consider applying it to clothing instead of skin. ⚠ CAUTION: Read labels on DEET products carefully. Wash hands thoroughly after touching DEET repellents. Never apply them to children's hands or faces.

— Wash repellents, natural or otherwise, off your skin as soon as you come indoors.

— Food is a lure. To keep insect invaders to a minimum in your home, store unrefrigerated foods in sturdy containers with tight-fitting lids. Clean up spills and crumbs from countertops and wipe down greasy cooking areas with natural cleaners (see pages 239–241).

— If you need help distinguishing insect pests from their helpful cousins, visit your library to pick up insect identification guides.

— Don't kill spiders. They eat flies, ants, and other insect pests.

outside in the sun. Brush thoroughly, especially along seams. If possible, wash in hot water or have them dry-cleaned (choose cleaners that use environmentally friendly dry-cleaning processes). Alternatively, put in the freezer for several days. Once clothes are clean, keep moths away by suspending herbal sachets in closets and slipping into drawers (see recipe).

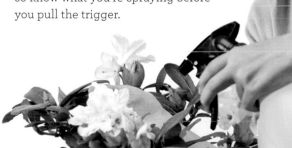

- **Dispatch Sugar-Eating Ants** Mix about 1 cup powdered (confectioners') sugar with 2 to 3 tablespoons borax. Distribute in small mounds along paths ants seem to be following, or put some in a small container with holes for access and place along the path.

⚠ **CAUTION:** Keep pets and small children away from this bait, as borax is harmful if ingested.

- **Make a Roach Trap** Put a few pieces of cut-up apple or potato inside a quart or pint canning jar (narrow neck types are best). Coat the inside of the jar's neck with petroleum jelly. Place the jar inside a cabinet where you've seen evidence of roaches. Attach one end of a piece of masking tape to the outside of the jar's top and the other end to the cabinet floor (this will give roaches a "ladder" to climb.) Attracted by the bait, roaches will climb the tape, fall into the jar, and not be able to get out. Check every morning, dispose of captives, and re-bait.
- **Drown 'Em** Pour a cup or two of boiling water down holes where you see ants coming out around your house's foundation. Alternatively, pour in a similar amount of white distilled vinegar or lemon juice.

▶ | IN YOUR GARDEN

Controlling pests in the garden is largely about getting to know who your enemies really are. It has been shown that only about 5 to 15 percent of the bugs and other insects in the average yard are pests. The rest are either neutral or helpful visitors or residents. Small-scale insect invasions can usually be handled by employing safe, natural controls.

Garden Gambits

- **Do a Quick Pick** Unless you have a very large garden, it's often possible to remove many insect pests by hand. Early in the morning, before insects have warmed enough to make a fast escape, walk among the plants. Take a small, lidded container with you. Look for signs of damage and pick or knock off culprits you spot into the container. Repeat daily.
- **Use a Hand Vacuum** You can vacuum small insect pests, such as sap-sucking aphids, from leaves with a hand vac. Use relatively low suction to avoid damaging the leaves.
- **Try a Jet Stream** A hard stream of water can dislodge many leaf-eating pests. True, this doesn't kill them. But the insects expend energy climbing back up again, and while on the move, they are exposed to their natural predators. Repeating this water treatment every morning will go a long way toward controlling an attack.
- **Spray On Soap** Ordinary liquid castile soap can be a powerful insecticide. Add about a tablespoon of liquid castile soap to a quart-size plastic spray bottle and fill with water. Shake well to mix. Spray on pests as needed. Note, however, that soap is not selective. It can potentially kill any insect, so know what you're spraying before you pull the trigger.

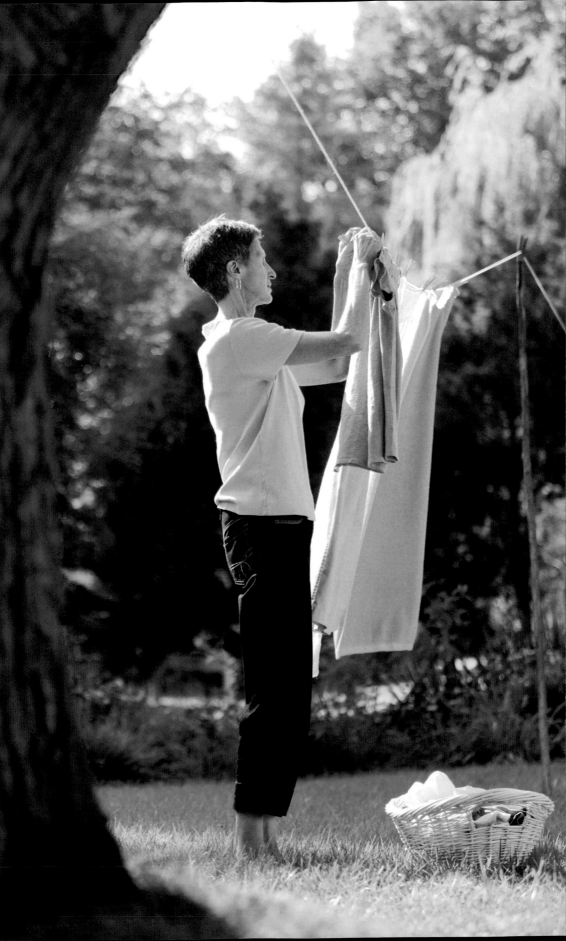

Laundry Care

14 NEW HABITS TO HANG ON THE LINE

Can you tell when your neighbors are doing laundry by the cloying smell of dryer sheet "perfume" wafting through the air? You might want to close your windows. Researchers at the University of Washington recently showed that air vented from dryers in which scented dryer sheets are tumbling around with the clothes contains hazardous chemicals, including some, such as benzene and acetaldehyde, that are classified as human carcinogens. Doing laundry may seem like a simple, albeit tedious, task. But its environmental impact is huge. Even using high-efficiency washing machines, washing clothes consumes enormous amounts of water and energy.

And the sudsy water that jets down the drain contains a lot more than dirt. Depending on the type of laundry detergents, bleaches, brighteners, softeners, and stain removers used, that wastewater likely contains a host of petrochemicals, synthetic fragrances, chemical whiteners, and other decidedly unnatural and unhealthful ingredients. Some of these chemical compounds, or the substances formed when they break down, are hormone disruptors, irritants, carcinogens, and neurotoxins. They can get into waterways and groundwater. The good news is that it's possible to clean clothes simply and safely, without polluting your home or the environment.

▶ | LAUNDERING

Just coming into contact with many commercial laundry products—before even using them—can pose health risks. Most laundry powders, for example, contain surfactants (chemicals that make surfaces absorb water to enhance cleaning) that can trigger contact dermatitis, respiratory irritation, eye irritation, and, if ingested, nausea, vomiting, and diarrhea. Synthetic fragrances are a source of hormone-disrupting phthalates, chemicals known to trigger asthma and other respiratory problems in some people. The components of synthetic fragrances are persistent, too. They hang around in the laundry room and can linger in clothes for weeks, which can lead to respiratory distress, headaches, and allergic reactions. Natural laundry solutions can go a long way toward reducing the amount of chemicals and toxins that you and your family come in contact with.

A Laundry List of Options

■ *Make the Switch* Nearly all modern laundry-cleaning products are detergents rather than soaps. (Soap consists of natural animal fats and/or plant oils combined with some form of lye, usually sodium hydroxide. Soaps contain natural surfactants, substances that lower the surface tension of water and make it easier for oils and dirt to be washed off fabric. Most common detergents are synthetic surfactants, many of which are derived from petroleum.) In general, soaps are better for the environment, and it is possible to make your own laundry soap (see recipe on next page). The problem is that in hard water, soap creates a scum known as soap curd that gets into fabric and can turn it gray (it's also what forms a ring around the tub). So, unless you have very soft water, your best bet is to swap detergents for more natural options that contain plant-derived rather than petroleum-derived

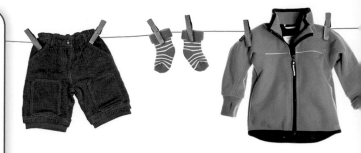

HOMEMADE LAUNDRY SOAP

1 cup shredded bar soap (for example,
   pure castile bar soap)
½ cup washing soda
½ cup borax

Shred the soap using a hand or box grater (the finer the pieces, the easier and faster they will dissolve in water.) Mix the grated soap, soda, and borax together thoroughly and store in a glass jar with a tight-fitting lid. Use about ¼ cup, depending on the size of the load (if too sudsy, use less). Use the hottest water possible in the wash cycle to help the soap dissolve well, but rinse in cold water to reduce sudsing. To lessen the chance of soap scum forming, add baking soda (about ¼ cup) to the water in the washing machine several minutes before adding soap and clothes.

surfactants. Natural food stores carry these healthier, safer laundry products. But read the labels carefully before you buy. Reputable brands will state specifically that the detergent contains natural surfactants that are plant derived (or "botanically" derived) and will often give the plant source.

■ *Choose Fragrance-Free* Some very hazardous chemicals lurk behind the innocuous word "fragrance" in commercial laundry powders and liquids. Some natural laundry detergents add natural scents, typically citrus or other essential oils. But even these can cause allergic reactions in some people. The safest approach is to choose fragrance-free products. Clean laundry doesn't need to smell anything other than clean.

■ *Avoid Dyes* Along with fragrance-free, look for "dye-free" on the label. A good natural detergent will state clearly that it contains no dyes.

■ *Look for Biodegradable* The synthetic surfactants, as well as other ingredients, in many commercial detergents tend to persist in the environment; in other words, they are not biodegradable. Good natural detergents contain biodegradable ingredients. Choose those that state they will biodegrade in less than a year.

▶ BOOSTERS & WHITENERS

Commercial detergents commonly add optical brighteners to their products to help make whites look whiter and bright colors look brighter. Yet studies show that some of these chemicals may cause skin irritation and allergies in some people, and can be toxic to fish and other aquatic organisms. There are simple steps you can take to help boost natural detergent's cleaning power to get "whiter and brighter" naturally.

Bright Ideas

■ *Presoak* Lemon juice has mild bleaching properties. To help brighten clothes, add one cup freshly squeezed lemon juice to ½ gallon water in a bucket. Let clothes soak in this solution overnight.

■ *Rinse With Lemon Juice* To whiten clothes during washing, add the juice of a large lemon (about ½ cup) to the rinse cycle. The whitening power of lemon juice tends to work best when clothes are exposed to sunlight, so this is a good option if you hang your washing outside to dry.

■ *Remove Odor* A natural approach to removing odors and stains from the underarms of shirts is to spray full-strength white distilled vinegar on the area a few minutes before washing. (Test in a small area when treating delicate or synthetic fabrics.)

- **Go With Minerals** For clothing that can be washed in very warm to hot water, try adding ¼ to ½ cup washing soda to the wash cycle, along with a natural detergent.

▶ SOFTENERS & DRYING AIDS

A static charge builds up when two dissimilar materials are rubbed together. When clothes tumble in the dryer (usually a combination of different kinds of fabrics), static can build up that makes clothes cling to each other or other surfaces. Commercial fabric softeners, either liquids or dryer sheets, promise soft clothes that are free of static cling. But both types of products contain chemicals known to be toxic after prolonged exposure. Prolonged exposure is almost a given when using commercial fabric softeners, because they are designed to stay in clothing for extended periods of time. Soften clothes safely with these natural solutions.

Soft & Sweet

- **Add Vinegar** White distilled vinegar helps remove detergent residue from clothing and makes an effective fabric softener substitute that will reduce static cling. Simply add ¼ cup undiluted white vinegar to the rinse cycle.
- **Substitute Soda** Baking soda also helps soften clothes during washing. Add ¼ cup during the rinse cycle. (Use either baking soda or vinegar, but not both; added together, they will neutralize each other.)
- **Try Natural Tumblers** Some companies have introduced knobby plastic balls as an alternative to dryer sheets. These plastic balls are not a safe substitution. They are typically made from polyvinyl chloride, a plastic that can release hormone-disrupting phthalates. Look for all-natural felted wool dryer balls that help separate clothing tumbling in the dryer without releasing toxic chemicals.
- **Look for Natural Fabric Softeners** Some of the same companies that manufacture natural, plant-derived laundry detergents have developed liquid fabric softeners that rely on plant ingredients and natural essential oils to soften clothing. Look for them in natural food stores.
- **Add Your Own Fragrance** If you love the idea of clothes coming out of the dryer with a nice fragrance, add a drop or two of pure lavender essential oil (or your favorite essential oil) to a square of cotton cloth and toss this into the dryer with wet clothes.

---

good to know: ABOUT LAUNDRY CARE

- Save energy by washing in cold water whenever possible, and hanging clothes outside in the sun to air-dry. One caution for line-drying: If you or family members have serious allergies, avoid line-drying (especially sheets and towels) during pollen season.
- If a piece of clothing isn't dirty but has picked up odors, perhaps from your having traveled or eaten in a restaurant, hang it outside to air out rather than washing it. Turn it inside out to prevent sunlight from fading the fabric.
- Save water by hand-washing small loads, using a natural, plant-based detergent.
- Get a good clothes brush or lint brush. Instead of washing clothes that have picked up dust, pet hair, or lint, brush them to take care of the problem.
- Always wash new clothing before wearing to remove the "new" smell. That smell likely comes from finishing agents such as wrinkle protectants, stain guards, and fire retardants. These treatments are chemical based, and some of the chemicals used are health hazards.

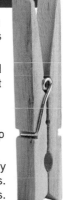

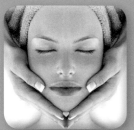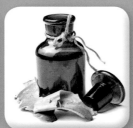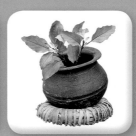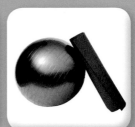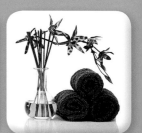

healing tr

aditions

Traditions

12 OF THE WORLD'S WISEST HEALING WAYS

If you've ever done yoga, had an acupuncture or acupressure treatment, or sat quietly trying to focus your attention on your breathing as a part of meditation, you've tapped into some of the world's oldest healing traditions. Compared to the modern medicine practiced in much of the Western world, many ancient healing systems, such as Ayurveda and traditional Chinese medicine have far deeper roots, stretching back millennia.

In these forms of traditional medicine, illness isn't viewed solely as the malfunctioning of cells, tissues, or organs, but as an imbalance in the vital, universal energy that flows through all living things. The path to health involves rebalancing this vital life force, which can be achieved through many means.

A Wealth of Health Practices

This chapter introduces you to a dozen of some of the most well-known and widely practiced healing traditions from around the world. Acupressure is an ancient traditional Chinese healing practice in which gentle but firm pressure is used to stimulate and balance the flow of vital energy. Aromatherapy involves using aromatic essential oils extracted primarily from plants to cleanse, enhance mood, and promote healing. Ayurveda, from the Indian subcontinent, is one of the oldest recorded

healing traditions and encompasses a complex system of diet and lifestyle, as well as exercise, the use of medicinal herbs, meditation, relaxation, and breathing techniques for cleansing and rejuvenating. Breath therapy—controlled, focused breathing—is integral to many healing traditions, often as part of meditation. Both hydrotherapy and massage are likely as

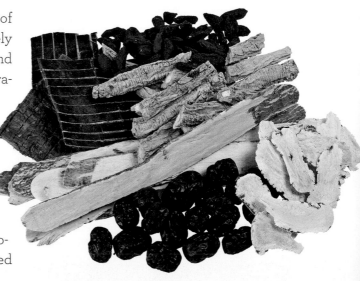

old as human culture, but became somewhat formalized as healing techniques over the past few centuries. Qigong (chee gung) is a healing form of exercise, one of several fundamental aspects of traditional Chinese medicine—like Ayurveda, one of the oldest extant healing traditions, practiced by millions of people worldwide.

Shiatsu is a Japanese-based form of therapeutic massage with roots in traditional Asian medicine, but developed relatively recently, in the early 20th century. Reflexology, too, is a fairly recent—and quite controversial—alternative approach to healing that came on the scene in the early 1900s. Finally, there is yoga. Familiar to many Americans as a therapeutic form of exercise and stress release, yoga is an ancient healing system that originated in India thousands of years ago.

Integrating Old & New

These healing traditions can all be loosely classified as alternative. Unlike conventional (Western) medicine, which is based on scientific evidence, alternative approaches to healing tend to be grounded in historical or cultural traditions. Because rigorous, well-designed scientific studies of alternative therapies are sparse, the effectiveness and safety of these approaches to healing are uncertain. The healing traditions touched upon in this chapter may have much to offer, but should never be used as a substitute for conventional medical treatment of any illness, injury, or disease.

THE ANCIENT ARTS OF HEALING

Long before there were modern drugs, operating rooms, and sophisticated diagnostic equipment, people around the globe sought to understand the cause of sickness looking to the heavens, the earth, and within for healing. Our ancestors developed a sophisticated understanding of plants used for medicine. Some of these gave rise to powerful modern medicines such as morphine, aspirin, digitalis, codeine, and quinine. For thousands of years, healers in what are now China and India prescribed acupuncture, herbal medicines, dietary interventions, massage, meditation, and physical exercises such as yoga, tai chi, and qigong to restore harmony in the sick and prevent disease in the healthy.

Many of these ancient approaches are being subjected to rigorous scientific evaluation, and a growing number of studies show that they can contribute to our health in meaningful ways. Meditation, focused breathing, and aromatherapy help calm and center us, reducing the negative effects of stress. Massage can relieve pain and ease anxiety; acupuncture is highly effective for a wide variety of conditions; and yoga, tai chi, and qigong provide a gentle form of exercise for both young and old. Alongside the wonders of modern medicine, which tends to focus primarily upon the body, these ancient systems attempt to treat the *whole person*—body, mind, and spirit.

Tieraona Low Dog, M.D.
Author, clinician, and educator on integrative medicine and native healing traditions

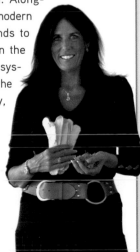

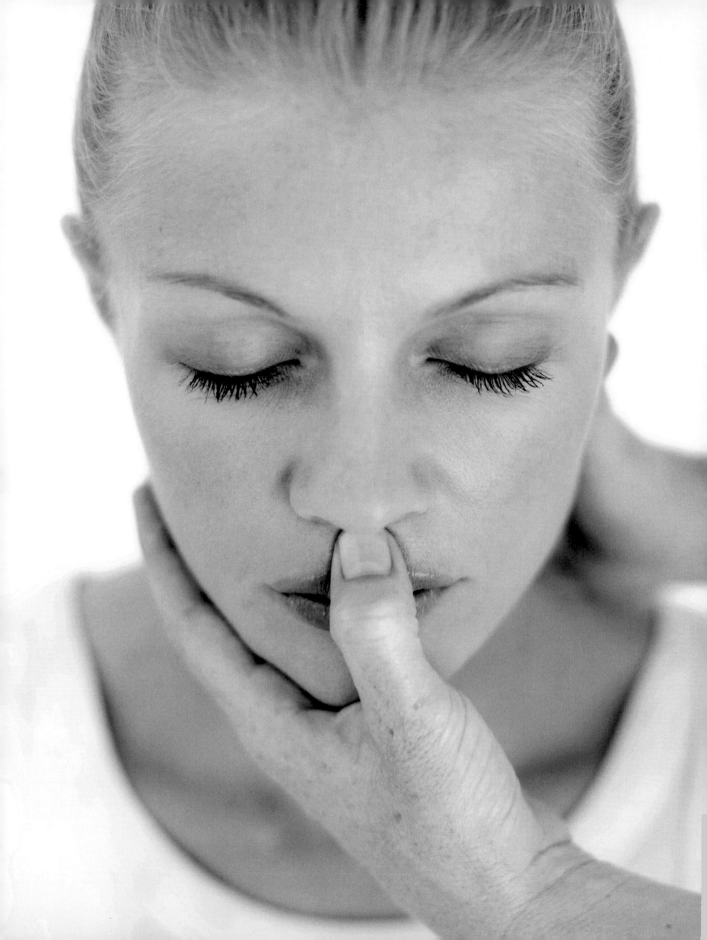

Acupressure

7 POINTS ON USING PRESSURE

Acupressure is an ancient traditional Chinese healing technique. It's similar to—and very likely predates—acupuncture, in which tiny needles are inserted into the skin at different points around the body. In acupressure, gentle, firm finger pressure is used instead of the needles. Both acupressure and acupuncture share the same goal: to stimulate and balance the flow of *qi* or *chi* (pronounced chee), believed by Chinese medical practitioners to be the body's own fundamental healing energy. Worldwide, many health care professionals recognize the use of acupressure and acupuncture for relieving pain and treating certain ailments, though the mechanism by which these therapies work is still subject to considerable scientific debate.

The idea of qi is a fundamental concept in traditional Chinese medicine. This life-sustaining energy is believed to flow along specific paths or channels in the body called meridians, almost like electricity flows along metal wires. In a healthy person, qi is thought to travel freely along the meridians to all the body's major organs and systems. When qi is inhibited or blocked, it becomes imbalanced, and illness results. Fundamental to acupressure is the belief that it's possible to change the flow of qi, and thereby help rebalance it, by applying pressure to places on the skin that overlie the meridians. In other words, pressing on key acupressure points can restore the free flow of qi along the meridians to the organs and body areas they connect, and thus help restore health.

As a supportive therapy, acupressure may offer some people relief from many everyday aches and pains, particularly those that involve muscles, tendons, ligaments, and other soft tissues. It may also help ease headaches, arthritis pain, sports injuries, constipation and other digestive problems, insomnia, poor circulation, tension, and stress. A limited number of clinical studies on the effects of acupressure indicate it may be a helpful addition to treatments for certain diseases and conditions. For example, in a recent study on patients with type-2 diabetes, acupressure—used in conjunction with hypnotherapy and meditation (see page 279)—helped reduce blood sugar levels after ten days. Other studies indicate that acupressure can be beneficial for easing pain, including menstrual pain, relieving nausea and vomiting in certain situations, such as following some types of surgery, and also for improving sleep. One of acupressure's great advantages as a natural remedy is that you can do it (at least to some extent) on yourself; the only tools needed are your hands. And because acupressure is not an invasive technique, it's usually safe for most conditions (see cautions on next page).

▶ | THE BASICS

In traditional Chinese medicine, 20 meridians are recognized; however, most acupressure work centers around 14 meridians along which are more than 300 acupressure points. Many acupressure remedies involve combining pressure points near the problem area with other points that don't seem to have any connection at all. According to the ancient philosophy behind the treatment, the meridians connect the points, allowing qi to flow between them. It's

RELIEVE HEADACHE PAIN

Using the thumb and forefinger of one hand, feel for a tender area in the slightly meaty area in the "webbing" between the thumb and forefinger of the other hand. When you've located it (you may be surprised at just how sensitive it is when you have a headache!), squeeze very firmly (enough to almost be painful, but not quite) with a slow, rhythmic pumping action—squeezing for one or two seconds, then releasing and repeating. After doing this on one hand for about a minute, switch to the other hand. Use in conjunction with other natural headache remedies (see pages 31–32) as desired.

⚠ **CAUTION:** Pregnant women should not use this technique.

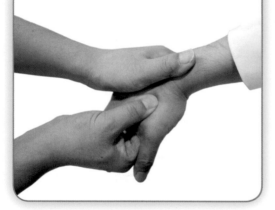

important to note that not all Western medical practitioners believe that there are energy meridians in the body. Some credit results of acupressure treatments to other, more tangible factors, such as improved circulation, release of muscle tension, and the possible stimulation of natural mood-affecting and pain-relieving substances in the body, such as endorphins. Interestingly, however, at least one study has shown a relationship between acupuncture points and meridians and planes of connective tissue that extend through parts of the body.

▶ | PUT INTO PRACTICE

Despite the fact that there are hundreds of acupressure points, it's possible to help relieve some common, everyday health complaints

yourself by utilizing just a few of them. These points are primarily in the hands, wrists, legs, feet, and on the face. To apply pressure to an acupressure point, use only your hands. In most cases, fingers are the easiest and most effective parts of the hand to use. But you may find that applying pressure with knuckles, thumbs, or the palm or heel of the hand works better for you. As a general guideline when performing acupressure, the amount of pressure you exert should be very firm but not painful. This can be a fine line, but use common sense; if it really hurts, you're pressing too hard.

It's also generally a good idea to go slowly. Begin with gentle pressure on an acupressure point and increase pressure gradually until it's quite firm. Hold the pressure constant for the recommended amount of time. Then gradually release it, taking about as long to ease off as you did to bear down. As you're performing the technique, remember to breathe and try to keep other parts of your body as relaxed as possible.

⚠ **CAUTION:** If you have cancer, arthritis, heart disease, or any chronic conditions, talk with your health care provider before trying any acupressure therapy. Because pressing on certain acupressure points can sometimes trigger uterine contractions, pregnant women should have acupressure performed only by a licensed practitioner and should not self-treat.

How to Press the Point

■ *Ease Motion Sickness* If motion-caused nausea strikes when you're on the water or in a vehicle, try one or all of these simple techniques. First (and easiest), simply grab your earlobes and gently but firmly pull down on them for a few seconds. Repeat several times. A second option: Using your index finger, press the indented spot directly above the "bow" in your lips (and beneath the septum of your nose). Hold firm pressure for 30 seconds, then release. Repeat every few minutes. Third, use your thumb to press on a spot on the center of the inside of your forearm about three finger-widths above the crease at your wrist. The spot is between the tendons (you'll feel them under the skin). Press firmly for

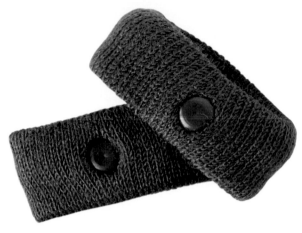

about 20 to 30 seconds. Release and wait for a minute, then repeat. Continue as long as needed. Combine any of these techniques with other natural remedies for motion sickness, such as eating ginger (see pages 95–96).

- **Try a Wrist Band** A number of commercial wrist bands are available, both in stores and online, that use the principles of acupressure as a treatment for nausea, air sickness, or morning sickness. These bands fit your wrist and lower arm snugly and have protruding buttons, usually made of plastic, that should be adjusted to press against the spot just above your wrist, as described in the previous paragraph. While you can target the pressure of your fingers and thumbs better, wrist bands (worn on one or both wrists) may be easier for long spans of time.

- **Relieve Headache and Neck Tension** Using either your thumbs or your index fingers, find the bony bumps just behind your ears on the back of your head (known medically as the mastoid processes). Press firmly into these bumps, holding for about 30 seconds. Release and repeat. Breathe slowly and evenly as you press and release; avoid holding your breath. This acupressure technique is also good for releasing tension in the neck, because the mastoid processes act as attachment points for several neck muscles.

- **Treat Constipation** As an adjunct to common natural remedies for constipation (see pages 28 and 92), place your index and middle fingers on the side (the outer side) of one of your legs, about three inches below the outer edge of the kneecap. Apply very firm pressure for five seconds, and then release. Wait a couple of breaths, and repeat. Do this five times on one leg, and then repeat the same procedure on the other leg.

- **Relax Wrists** If you work at a keyboard all day, your fingers, wrists, and lower arms can become stiff, cramped, and tense. Relieve this tension by placing your right index finger on the outside (top) surface of your lower left arm about two inches above the wrist crease and in between the two bones (the radius and ulna). Press firmly on that point for one or two minutes. Then switch arms.

- **Soothe Sore Feet** To relieve pain in your feet or toes, grip the webbing between your little toe and the toe next to it. Slide your fingers inward, until you feel a V or notch where bones come together. Within that notch is an acupressure point. Apply firm, steady pressure (the point will likely be quite sensitive) for one to two minutes, and then release. Repeat on the other foot (or do both feet simultaneously).

good to know: ABOUT ACUPRESSURE

- Avoid using acupressure points near an injury, serious skin irritations, or breaks in the skin, ulcerated sores, or varicose veins.
- People who have recently suffered a stroke should avoid acupressure treatments until given permission to do so by their medical doctor.
- Acupressure should never be substituted for medical consultation or advice or prescribed medical treatment.

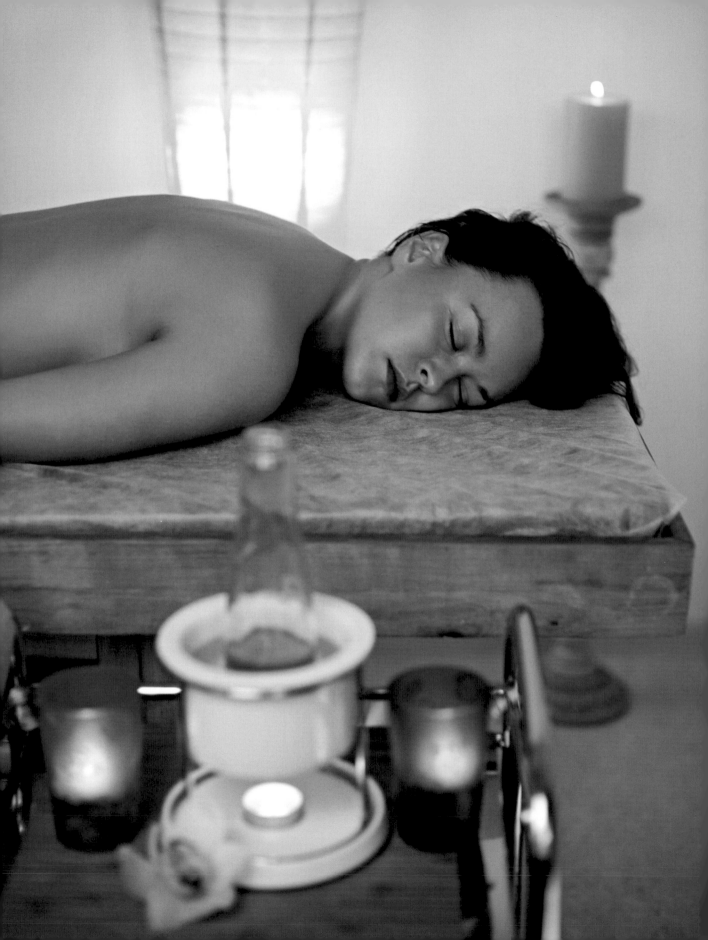

Aromatherapy

9 IDEAS FOR FOLLOWING YOUR NOSE

Hippocrates—the fifth-century B.C. Greek physician often called the father of Western medicine—is credited with saying that the way to health is to have an aromatic bath and a scented massage every day. For most of us, that sounds like a delightful luxury. Yet throughout most of recorded history, aromatic plants and their oils were revered for their healing, cleansing, and mood-enhancing properties. The use of aromatic essential oils for healing, known as aromatherapy, has ancient roots. The stylized paintings and hieroglyphics that decorate Egyptian tombs bear witness to the fact that aromatic plants, oils, and resins were so highly prized that they were offered as gifts to the gods and used to embalm the dead bound for the afterlife.

The most famous ancient Egyptian fragrance was called *kyphi,* which translates as "welcome to the gods." Egyptian high priests used plant oils in their role as healers to the pharaohs for treating nervous and mental conditions. Some of those oils came from India and China, where there is strong evidence to suggest they were employed therapeutically in those lands many centuries before the Egyptian pharaohs came to power.

The Greeks and Romans also held aromatic plant oils in high regard, attributing their heavenly scents to divine origins. In Arabia, the art of aromatics flourished. The Persian physician, philosopher, and alchemist Hakim Abu Ali Abdulah Husayn Ibn Sina (known in the West as Avicenna) improved on primitive distillation techniques and succeeded in producing remarkably pure plant essential oils around A.D. 1000. The production and use of essential oils spread throughout Europe during the Middle Ages and continued to grow in popularity during the Renaissance. By the 18th century, nearly every European herbalist and many physicians used essential oils as an integral part of their healing practice. For a while during the late 1800s and early 1900s, the development of synthetic drugs eclipsed the

259

AROMATHERAPY

good to know: ABOUT AROMATHERAPY

- Always follow recommendations about diluting essential oils with carrier oils. Sweet almond oil is one of the best carrier oils because it is neutral and nonallergenic for most people.
- Look for language indicating purity on bottles of essential oils. Ideally, a label should state that a product is a "pure plant essential oil." Be wary of phrases such as "perfume oil" and "fragrance oil" on a label—it's a clue the product is likely a synthetic oil; synthetic oils should not be used for therapeutic or aromatherapy applications. Purchase essential oils from well-known, reputable companies to avoid products that have been diluted with synthetic chemicals.
- Always store essential oils in a secure place where children cannot access them, in bottles with single-drop dispensers.

use of plant essential oils in medicine. But in the 1920s, French chemist René-Maurice Gattefossé revived interest through his scientific study of the oils' therapeutic properties. It was Gattefossé who originated the term *aromathérapie*, which became the title of his first book.

▶ | THE BASICS

The philosophy underlying aromatherapy is that plant essential oils can help restore health to the body and harmony to the mind. Essential oils are pure, concentrated extracts of aromatic plants, taken from a wide array of sources, including flower heads and petals, leaves, stalks, bark, seeds, gums, and resins. Making essential oils is no small task. It takes about 60,000 rose blossoms to produce a single ounce of rose essential oil, and an astounding 8 million handpicked jasmine blossoms—plucked in the early morning of the first day they open—to produce 2.2 pounds of jasmine oil. There are hundreds of essential oils in general use in the cosmetic, pharmaceutical, and perfume industries, and among professional aromatherapists. Each essential oil has a particular fragrance, a distinct chemical composition, and a unique set of physical and therapeutic properties. Essential oils are highly volatile (they evaporate quickly), and they exert their effect on the body in two fundamental ways. They can be inhaled to stimulate olfactory centers in the brain. And they can be absorbed through the skin. In their pure state, however, essential oils are too highly concentrated to be applied to skin directly; they are always diluted in a base, or carrier oil, so that they can be massaged into the skin in a safe manner and at a safe dose.

CLEAR SINUSES

3 drops rosemary oil
1 drop peppermint oil
1 drop eucalyptus oil
4 cups of boiling water

Place 3 drops rosemary, 1 drop peppermint, and 1 drop eucalyptus essential oil in a large heat-proof bowl on a table. Add 4 cups just-boiled water. Sit in a chair and drape a towel over your head and shoulders. Lean over the bowl and inhale a shallow sniff of the scented steam. If this feels good, continue inhaling, keeping your face at least 12 inches above the surface of the water. ⚠ **CAUTION:** People with asthma or reactive airway diseases, or who are allergic to rosemary, peppermint, or eucalyptus, should not do this. It is also not appropriate for children under the age of three.

▶ | PUT INTO PRACTICE

The practice of aromatherapy as a healing art is just that: an art that can take years of training and practice. However, you can access some of the therapeutic properties of essential oils by making simple aromatherapy treatments at home. You can use essential oils by adding them to bathwater, diffusing them into the air of a room, inhaling them in steam, mixing them into carrier oils for a massage, creating healing compresses, or making your own unique and natural perfume. And depending on the characteristics of the oils you choose, the results can be relaxing, soothing, stimulating, refreshing, energizing, and much more.

⚠ **CAUTION:** Never take essential oils internally; avoid getting them in your eyes. Do not use undiluted essential oil on bare skin; always dilute with a carrier oil when applying topically. Because most essential oils are derived from plants, they may cause sensitivity or allergic reactions in people who are sensitive or allergic to the plants from which the oils came.

Hints for Scents

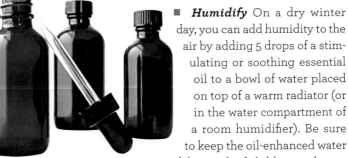

- **Refresh Tired Feet** Rejuvenate tired feet with an essential oil footbath. Pour 1 quart of warm water into a large bowl or plastic tub (large enough to accommodate both feet), then add 5 drops of peppermint essential oil, and disperse with your fingertips. Soak feet for ten minutes, periodically clenching and then extending your toes outward while underwater. Rosemary or thyme essential oil can be substituted for peppermint. For a soothing footbath for sore feet, use lavender oil.

- **De-stress in the Tub** While running a tub full of very warm water, add 5 to 10 drops of one of the following for a wonderfully relaxing soak: lavender, geranium, neroli, jasmine, or ylang-ylang. You can also use a combination of these oils, as long as you make sure the total number of drops doesn't exceed ten. If you're feeling indulgent, splurge on rose essential oil, which is one of the most expensive essential oils. Close the bathroom door to hold the fragrance in the room and soak in your aromatic tub for about 15 minutes.

- **Relieve a Headache** Mix 3 drops lavender oil and 2 drops peppermint oil in 1 ounce sweet almond or sesame oil and mix well. Massage the essential oil/carrier oil mixture around your temples (avoid the eye area) and the base of your skull for several minutes. Keep eyes closed and breathe deeply.

- **Ease an Aching Back** For mild lower back pain, combine 5 drops rosemary, 3 drops peppermint, and 2 drops chamomile essential oil with 2 teaspoons sweet almond or another carrier oil. Mix well. Use this oil to gently massage the lower back.

- **Make a Compress** Add 5 drops lavender or chamomile essential oil to 1 cup cool water. Saturate a small soft cloth in the solution, squeeze out excess, and lay over a blister, scrape, or sunburn to soothe irritation and soreness.

- **Humidify** On a dry winter day, you can add humidity to the air by adding 5 drops of a stimulating or soothing essential oil to a bowl of water placed on top of a warm radiator (or in the water compartment of a room humidifier). Be sure to keep the oil-enhanced water out of the reach of children and pets.

- **Scent a Room** In a plastic spray bottle, combine 10 drops lavender essential oil (or another oil you like) with about ½ cup water and 1 tablespoon vodka. Mix well. Mist a little of this mixture into the air to infuse the room with fragrance.

- **Create a Body Oil** Make your own scented body oil by adding 10 to 12 drops of your favorite essential oil to 2 tablespoons of a neutral carrier oil, such as sweet almond oil (this is a 2 percent solution). Store in a glass jar with a tight-fitting lid. Apply to damp skin after a shower or bath.

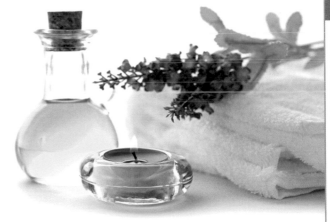

⚠ **CAUTION:** Always do a skin patch test first before using a particular essential oil or oil blend; apply a drop or two of a diluted essential oil on a small area of skin in an inconspicuous place (such as the inner arm) and watch for signs of allergic reaction over 24 hours. Certain essential oils, including but not limited to angelica, bergamot, lemon, lime, and orange, can induce or increase photosensitivity in skin. Do not use essential oils on babies or young children. If you are pregnant, consult your health care provider before using any essential oil.

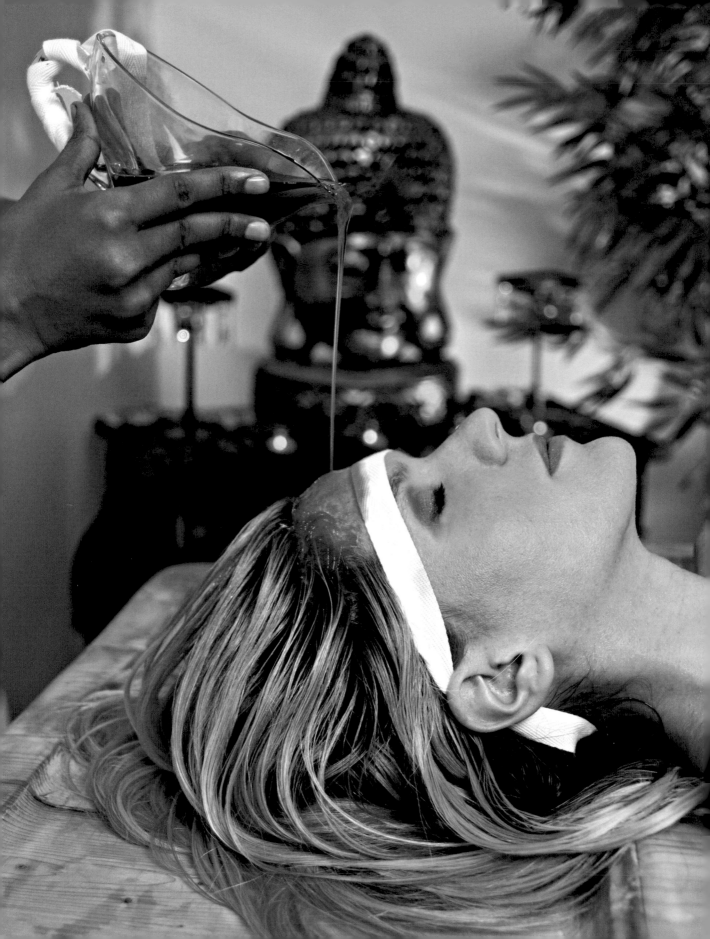

Ayurvedic Medicine

8 WAYS TO RESTORE LIFE'S BALANCE

I f you've ever watched an acrobat walking the high wire, you have seen balance made manifest. Eyes are focused. Breathing is controlled. Muscles are contracting and relaxing in harmony and with utter precision. And above all, the mind is completely aware of the body and its place in the space it occupies at that moment in time. Ayurvedic medicine, or simply Ayurveda, is all about balance. This ancient medical system aims to integrate and balance the body, mind, and spirit to promote wellness and prevent illness.

Ayurveda originated in India perhaps as long as 5,000 years ago. Along with traditional Chinese medicine (see pages 295–297), it is one of the world's most ancient medical systems. The name *Ayurveda* is a Sanskrit word meaning "the science of life and longevity." Ayurvedic practice predates written records, but roughly 2,000 years ago, the fundamental tenets of this "science of life" were recorded in two books: the *Charaka Samhita* and the *Sushruta Samhita*. Those books established the principles and goals of Ayurveda, which are to restore and maintain health by balancing the body's three fundamental life forces or energies—called *doshas*—and to create harmony between the mind, the body, and the universe.

▶ | THE BASICS

The doshas are known by their Sanskrit names: *vata, pitta,* and *kapha.* According to Ayurvedic teachings, vata, pitta, and kapha are present in every person (as well as everything else in the universe). Each person has a different mix of doshas, however; typically one is dominant, one secondary, and one less prominent. Just as each of us has a unique fingerprint, every individual according to Ayurveda has a unique "energy print," which is their particular balance of the three doshas. When this unique and innate balance of doshas becomes unbalanced—by stress, poor diet, bad habits, loss, anger, and countless other influences—physical, mental, or emotional illness can result. The key to healing in Ayurvedic medicine lies largely in rebalancing one's doshas.

good to know: ABOUT AYURVEDIC MEDICINE

— Ideally, choose an Ayurvedic practitioner who is also trained in Western medicine. If that's not possible, then coordinate Ayurvedic consultations with your regular health care provider.

— If you have an acute or chronic medical condition, consult your primary health care provider before making any changes to your treatment regimen.

— Be aware of the potential for contamination of some Ayurvedic herbal preparations. In a recent study, Boston University School of Medicine researchers found that nearly 21 percent of both U.S.-manufactured and Indian-manufactured Ayurvedic medicines purchased via the Internet contained detectable levels of lead, mercury, and/or arsenic that exceeded acceptable U.S. standards.

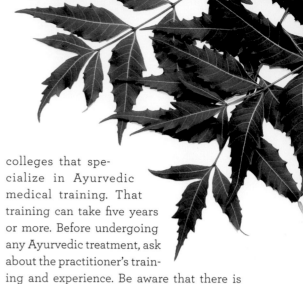

▶ | PUT INTO PRACTICE

Ayurveda is sometimes described as a holistic system of healing because it involves essentially all aspects of a person's life. Unlike Western medicine, where doctors identify a problem and may prescribe a pill or surgery to fix it, the Ayurvedic approach is more global in the sense that treatment encompasses diet, habits, and lifestyle, as well as exercise, the use of medicinal herbs, meditation, rest and relaxation, breathing techniques, and prescribed cleansing and rejuvenating procedures. All of these activities, taken together, are designed to restore balance, and therefore, health. And because lives and bodies are constantly changing, maintaining this health-promoting balance is a dynamic undertaking.

Ayurvedic medicine has a focus of active, personal responsibility for one's health, but it is not a do-it-yourself approach to illness. The following suggestions are intended only to provide information. Although some of the suggestions and recipes in this book are derived from an Ayurvedic approach to treating minor ailments, they do not represent Ayurvedic medicine any more than taking an aspirin would fully represent Western medicine.

⚠ **CAUTION:** Ayurvedic medicine uses many techniques, products, and substances for cleansing the body and restoring balance of doshas. Some of these products may not be safe and could be harmful if used improperly or without the careful guidance of a trained practitioner. Consult your health care provider prior to beginning any Ayurvedic treatment so that he or she can work with you to coordinate your medical treatments with those of Ayurveda. Make sure that any diagnosis of a disease or condition has been made by a licensed medical practitioner who is experienced at managing that disease or condition. Be aware that some herbs or herbal mixtures used in Ayurvedic medicine can cause side effects or interact with prescription drugs and may not be subject to U.S. standards for purity.

Avenues to Ayurveda

■ *Conduct an Interview* Choose an Ayurvedic practitioner with the same care you would choose any health care provider. In India, the home of Ayurvedic medicine, there are more than 150 undergraduate and 30 postgraduate colleges that specialize in Ayurvedic medical training. That training can take five years or more. Before undergoing any Ayurvedic treatment, ask about the practitioner's training and experience. Be aware that there is no national standard for training or certifying Ayurvedic practitioners in the United States. A few states have approved Ayurvedic schools as educational institutions but that is not necessarily a guarantee of quality. For more information, contact the National Ayurvedic Medical Association.

RESOLVING NEGATIVE EMOTIONS

In Ayurvedic medicine, negative emotions are believed to harm health, both when they are expressed and when they are bottled up. Patients are encouraged to resolve negative emotions using a meditative technique similar to the following one:

Suppose the negative emotion you are feeling is jealousy. In a quiet place, sit comfortably on the floor or in a chair with your feet on the ground and your arms relaxed at your sides. Close your eyes. Inhale slowly and deeply while letting yourself feel jealousy. Allow yourself the freedom to let that strong emotion express itself fully inside your mind. Concentrate on how it makes you feel physically and emotionally and how it draws energy from you. Look at it like an observer and try to see your jealousy for what it is: an emotion triggered by something outside yourself. Then slowly exhale. Continue this process—slowly breathing into the emotion, exploring it calmly in your mind, and then breathing out with this new perspective. After a while, the strong feeling (in this case, jealousy) should begin to dissipate.

Determining Doshas Ayurvedic practitioners typically begin their work with a patient by assessing that person's unique blend of doshas. This is usually done by asking detailed questions about diet, behavior, lifestyle, recent illnesses, and symptoms of current problems or issues. For instance, signs that vata is out of balance might include dry skin, constipation, joint pain, and insomnia. A cold, cough, or congestion might indicate an aggravated kapha, whereas heartburn, nausea, hives, or a rash might point to too much pitta. The practitioner will likely note many of a patient's physical characteristics and carefully analyze pulse patterns. (Each dosha is believed to produce a particular type of pulse.)

Reducing Impurities Once the doshas and their proportions have been identified, the practitioner suggests methods to rebalance them. One approach is through *panchakarma*, a multistep procedure for removing toxic impurities from the body. Panchakarma often includes drinking prescribed amounts of ghee (clarified butter) for several days, followed by oil massages and possibly steam baths. The final step is to remove built-up toxins, typically through enemas, cleansing the nasal passages with certain solutions and oils, or other types of purging.

Treating Symptoms To relieve symptoms and encourage the body to restore itself to health, Ayurvedic practitioners may suggest dietary changes (sometimes a person is encouraged to eat only certain types of foods), lifestyle changes, breathing exercises, and meditation, as well as tonics and herbal

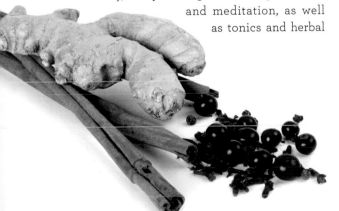

preparations. Sometimes herbs are mixed with metals or other substances according to recipes in the ancient Ayurvedic texts.

Promoting Mental Health Mental and spiritual health are as important to Ayurvedic medicine as physical health; all are part of the same whole. In addition to dietary and lifestyle changes, Ayurvedic practitioners may help train patients in techniques such as meditation that reduce stress and worry and encourage the resolution of negative emotions.

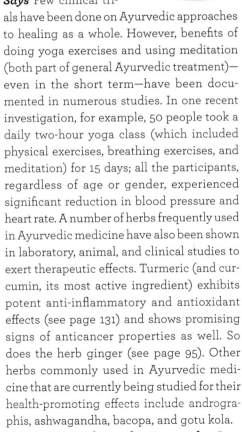

What the Science Says Few clinical trials have been done on Ayurvedic approaches to healing as a whole. However, benefits of doing yoga exercises and using meditation (both part of general Ayurvedic treatment)—even in the short term—have been documented in numerous studies. In one recent investigation, for example, 50 people took a daily two-hour yoga class (which included physical exercises, breathing exercises, and meditation) for 15 days; all the participants, regardless of age or gender, experienced significant reduction in blood pressure and heart rate. A number of herbs frequently used in Ayurvedic medicine have also been shown in laboratory, animal, and clinical studies to exert therapeutic effects. Turmeric (and curcumin, its most active ingredient) exhibits potent anti-inflammatory and antioxidant effects (see page 131) and shows promising signs of anticancer properties as well. So does the herb ginger (see page 95). Other herbs commonly used in Ayurvedic medicine that are currently being studied for their health-promoting effects include andrographis, ashwagandha, bacopa, and gotu kola.

Learn More About the Ayurvedic Diet Ayurvedic medicine classifies all foods according to their spiritual forces—pacifying or aggravating, for example—and offers a way to determine the most well-balanced diet for a given body or personality type. Entire books are available on the subject.

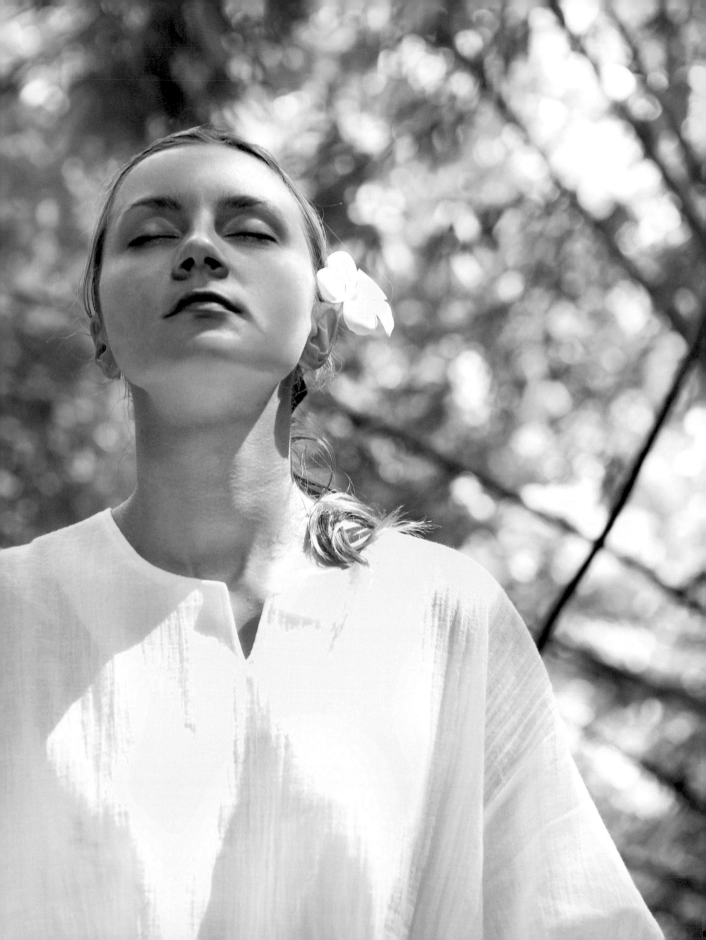

Breath Therapy

8 PATHS TO DEEPER BREATHING

Your body is composed of trillions of cells. Right now, each and every one of those cells is carrying out a fundamental life process called cell respiration. Molecules of sugar are broken down, with the help of oxygen, to release the energy they contain. That energy powers everything cells do, and by extension, everything you do. Something more happens during cell respiration, though. Water and carbon dioxide are produced as by-products of the reaction. Your cells can use the water. But the carbon dioxide is a waste product. In fact it's toxic to cells in high enough concentrations, so they need to get rid of it as fast as it's made. Cells do this by releasing carbon dioxide into your blood, which carries the gas to your lungs, where—with each exhalation—you expel it. When you inhale, you draw in oxygen that's carried via the blood to cells to keep the cell respiration process going, constantly, and without fail.

Drawing in oxygen and getting rid of carbon dioxide is what breathing is all about. Those inhalations and exhalations that help bring in the good air and get rid of the bad are healthy and natural. Yet how often do you find yourself taking a sudden deep breath—and realize that you've been holding your breath or breathing very shallowly for quite some time? Many of us tend to breathe in unnatural, constricted ways as we sit hunched over our desks or slouched in chairs. We take short, shallow breaths and release the air we inhale before it even has a chance to reach the bottom of our lungs. Shallow breathing can be triggered by stress, but it can also become a habit over time. Breath therapy is about learning to breathe more naturally. It's also about using breathing to reduce stress, influence your thoughts and emotions, and reconnect with the natural flow of life.

▶ | THE BASICS

Breath therapy, or breathwork as it's sometimes called, combines exercises and techniques from yoga (see pages 299–303), tai chi, and other traditional healing therapies as well as some from conventional medicine. Breathing is a natural body function that we can control and regulate, and regular, mindful breathing can support health in many ways. Breath therapy can help reduce stress (take a deep breath right now, release it, and notice how you feel), ease pain, and promote relaxation. It can be useful for people with certain health conditions, including respiratory disorders. In one study of patients with stable, mild to moderate asthma, those who received breath training experienced notable improvement in controlling their symptoms. Another study has shown that breath therapy can help reduce the symptoms and severity of panic attacks.

▶ | PRACTICE

There are many approaches to breath therapy. Some focus on breath awareness in which a person learns to observe the movement of air in and out of his or her body, and in doing so, to become aware of restrictions and imbalances in breathing. Another approach is focused breathing, in which breathing is consciously directed toward a particular part of the body for healing. Controlled breathing—an approach often used in yoga—includes taking fast breaths, slow breaths, and even holding breaths, all as a means of promoting physical, mental, and spiritual health. Trying new breathing techniques may feel awkward at first, but it becomes easier with regular practice. And, you might be surprised by how much more aware of your breathing you become.

Breathe Better

- *Fill Your Lungs* The Three-Part Breath, sometimes called the Complete Breath, is a technique designed to draw air deep into the lungs. It is good for stress relief and promoting relaxation, as well as improving focus and concentration. You can perform this exercise standing, sitting, or lying down, but when first learning the technique, it's probably easiest to sit on the edge of a chair with feet flat on the ground. First, inhale slowly, breathing only through your nose, and allowing your stomach muscles to relax and your belly to expand. Second, continue inhaling, letting air fill your lungs in the

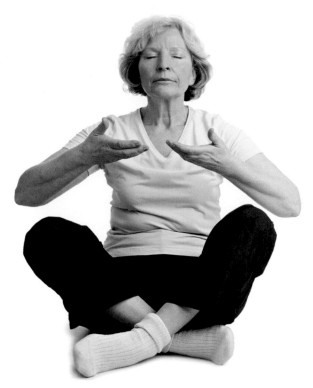

center of your chest. Third, continue inhaling a little more so you can feel air filling the top parts of your lungs higher in your chest. Immediately begin breathing out, slowly, from the top down. Exhale from your upper chest, then your middle chest, and finally your belly (contracting your abdominal muscles will help push the last of the air out). Try to take as long breathing out as you do breathing in. Start with five repetitions of this technique once a day and see if you can work up to five or even ten minutes of focused breath practice.

⚠ **CAUTION:** If you feel dizzy at any time performing this breathing exercise, stop, relax, and breathe normally.

- *Alternate Nostrils* Alternate nostril breathing is a yoga breathing exercise considered calming to the mind. Sit in a comfortable position. Gently close your right nostril with your right thumb. Inhale through your left

CREATE A FLOW ROOM

Psychologist and author Mihaly Csikszentmihalyi describes the experience he calls "flow" as the state of engagement in which you're experiencing your talents, optimally challenged, consummately interested, and able to let time melt away. Create a room that will promote such flow. Place a large table in the middle of the room to accommodate the whole family's projects. Make it a room where it's easy to play an instrument, take part in a hobby, read a book, or play a game. Lose the clock, TV, computer, or other gadgets. Make it the most appealing room in the house so you'll be drawn to spend time in it and experience blissful flow.

–Dan Buettner
Author and lecturer on longevity

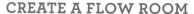

good to know: ABOUT BREATH THERAPY

- If any breathing exercise makes you feel nauseous, tense, dizzy, or uncomfortable, stop doing it and breathe normally.
- If you have recently had surgery, wait until you are completely healed before doing any breathing exercises that might stretch the tissues around the area of your surgical incision. Get your doctor's approval before proceeding.

nostril for four seconds. Close the left nostril with your ring finger and at the same time remove your thumb from the right nostril. Exhale through the right nostril for eight seconds. Inhale through the right nostril for four seconds, and then close the right nostril with your right thumb and remove your ring finger from the left nostril. Exhale through the left nostril for eight seconds. Repeat twice more.

⚠ **CAUTION:** Do not practice this breathing exercise if your nasal passages are blocked from congestion, allergies, or for any other reason.

■ **Relax With Wu** This Chinese technique, Wu breathing, is performed while lying down. Place a small pillow under your head, keep your arms resting at your sides, and let your legs relax and toes fall out to the sides. Place the tip of your tongue where your front teeth meet the gum. Begin breathing naturally through your nose, imagining the air flowing into your nose and rising to the top of your head on the inhalation, and then moving down to the center of your belly on the exhalation. Continue like this for 20 minutes, keeping your focus on the flow of air.

■ **Do a Count** The 4-7-8 Breath is an exercise that author and physician Andrew Weil, who played a major role in establishing the field of integrative medicine, recommends for reducing stress. Sit in a chair with your back straight. Place the tip of your tongue where your front teeth meet the gum and keep it there as you exhale completely through your mouth, making a whooshing sound (you'll probably need to purse your lips slightly).

Close your mouth (keep your tongue in place) and inhale through your nose while counting to 4. Hold this inhalation while you count to 7. Then exhale completely through your mouth again (with tongue still in place) for a count of 8. Repeat this 4-7-8 routine three more times. Practice twice a day.

■ **Promote Deeper Breathing** If you tend to be a shallow breather, try this simple exercise to help retrain your body to breathe more deeply and exhale more completely. Take a deep breath in through your nose, let it out naturally, and then squeeze out a little more air. You'll do this by contracting the muscles between your ribs. Doing this regularly will help strengthen those muscles and may help you breathe more deeply over time.

■ **Try 20** The 20-Cycle Breath can be a simple way to lift mood or improve concentration. Simply take four short continuous breaths (don't pause between the inhalation and the exhalation) and then take one long, deep extended breath. Repeat five times.

⚠ **CAUTION:** Limit rapid breaths to five- to eight-second intervals, as there is a risk of hyperventilating with prolonged rapid breathing.

■ **Strengthen Your Diaphragm** Years of poor posture, snug waistbands, and habitual breath holding can lead to a weak diaphragm—the sheet of muscle that underlies your lungs and works to help you inhale by contracting. Try this simple exercise to strengthen it: Lie on your back in a comfortable position. Lay a soft one- to two-pound weight (a bag of rice works well) across your belly. Perform several rounds of the Complete Breath exercise. Each time your belly expands to help fill your lungs deeply with air, your diaphragm will have to work a little harder than normal because of the added weight. The diaphragm will become stronger over time.

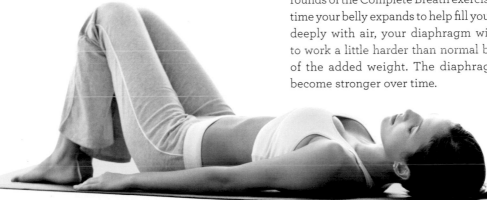

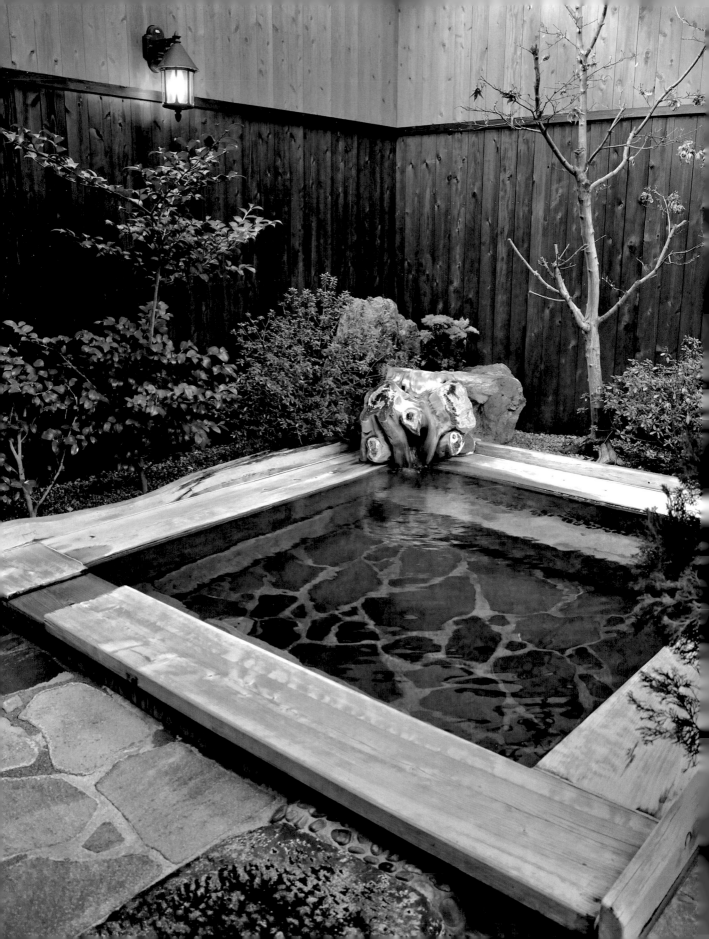

Hydrotherapy

8 WAYS TO NAVIGATE BETTER HEALTH

I f you've ever singed a finger, your first (and correct) instinct might have been to plunge it into cold water. That simple act was a form of hydrotherapy—the use of water for healing purposes. Water in all its forms underlies this ancient therapeutic approach to treating injuries and ailments, from steam and water vapor to hot or cold liquid water to ice. Egyptian, Greek, Roman, Hebrew, and Celtic societies all used water for medicinal purposes, sometimes in conjunction with herbal medicine. The Greeks and Romans were particularly fond of hot and cold baths, and the process of bathing was an elaborate physical and social ritual.

Archaeological excavations reveal that some Roman baths were enormous, many-roomed structures in which bathers first took a lukewarm bath in the *tepidarium,* then soaked in very hot water in the steamy *caldarium,* and finished with an invigorating, pore-tightening plunge in the *frigidarium.* As Roman legions crisscrossed Europe and England, they constructed their beloved baths along the way. Some European spas are located near a few of these ancient sites.

Modern hydrotherapy can trace its roots to 19th-century Austria, where Vincent Priessnitz, a farmer turned naturopathic healer, developed a system of natural therapies that involved various water treatments for stimulating circulation, purifying the body, and promoting healing. Priessnitz and the Graefenberg spa he founded became household names in Europe. Water cures based on Priessnitz's approach made their way to the United States by the 1840s. (Of course, some Native American tribes had been practicing hydrotherapy for centuries, by using sweat lodges and bathing in natural hot springs.) In the late 1800s and early 1900s, Priessnitz's hydrotherapy techniques gained acceptance in the United States. Cold-water sprays, friction rubs, and other water cures were common treatments for pneumonia and typhoid, and many hospitals used hydrotherapy to treat medical and surgical cases as well as mental illness. When President Franklin D. Roosevelt, whose legs were paralyzed by polio, bathed in a natural

hot springs in Georgia in the 1920s, he experienced so much improvement that he became a hydrotherapy advocate and brought worldwide attention to this therapy.

▶ | THE BASICS

The idea behind hydrotherapy is fairly simple. Applying warm or hot water to a part of the body relaxes muscles and expands blood vessels, temporarily increasing circulation in that area. Applying cold water has the opposite effect: Muscles contract and vessels constrict, reducing circulation and also inflammation and swelling. By applying hot and cold treatments, it's possible to direct blood flow to some extent to nourish cells with oxygen and nutrients, remove toxins, and promote healing of damaged tissues. Typical hydrotherapy treatments include contrast baths (alternating hot baths with cold ones or bathing one body

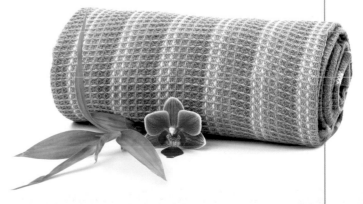

part in cold water while another is submerged in hot), high-pressure hosing with cold water, cold-mitten friction rubs, and hot or cold body wraps. Hydrotherapy can also take the form of whirlpool baths and steamy saunas as well as hot or cold compresses and steam inhalation. Physical and sports therapists also widely use some forms of hydrotherapy.

▶ | PUT INTO PRACTICE

Although some hydrotherapy treatments are best carried out by professionals, there are easy and inexpensive water therapies you can do at home. Besides hot and cold water, about the only thing you'll need is a shower or bathtub, basins large enough to accommodate hands and feet, and towels and washcloths. You may find that you're already using some hydrotherapy techniques in your daily life without even knowing it.

> ⚠ **CAUTION:** Hydrotherapy is not a substitute for medical care in treating any injury, medical condition, or medical or mental illness. Pregnant women and people with diabetes, heart disease, cancer, multiple sclerosis, high or low blood pressure, Raynaud's disease or phenomenon, bladder or rectal irritation, pelvic inflammation, sciatica, arthritis, and other chronic or acute health conditions should not use hydrotherapy treatments without a medical doctor's advice and consent.

Water Works

- ***Drink Sufficient Water*** The most fundamental hydrotherapy treatment—and one doctors and other health professionals widely recognize—is to keep your body well hydrated by drinking plenty of clean, fresh water every day. How much is enough? A common recommendation is to drink six to eight eight-ounce glasses a day. An alternative (possibly easier to incorporate into your lifestyle) is to drink a glass of water with each meal and one between each meal. Also drink water before, during, and after exercise.

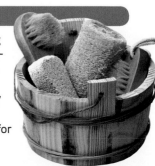

- ***Treat a Bruise*** Alternating hot and cold compresses can help speed healing (and fading) of a bruise. You'll need two washcloths and two large bowls or basins, one with hot water (not so hot that it could burn your skin) and the other with cold water with a few ice cubes in it. Place a washcloth in each bowl. Wring out the hot water cloth and hold over the bruised area for three minutes. Quickly switch to the cold cloth (wring out excess water) and apply for 30 to 60 seconds. Repeat this procedure—hot cloth for three minutes, cold cloth for 30 to 60 seconds—three to four more times, ending with the cold application. The idea is to create a sort of pumping action in which blood vessels are relaxing and constricting due to the application of heat and cold to help improve circulation and flush accumulated fluids from the tissues.

- ***Fight a Cold*** If a cold has you feeling achy, you might try a cold body wrap to help relieve some of the symptoms. You'll need two large bath towels (one should be relatively thin), a basin of cold water (large enough to accommodate a bath towel), and a thick warm robe or blanket. Assemble these items in the bathroom near the tub or shower. Put the thin

---

good to know: ABOUT HYDROTHERAPY

- Hydrotherapy can be helpful in relieving minor aches and pains, reducing swelling and inflammation, and promoting relaxation. A few studies conducted on hydrotherapy for lower back pain suggest it might be helpful but more research is needed.

- Available scientific evidence does not support claims that hydrotherapy can cure any disease.

- Hot immersion baths and hot sauna treatments are not recommended for pregnant women, the elderly, or young children.

towel in the basin of cold water and swish around until thoroughly saturated. Begin by taking a comfortably hot bath or shower for five minutes. Moving quickly, towel your body dry (with the dry towel), and then wring out the towel in the basin and wrap it securely around your torso (it should reach from your armpits to your pelvic area). Immediately wrap yourself snuggly in the robe or blanket. Lie down (add another blanket if you need it) and relax for 20 minutes. Remove the towel and pat yourself dry. If you can, crawl back under the covers and rest. If you can't, dress warmly. Try doing this wrap once or twice a day during your illness.

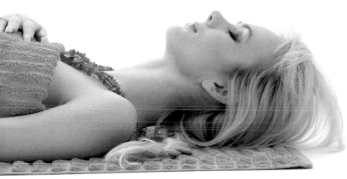

- **Rub Away Fatigue** Immediately after taking a hot bath or shower, dip a washcloth into cold water and wrap it around your fist; grip the ends so it will stay on your hand, like a mitten. Using vigorous circular motions, rub the cold washcloth over one of your arms, starting at the fingers and moving up toward your shoulder. If the cloth warms before you finish, dip in the cold water again. Dry the arm thoroughly and vigorously. Repeat the same procedure on your other arm, your legs and feet, and your chest, abdomen, and buttocks.

- **Soothe a Sunburn** A tepid bath, laced with tea and vinegar, may help calm a sunburn's pain and "heat." Make strong black tea by adding 3 tea bags to 2 cups just-boiling water. Let steep 10 to 15 minutes. Begin running a bath with tepid water (not hot, not cold). Add 1 cup of the tea and 1 cup pure apple cider vinegar to the tub as it fills. (If the odor of vinegar seems unpleasant, add up to

5 drops lavender essential oil, which has skin-soothing properties; see page 101). Ease into the tub and soak for 15 to 20 minutes.

- **Submerge Your Feet** Using hot and cold footbaths can help stimulate circulation in the feet and legs. Fill one basin with comfortably hot water and the other with cold water. Sit in a chair with the tubs side by side in front of you. Start by soaking your feet in the hot-water tub for 60 seconds and then plunge them into the cold-water tub for 20 to 30 seconds. Repeat three to four more times.

- **Go Aquatic** Pool therapy, or aquatic therapy, is a form of hydrotherapy. Aquatic therapy involves doing various forms of exercise or controlled movements in either the shallow or deep end of a pool (with a flotation aid). Aquatic therapy uses water's viscosity ("thickness") to provide resistance to body movements and so stimulate and strengthen muscles; water also provides buoyancy to reduce stress on joints. Warm-water pool therapy helps to relax muscles and blood vessels, increasing blood flow. Aquatic therapy is often recommended for people with arthritis and fibromyalgia as well as those recovering from many types of surgery. Studies have shown that aquatic therapy can also be beneficial for people with multiple sclerosis, cerebral palsy, and Parkinson's disease. Slow-movement therapies, such as "aqua chi" (tai chi–based exercises performed in a pool) can be very relaxing and are good for improving balance, flexibility, and coordination.

- **Listen to Water** One of the simplest forms of hydrotherapy is to find a place where you can rest comfortably and listen to the sound of flowing water. In a city, find fountains; in the country, find babbling brooks and rippling streams. Going outdoors is in itself a therapy, and listening to the calm sound of flowing water enhances the experience.

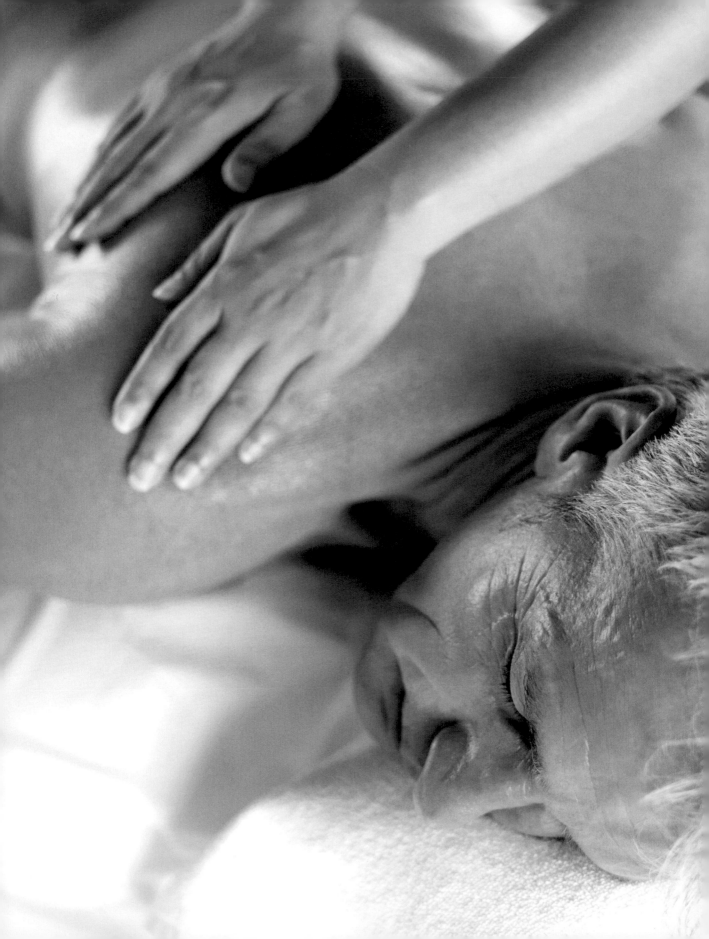

Massage Therapy

4 RUBDOWN RELAXERS

Although there's no proof, massage is quite likely the world's oldest healing therapy. It's almost instinctive that when our heads ache, our joints are tender, or our stomachs are churning, we rub them. We stroke and knead and ply the sore parts of our bodies to make them feel better. And very often, it works. Every culture throughout history has used massage, in some form or another, as part of its approach to healing. Hippocrates, the ancient Greek physician who so greatly influenced Western medical philosophy, had this to say about "rubbing," as massage was called in his day: "The physician must be experienced in many things, but assuredly also in rubbing."

The form of massage we're most familiar with in the Western world, often called Swedish massage, had its start in Europe in the early 1800s with a Swedish gymnast, Per Henrik Ling. Ling brought together some of the manipulation techniques now associated with massage (many with ancient roots) and incorporated them into a program of exercise he called medical gymnastics. But it was a Dutch practitioner, Johan Georg Mezger, who organized some of Ling's techniques for passively manipulating muscles and soft tissues into the four types of massage movements (with French names) that are integral to Swedish massage: *effleurage* (stroking), *petrissage* (lifting, rolling, and kneading muscles), *frictions* (deep, firm, circular motions), and *tapotement* (beating and tapping). This form of massage became widely accepted as a beneficial adjunct to medicine by doctors in Europe and America during the 19th and early 20th century. By the mid-1900s, however, the connection between massage and conventional medicine in the United States loosened, and massage therapy began establishing itself as a separate vocation. Today you're likely to find massage therapists who offer many variations of Swedish massage, including deep tissue, sports, trigger point, neuromuscular, Rolfing, and others.

Most of these forms of massage therapy focus on rubbing, kneading, and soft tissue manipulation to relax muscles, increase flexibility, and improve circulation. Shiatsu (see page 291), reflexology (see page 287), and other techniques take a different approach, working primarily with pressure points in the body to promote healing and maintain health.

▶ | THE BASICS

Most people would probably agree that massage therapy can be deeply relaxing. Scientific studies show that massage can reduce muscle tension, lessen stress and anxiety, and provide relief from pain (including chronic back and neck pain). There is also some evidence that massage can relieve pain and improve mood in some cancer patients. Some research suggests that it might also improve circulation, increase mobility in joints, reduce swelling and inflammation, and help with mild depression. Several theories have been suggested as to why massage may make people feel better, including the possibility that it blocks pain signals to the brain, stimulates the release of certain chemicals in the body such as endorphins, or brings about beneficial changes in body position and mechanics. None of these theories has been fully tested. Nevertheless, many people find massage can help with common health complaints, and when administered by a qualified and experienced massage therapist, can be a useful tool for maintaining and promoting health.

▶ | PUT INTO PRACTICE

Always use an experienced therapist. To find one, start by calling or emailing the American Massage Therapy Association, which can provide you with a list of qualified, licensed massage professionals in your area, including those who specialize in particular techniques. Before deciding on a therapist, call or visit them. Ask questions about training, years of experience, and the types of massage they are certified to perform. A well-trained massage therapist will ask you questions, too, about your medical history, symptoms, injuries, or physical problems and limitations, as well as your desired results.

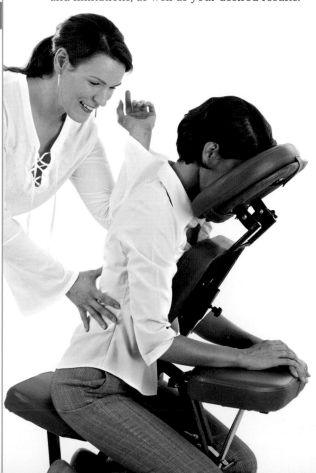

They may also perform an evaluation to locate tense or painful body parts and determine how much pressure they can exert and still remain within your comfort range. Typically, people lie on a massage table to have a massage, although certain types of massage can also be done with the patient sitting in a specially designed massage chair.

Nothing can quite match the benefit and enjoyment of getting a massage from an expert massage therapist. But there are self-massage techniques you can use at home. You'll never be able to give yourself a full back massage, of course, but using some of the following techniques you should be able to release tension, loosen cramped muscles, and ease away some stress. To perform any of these techniques, find a quiet place that is neither too hot nor cold. Start with clean skin and hands; self-massage after a bath or shower is ideal. Sit comfortably. Use a little sweet almond oil as a lubricant so that your fingers will slide easily over your skin. Be aware that any oil can stain fabric.

⚠ **CAUTION:** Do not have massage therapy, or perform self-massage, if you are pregnant, have any type of pain, have circulatory problems, heart disease, high blood pressure, a severe sprain or other injury, severe bruising, open wounds, infections, or contagious skin conditions or diseases without first consulting with your health care provider.

Massage Messaging

- ***Release Facial Tension*** Dip the tips of the index, middle, and ring fingers of each hand in a small amount of oil. Rub hands together briefly to spread it evenly. Holding the three fingers together on each hand, make tiny, slow circles on your face, applying gentle pressure with the flat pads of the fingertips. Start at your chin and steadily work upward along the jawline on either side of your face. Continue upward from the angles of your jaw to your temples. Move your fingers to either side of your nose and continue massaging in small circles under and around your cheekbones and then up toward the tops of your ears. Move your fingertips to the bridge of your nose. Massage along the bony ridges

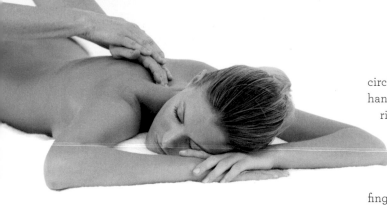

above your eyes, moving from the center outward, roughly following the line of your eyebrows. (Keep eyes closed.) Move up to the center of your forehead and massage outward toward your temples in the same fashion. Repeat this several times, moving higher on your forehead each time, until you reach the hairline.

- **De-stress Shoulders** Dip the fingertips of one hand in a little oil. Reach for the area between your left shoulder and your neck with your right hand. (Use your left hand to support your right arm at the elbow). Firmly squeeze and knead the large band of muscle and tissue that runs between your neck and the end of your collarbone (you'll feel the bony bump). Massage slowly back and forth for a minute or two, and then switch sides and arms.

- **Help Your Hands** Using the thumb and index finger of your right hand, gently squeeze and knead the fleshy areas between the fingers and thumb of your left hand. Then squeeze each finger with a sort of rolling, rocking motion, working from the knuckle toward the fingertip. Pull outward gently as you do this, giving each finger and the thumb a little stretch. Finally, using your thumb, make firm

circling motions all over the palm of your left hand. Repeat the same procedure on your right hand, massaging with the fingers of your left. When you've finished massaging both hands, make a tight fist with each hand and hold for five seconds. Release and then extend the fingers of each hand, spreading them apart as far as comfortable. Hold for five seconds. Release, and end by shaking both hands gently from the wrists for a moment or two, keeping your hands completely relaxed.

- **Relax Your Lower Back** Do this whenever you feel tension in your lower back or you've been sitting for a long time. Stand up and place your thumbs on either side of your lumbar vertebrae (the bones that make up your lower back); let your fingers wrap around your hips, pointing forward. Gently press your thumbs into the muscular tissue on either side of the spine, being careful not to press on the vertebrae themselves. Make tiny circular motions with your thumbs (circles about a half inch in diameter). Gradually move your thumbs upward along the spine, moving in increments of about an inch at a time. Continue upward as far as you can reach and then gradually massage downward, again moving slowly, in very small increments. If you encounter a sore spot at any point, massage with less pressure but don't skip it. When you're finished, arch your lower back slightly and then flex forward slightly. Take a deep breath and exhale, letting tension release.

good to know: ABOUT MASSAGE THERAPY

- It is easier to give a comfortable self-massage with nails that are fairly short and filed smooth.
- You should feel comfortable with a massage therapist. If you don't like the mannerisms or personality of a therapist, find someone else.
- Never be afraid to tell a therapist that something is causing discomfort or pain, or that too much (or too little) pressure is being applied. Speak up immediately.
- If you are hesitant about the idea of having a full-body massage, try a foot massage first.

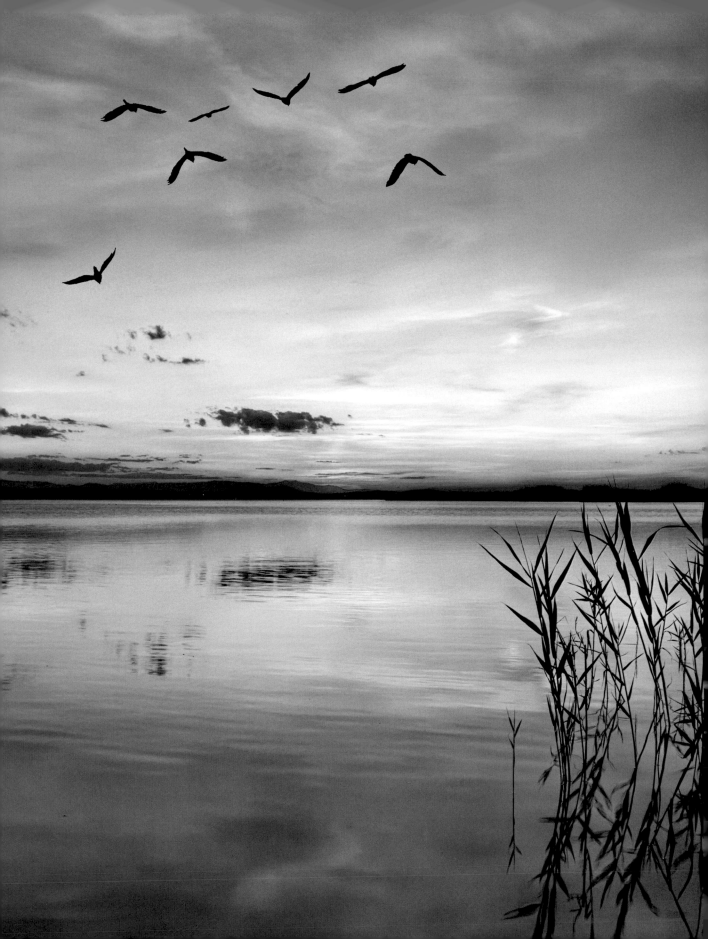

Meditation

5 WAYS TO CLEAR THE HEAD

Achieving stillness. Intense inward concentration. Connecting with a higher power. Peace of mind that heals. Resting the mind in silence and space. There are probably as many definitions and descriptions of meditation as there are types of meditation and paths to reach the meditative state. And perhaps that shouldn't be surprising. Meditation has been practiced since antiquity, and has had thousands of years to evolve. The origins of meditation lie primarily in ancient Eastern religions and spiritual traditions, where meditation was (and still is) used as a way to deepen understanding of the sacred and mystical forces of life.

Increasingly, though, meditation has come to be regarded as a mind-body practice that is part of complementary and alternative medicine. People meditate for many reasons, but some of the most common benefits and helpful results of meditation include stress reduction, relaxation, calmness and concentration, psychological balance, coping with illness, insomnia, and general health and well-being. A 2007 National Health Interview Survey revealed that nearly 20 million adults in the United States used meditation for health purposes.

Considerable research has been carried out on meditation and its effects on the body and the mind. The fact that meditation can reduce stress and promote relaxation is well documented. Certain studies have also shown that meditation causes measurable changes in brain wave patterns, and stimulates the parts of the brain involved in memory, learning, and emotion. The practice actually increases the density of gray matter in these brain areas.

Other studies have shown that meditation can stimulate the immune system to fight infection, increase empathy, improve mental processing of information, lower blood pressure, reduce symptoms associated with digestive ailments, and ease mild depression. There is also some evidence that certain types of meditation may be helpful to people who are trying to quit smoking and to those who are struggling with other types of addictions.

▶ | THE BASICS

There are many styles of meditation, but Transcendental Meditation, concentrative meditation, and mindfulness meditation are among the most common. The late Maharishi Mahesh Yogi based Transcendental Meditation on meditation techniques used in the ancient Vedic tradition of India; he introduced the practice to the United States in the 1960s. In Transcendental Meditation, you repeat a sound, or mantra, over and over. The constant repetition creates an almost hypnotic focus of attention on the sound, and as a result, you're able to transcend thinking and experience a deep state of restfully alert consciousness. Concentrative meditation involves using an object such as a candle flame, some type of picture or image, or a sensation such as breathing, to focus the mind. Each time your mind begins to drift and concentration slips, you refocus your attention on the object, image, or sensation, which helps restore the meditative state. Unlike Transcendental Meditation and concentrative meditation, mindfulness meditation doesn't foster the absence of thinking. Instead, you allow thoughts to move

GOD IS IN THE DETAILS

I've had chef jobs that were very stressful—but during those hard days, one of my favorite routines was preparing or filleting the fish. Though it is exacting and delicate work, my mind focused and my hands became my thoughts. It was the most peace I had in a decade of work. The same is true with the detail work of shelling beans, making ravioli, chopping vegetables, or making dough. These are pleasant acts that accomplish a necessary task and use time well—an important justification for people in a busy world.

–Barton Seaver
Chef and sustainable food expert

through your mind. But rather than thinking about those thoughts (and letting them draw you down random paths), you observe your thoughts, and the feelings and sensations that accompany them, in a nonjudgmental way. In short, you become intensely aware of everything going on within and around you. According to practitioners, this helps you gain new perspectives, and over time, trains you to place your attention where you want it to be, and to guide your thoughts and emotions in more productive and healthy directions.

People tend to reap the most benefits from physical exercise when they do it regularly. The same is true for meditation. In some respects, it is like any skill; the more you practice the better you get at it, and the easier the practice itself becomes. Many experts recommend meditating twice daily, for 10 to 20 minutes each time. Relaxation and breathing exercises (see pages 267–269) can help ease you into the frame of mind to enter a meditative state. Meditation is not easy; you may be surprised just how challenging it can be to clear your mind of the steady stream of thoughts and worries that typically run through our minds all day long (and sometimes, into the night). If a particular form of meditation doesn't seem to work for you, try a different one.

▶ | PUT INTO PRACTICE

Serious students of meditation often work with an experienced teacher. But if you're just beginning—or are just curious—there are many simple techniques that you can try on your own. It's best to practice meditation in a quiet place with as few distractions as possible. Sit in a comfortable chair or on cushions on the floor; lean up against a wall if your back needs support. You can also lie down, if that helps you to relax more completely.

Mind Modes

■ *Focus on Your Breath* Set a timer (something with a gentle beep rather than a blaring alarm) for 10 to 20 minutes. Close your eyes and begin to focus on your breathing. Observe each inhalation and exhalation with your mind. Give your complete attention to the air moving into and out of your body. Don't try to alter your breath in any way. Simply observe what's happening: the rhythm, any changes, occasional pauses, the sound of the breath, the feeling of the moving air. Each time your focus starts to drift away from your breathing (and it will) or you're distracted by something—a dog barking, an itchy nose, suddenly remembering a task you need to do— gently bring your attention back to your breath. Don't chastise or judge yourself for mentally wandering. Simply refocus on your breathing and try to keep concentrating on it, and only it. When the alarm goes off, slowly open your eyes and take in your surroundings. Note how you feel and resume your day. Repeat this practice every day. After a few days, you may not need the alarm.

- **Chant** Make yourself comfortable and set a timer (see the previous paragraph) for 10 to 20 minutes. Close your eyes, inhale normally and as you exhale, whisper the word calm (or simply say it to yourself in your head.) Draw out the word for the entire exhalation, and as you do, imagine stress or worry leaving your body with the exhaled air. Inhale again, and as you breathe out, repeat the mantra: calm. Keep doing this, breathing in normally, repeating the word with each exhalation, and focusing on the sensation of stress or worry exiting your body. Note how you feel at the end of the prescribed time. (If the word "calm" doesn't seem right for you in this meditative practice, experiment with other words—or try the following technique.)

- **Focus on Touch** If you find it difficult to concentrate on the sound of a word (either verbalized or in your head), try focusing your attention using your sense of touch. Rosary and prayer beads have long been used as a focal point for meditation. Find one or two small, smooth, rounded stones that appeal to you in some way. Begin your meditation by breathing normally, with eyes closed and either rolling the stones gently together in one hand or passing them back and forth from hand to hand. Focus all your attention on the feel of the stones—their smoothness, their coolness, their weight, and the sensation of their movement. When your attention wanders, simply bring it gently back to the stones.

- **Descend Into Water** Another option for meditation involves visiting and exploring a place or setting and all its details in your "mind's eye." Descending into water is one option. For example, as you close your eyes

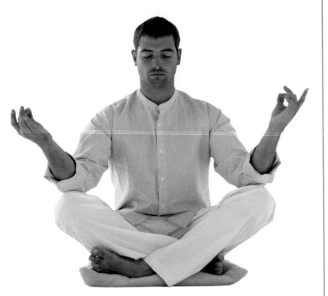

and begin your meditative session, picture a deep pool of water, with the sunlight glinting off its surface. Now see yourself take a coin and toss it into the water. Follow the coin with your mind. Watch it tilt from side to side as it descends through the clear water, going deeper and deeper and deeper, until it finally comes to rest on the bottom of the pond. Imagine how the coin feels lying there, cool and still and quiet. Explore that feeling, making it your own.

- **Be Mindful** Set a timer for ten minutes, if you wish. Sit comfortably, close your eyes, and take three slow, deep breaths. Release any tension you might be holding in your neck or shoulders. Concentrate on breathing, keeping your mind clear and free of thoughts for about ten breaths. Then let a single question form in your consciousness, such as "How do I feel?" Observe the answers that come into your mind in response to that question. They could reflect how you are feeling physically, mentally, or emotionally. Let the responses come without trying to analyze or guide them along a certain path. Simply observe them in a calm and peaceful way. If you find your thoughts straying, gently repeat the question to yourself and refocus your attention until the time is up. Repeat this practice daily with the same question. The responses that emerge from your subconscious can be very enlightening.

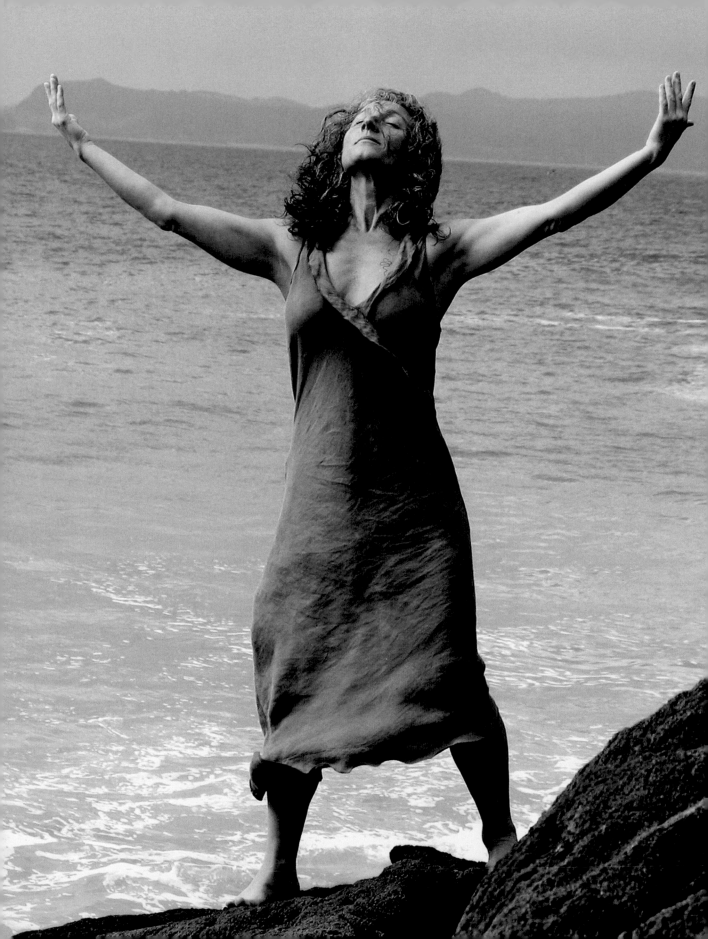

Qigong

3 LINKS TO YOUR LIFE FORCE

Qigong (pronounced chee gung or chee kung) is a healing form of exercise practice that is one of the four main branches of traditional Chinese medicine (the others are acupuncture and moxibustion, therapeutic massage and bonesetting, and herbal medicine—see pages 295–297). The *qi* in qigong refers to the concept of qi as the life force or vital energy, which TCM followers believe flows through all living things. *Gong* means work, cultivation, or practice. Qigong, then, can be described as a way of cultivating or building up qi, the fundamental energy of life. Unlike many forms of exercise Westerners practice, where the goal is to burn off energy, the aim with qigong is to generate, store, and reinforce energy within a person's body and mind. Strengthening personal qi is believed to foster physical health as well as a higher intellectual and spiritual state of mind.

Qigong is not a single type of exercise but encompasses a wide variety of practices. Soft qigong exercises, for instance, tend to be quiet, gentle, and nonvigorous, emphasizing balance, strength, breathing, and relaxation. (Some people consider tai chi a soft qigong exercise system; others view it as a separate but closely related practice.) Hard qigong exercises are just the opposite; these practices incorporate powerful, vigorous movements and include traditional Chinese self-defense and martial arts techniques such as kung fu. Dynamic qigong involves exercises that emphasize constant, fluid movement of arms, legs, and other body parts. Finally, static qigong focuses on stillness and motionless meditation.

▶ | THE BASICS

Qigong exercise routines are remarkably diverse. Many are performed standing; others can be done while walking, sitting, or lying down. Some are gentle and slow, while others involve quick movements and are physically very demanding. Nearly all forms of qigong, however, involve certain body postures, a method of breathing to expand lung capacity and promote better circulation and distribution of oxygen to tissues and organs, and a quiet state of concentration or mental focusing.

Proponents of qigong claim it promotes good health by stimulating the flow of qi freely and easily throughout all parts of the body, calming and sustaining the major body systems. Other health benefits of qigong are said to be reduction in heart rate and blood pressure; improved circulation and oxygenation of cells, tissues, and organs; improved balance and coordination; and an increase in strength and flexibility. Although not a great deal of scientific research has been carried out on qigong's effects on health at this point, several studies support its use as a complementary and alternative medicine (CAM) to improve function and reduce fall risk, blood pressure, and depression in the elderly. At least one study has shown that qigong practice may help regulate immunity and metabolic rate. Much research remains to be done, however, before any major conclusions can be drawn.

▶ | PRACTICE

Some qigong exercises or exercise routines are designed to promote health in the body as a whole, helping to boost energy and prevent illness. Others are designed to have a specific effect on a particular organ, organ system, or other part of the body.

The best way to learn qigong exercises is under the guidance of an experienced teacher—ideally in person, but watching a good video or DVD can be instructive, too. The following outlined steps will give you only a taste of this ancient practice; use them as a springboard to further study and continued exploration.

⚠ **CAUTION:** In general, soft qigong is quite safe. However, talk to your health care provider before beginning qigong practice, or any new exercise program. Be sure to consult your doctor prior to beginning qidong if you are pregnant or have any type of health problem.

Going With the Flow

■ *Try a Meditative Practice* This simple exercise takes about five minutes:

• Begin by sitting cross-legged on the floor (you may want to support your back against a wall) or in a chair with your feet flat on the ground. Keep your back comfortably straight with your head in line with your spine, and your hands and arms loose, either cradled in your lap or hanging by your sides. Relax and breathe naturally.

• Close your eyes. Imagine a beam of energy or light (qi) coming down from the sky, piercing your scalp and traveling straight through your head, neck, chest, and torso, down to the center of the earth. Align your body with this beam.

• As you inhale, feel qi flowing from the beam of light into the central core of your body and filling it. As you exhale, feel energy flowing out toward your body's surface. Focus on this sensation for a minute or two.

• Mentally follow the beam of light traveling through your body to your lower abdomen, specifically to a spot about three inches below your belly button. In your mind's eye, visualize the beam of energy concentrating in this location, forming a brilliant, luminous ball.

• Focus your attention on this glowing ball of light within you, letting go of other conscious thoughts. Breathe naturally for a minute or two.

■ *Experience the Eight Pieces of Brocade (Ba Duan Jin) Exercise* This gentle, elegant, and deceptively simple qigong series of eight positions has been practiced in China for hundreds of years as an exercise to improve health.

• Begin in a comfortable standing position. Inhale (through your nose) while sweeping both hands above your head, with the palms facing upward, fingers pointing toward each other. Keeping your eyes on your hands, go up on your toes. Hold this position for two to three seconds. As you breathe out (through your mouth), lower your body and arms to the starting position. Repeat six times.

• Spread your legs and bend at the knees. Inhale and draw your hands up to chest level. Pretend you are drawing a bow, left arm forward

good to know: ABOUT QIGONG

— As you perform qigong exercises, always work at your own pace.

— Know your limits and don't exceed them. If an exercise or position seems strenuous, or puts a strain on any part of your body that seems uncomfortable or unacceptable, don't do it.

— When doing the Eight Pieces of Brocade exercise, do only those sections that you wish to do; it is not necessary to do all eight positions to derive benefits from the practice.

and right arm back, and follow your arms with your eyes. Exhale as you bring your arms back down to your sides. Now inhale and draw the bow on the other side. Exhale when you bring your arms down. Repeat this entire sequence (both sides) six times.

• Exhale and raise your arms to chest height, palms facing upward. Inhale and move your right hand upward, palm up, until your arm is fully extended. At the same time, move your left hand downward, palm facing down, until it is fully extended. Exhale, bringing arms back to chest height. Inhale, reversing the process: Extend your left arm up and right arm down. Repeat the entire process six times.

• Standing with arms hanging loosely at your sides or gently resting on your hips, inhale and pivot your head and torso to the right as far as is comfortably possible. Exhale and return to center. Inhale and pivot to the left, looking as far left as is comfortably possible. Repeat the entire process six times.

• Bend your knees slightly while resting your palms on your thighs. Lean forward slightly, and exhale while turning your head to the left and swinging your hips to the right. Inhale as you bring your head and hips back to center. Exhale and turn your head to the right while swinging your hips to the left. Exhale and return to center. Repeat the cycle six times.

• With your knees slightly bent, inhale and bend gently forward at the waist. If you can touch your toes, fine, but only bend as far

FENG SHUI FOR HOME & OFFICE

In the practice of feng shui, every living space is divided into sectors representing different aspects of our life and concerns. Those who engage in feng shui believe, for example, that focusing on the prosperity section of the home office will help bring success to work. To attend to this area, enter the office and look to the far left—that is the prosperity section of the room. Keep it fresh and vibrant. Birds bring life and energy to a space. If there is a window in that corner, attach a window bird feeder. Place some bird sculptures there, or a painting of a bird. Purple, blues, and reds are the colors of prosperity. Green is also appropriate, and a great place for a plant, or green curtains or window trim. If you are looking for fame and a good reputation, focus on the middle of the far left wall. Place reds and oranges there, along with other representations of the fire element.

–Annie B. Bond
Author and eco-friendly living expert

forward as it comfortable. Slowly begin to straighten and place your hands on your lower back. Exhale and bend gently backward from the waist; go only as far as is comfortable. Return to a standing position. Repeat the cycle six times.

• With knees bent and legs slightly spread, clench your hands into fists and bring them up to your waist. Keeping the palm-side down, alternate punching your fists outward, fully extending your arms each time. Imagine anger dwelling in your body being released with each punch. Repeat a complete right-then-left punch six times.

• Inhale and interlace your fingers as you put your hands behind your neck. Tip your head back slightly, cradling it in your hands, and slightly arch your back. Exhale and rise up onto your toes. Inhale as you go down and let your hands drop back to your sides. Repeat six times.

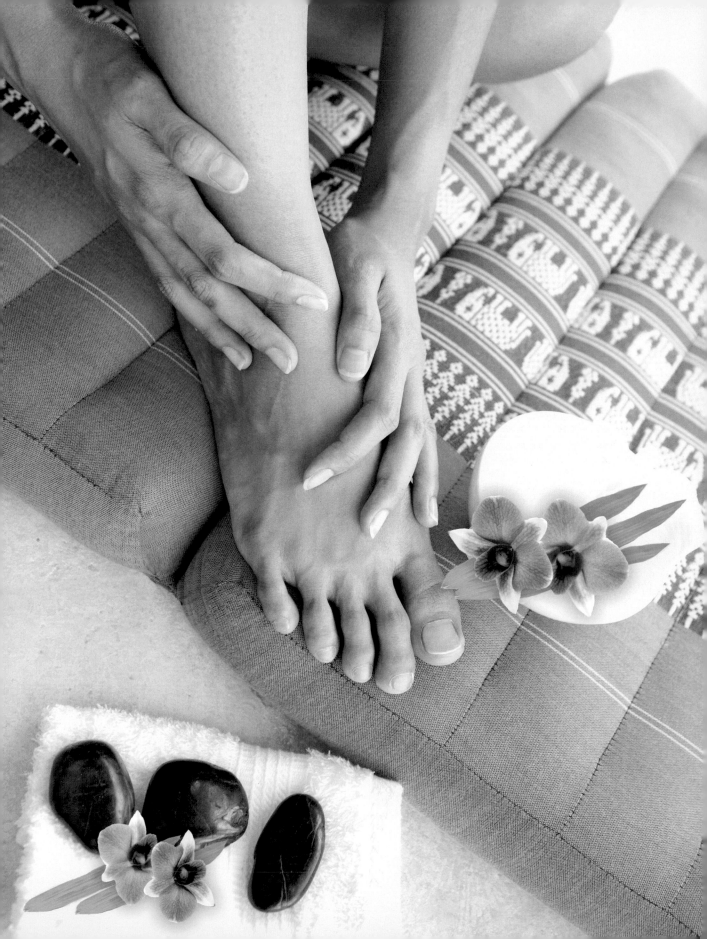

Reflexology

11 SURE-FOOTED STEPS TO BETTER HEALTH

I f you've ever had a foot massage, you know how deeply relaxing it can be. But reflexology, at least according to its proponents, is far more than a foot massage. Reflexology is based on a belief system, developed by several 20th-century practitioners, that the human body is divided into ten vertical "zones." Each of these zones is thought to correspond to a specific "reflex area" on the soles, tops, and sides of the feet (or hands), making the feet (or hands) a sort of map of the body. By putting pressure on or otherwise manipulating a particular reflex area, reflexology practitioners claim that they can stimulate organs, glands, and other body parts in the corresponding vertical zone and, in so doing, relieve stress and help prevent, alleviate, or correct health problems in a natural way.

Reflexology practitioners often trace the roots of their therapy back to ancient cultures in Egypt, China, and Rome. They sometimes draw parallels between reflexology and healing traditions such as acupressure (see page 255) that involves applying pressure to specific points to move or balance life energy, or qi, along pathways (meridians) that run between these points. It wasn't until the early 20th century, however, that modern reflexology came into being. Its early form originated with William H. Fitzgerald, an American ear, nose, and throat doctor who practiced in both the United States and England in the early 1900s. In 1913, Fitzgerald developed the vertical zone concept, and concluded that when pressure is applied to reflex areas in the feet, hands, face, and ears, it can bring about improvement in the functioning of internal organs or relief from pain. Fitzgerald published his ideas in 1917, calling his new approach to healing the "zone theory."

American physical therapist Eunice D. Ingham, though, is credited with popularizing what we now call reflexology. Ingham built upon Fitzgerald's zone theory, focusing almost exclusively on the reflex areas of the feet. In her first book, published in 1938, Ingham explained how she believed that the reflex areas were an exact mirror image of the organs of the body. She created detailed maps of these areas, indicating which spots to touch to affect which body parts. These reflexology diagrams are integral to reflexology practice today.

▶ | THE BASICS

In a typical reflexology session, a therapist systematically manipulates specific areas of the client's feet (some therapists work on the hands as well). Therapists use thumbs and fingers (and sometimes knuckles) to deeply massage reflex areas on the soles, sides, and tops of the feet. Ingham claimed that crystalline deposits of waste (calcium and uric acid) collect in the feet, especially around nerve endings. Reflexology therapists who hold this view say they can feel these tiny crystals as areas of "grittiness" and are able to identify specific health problems based on where the crystals are located. They then work to crush the crystals during treatment sessions to restore normal function. Other practitioners believe less in the idea of crystal accumulation and more in the concept of blocked qi-like energy; as they massage various reflex areas on the feet (and sometimes on the hands, face, and ears), impediments to energy flow are said to be removed in a way that rebalances vital energy and brings about healing.

There is no clear agreement as to what reflexology actually does (even among reflexology therapists). Scientific research has yet to reveal any anatomical link, via nerves, blood vessels, or otherwise, between various areas on the feet and the body's organs. A small number of studies suggest that reflexology may help relieve anxiety, nausea, and vomiting in cancer patients undergoing chemotherapy, and reduce symptoms of premenstrual syndrome (PMS) as well as pain associated with menstrual cramps. However, systematic reviews of controlled trials on reflexology's effects in 2009 and 2011 found no convincing evidence that the technique is a useful treatment for any medical condition. Nevertheless, reflexology's popularity has grown considerably in the past few decades as a noninvasive, alternative therapy. In the United Kingdom, for example, general practitioners with the National Health Service can now prescribe reflexology along with a number of other unproven alternative therapies. This is largely because, for many people, reflexology—like massage—does appear to provide relief from stress and certain types of pain.

⚠ **CAUTION:** Although reflexology is typically gentle and generally safe, it has not been shown to be effective in treating, curing, or diagnosing any disease. Reflexology should never be substituted for conventional medical care of an existing or suspected medical condition. Avoid reflexology on any area of broken skin, at the site of an infection, or where there is an injury or suspected injury. Consult your doctor before having any reflexology treatment if you have an existing medical condition, or have had reconstructive surgery of the feet, hands, or ears. Pregnant women and people who have arthritis, osteoporosis, heart problems, and thyroid disorders should not have reflexology except with the approval and consent of their health care provider.

▶ | A SPECIAL PRACTICE

To get a true sense of reflexology in action, you'd need to visit a certified or experienced reflexology therapist. Like massage (see page 275), it is difficult for individuals to perform most of the

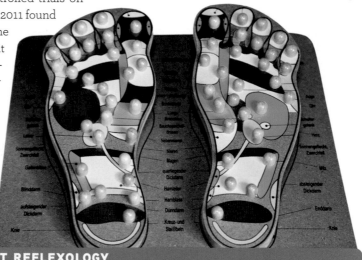

good to know: ABOUT REFLEXOLOGY

— Reflexology has not been scientifically proven to cure any medical condition or disease, despite claims you may see on the Internet.

— If you choose to receive treatment from a reflexology therapist, ask about that person's experience and training and if they are certified by the American Reflexology Certification Board. Be aware that neither certification nor licensing is required to practice reflexology in most states. Currently, only two states, Tennessee and North Dakota, have any laws pertaining to reflexology.

techniques associated with reflexology on themselves. As a home therapy, however, it is possible to try a few simple movements on your feet or hands as a means of providing gentle relaxation.

In the Zones

- **Consult a Map** Reflex areas are specific spots that have been mapped out on the soles, sides, and tops of the feet, both sides of the hands, and the ears. Charts depicting these areas are widely available in books and online. Use one, preferably of the feet or hands, to get acquainted with the reflex areas and what they are said to connect to in the body's vertical zones.

SMOOTH & SOOTHE

Some reflexology practitioners work on their clients' feet or hands without any lubricating substance. Others use powders, lotions, or oils to reduce friction. Lotions and oils also soothe dry or irritated skin.

For a fragrant oil blend to use when trying the reflexology self-treatment on this page, add 3 drops each of lavender, geranium, and chamomile essential oil to ¼ cup of a light, non-greasy carrier oil such as fractionated coconut oil or jojoba oil. If used on feet, don socks, as any oil can make feet slippery.

- **Give It a Try** What follows is a very simplified reflexology self-treatment to relax the hands and possibly improve circulation using the hands. Do not perform it if you have arthritis or a hand injury or infection.
  - Begin by firmly squeezing the tips of each finger and the thumb of the left hand using the thumb and index finger of your right hand (thumb on top, pushing on the nail; index finger below). Hold each squeeze for about three seconds. Do not squeeze hard enough to cause pain. Repeat the same procedure on the other hand.
  - Using the thumb and index finger of your right hand, squeeze the sides of the tips of the fingers and thumb on your left hand. Again, hold each squeeze for about three seconds. Repeat the same procedure on the other hand.
  - Grip the base of your left thumb with the thumb and index finger of your right hand. Vigorously rub the top and bottom surfaces of the thumb while moving from the base toward the tip. Repeat on all four fingers on the left hand as well. Repeat the same procedure on the other hand.
  - Grip the base of your left thumb and, this time, vigorously rub side to side and on the upper and lower surfaces while moving toward the thumb's tip. Repeat for all four fingers on the left hand. Repeat the same procedure on the other hand.
  - Grip the left thumb at its base and pull gently outward as your right finger and thumb slide along the skin toward the left thumb's tip. Repeat on all four fingers on the left hand and then the other hand.
  - Grip the fleshy webbing between the thumb and index finger of the left hand with the thumb and index finger of the right. Squeeze while moving the right hand away from the left, so your right finger and thumb slip off the webbing. Repeat on the webbing between the other fingers. Repeat on the other hand.
  - Use your right thumb to massage the back of your left hand, working thoroughly around each knuckle and between all the fleshy and bony areas. Repeat on the other hand.
  - Use your right thumb to massage the inside of the left wrist, at the point where the skin folds where hand and arm meet. Repeat the same procedure on the other hand.
  - Use your right thumb to massage all around your left palm. Repeat on your right.
  - Place your right thumb in the center of your left palm. Press firmly for about ten seconds, breathing deeply. Repeat on the other hand.

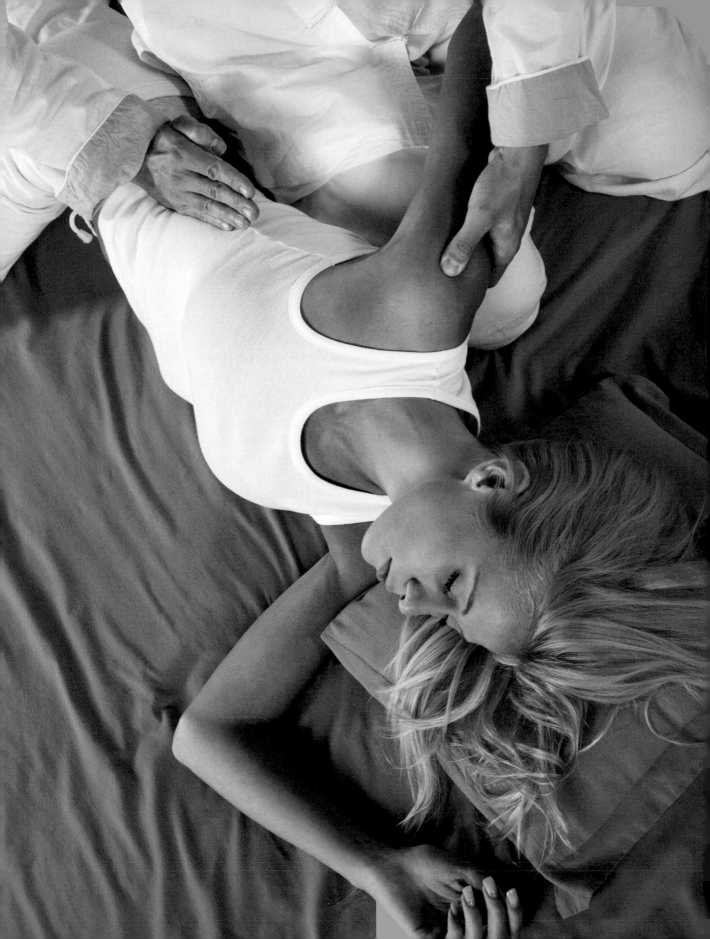

Shiatsu

15 MOVES TO FIND ENERGY WITHIN

Shiatsu is a Japanese-based form of therapeutic massage with roots in traditional Oriental medicine. The word "shiatsu" means "finger pressure" in Japanese. A shiatsu practitioner applies pressure with his or her fingers—and sometimes thumbs, hands, elbows, and knees—to massage and manipulate the body to adjust its physical positioning and direct its inner natural energy to promote health. This inner natural energy is called *ki* in Japanese (or *qi* in Chinese; see page 283). It is sometimes described as a vital life force that flows through the universe and all living things, where it regulates physical, emotional, mental, and spiritual well-being. Ki is thought to move through a person's body along special energy pathways, or meridians.

When ki is flowing along these meridians and throughout the body in a complete and natural way, the result is a healthy body and mind. When something interrupts the flow of ki, or causes it to become unbalanced, health is disrupted and illness may follow. Like acupressure (see page 255), shiatsu involves applying controlled force to special pressure points along energy meridians. In shiatsu, these pressure points are called *tsubo*. By using different shiatsu techniques, practitioners work to unlock blocked ki at these points, rebalance its flow through the body, and in so doing, restore or maintain health.

Shiatsu as we know it today had its start in the early part of the 20th century with a Japanese massage practitioner, Tamai Tempaku. Tempaku had studied older forms of Japanese massage and Chinese acupuncture, and was well versed in Western medical knowledge about human anatomy and physiology as well as European-style massage. In 1919, Tempaku published a book called *Shiatsu Ho* ("finger pressure therapy") in which he integrated elements from all these areas into the somewhat revolutionary concept of shiatsu. The technique quickly gained followers throughout Japan. Several students of Tempaku went on to develop their own styles of shiatsu. One of the most influential of Tempaku's students was Tokujiro Namikoshi, who founded the Shiatsu Institute of Therapy in the late 1920s, and the Nippon Shiatsu Institute in Tokyo in 1940. Following World War II, all forms of traditional Japanese medicine, including shiatsu, were temporarily outlawed by the occupying Allied forces—but later were allowed due to protests by the Japanese people. In 1953, Tokujiro Namikoshi's son, Toru Namikoshi, began teaching shiatsu at a chiropractic college in Ohio. Namikoshi, and the other Japanese practitioners who followed him to the United States, sparked the development and practice of shiatsu in America.

▶ | THE BASICS

There are different styles of shiatsu, including Zen shiatsu, barefoot shiatsu, macrobiotic shiatsu, Namikoshi style, Shiatsu-Do, and others. They all follow the same basic principle of applying pressure on particular parts and points of the body, but employ different techniques. For instance, some use stretching exercises whereas others focus on special breathing practices and meditation. But the goal is the same: to manipulate ki to improve the body's ability to heal itself and to promote overall health. Scientific research on shiatsu and its effects is still preliminary. People typically seek

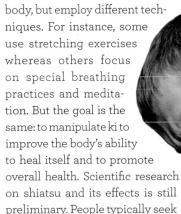

out shiatsu treatments for relief of neck, shoulder, and back pain, for headache relief, and for release of muscle tension and stiffness. Shiatsu is also used to reduce fatigue, aid in relaxation, reduce anxiety and stress, ease insomnia, improve digestion and circulation, and provide relief from arthritis pain and stiffness. Many people who have had shiatsu treatments for various conditions report that they feel more relaxed, more flexible, and have less pain.

A typical session with a shiatsu practitioner usually lasts 45 minutes to an hour. Unlike massage or similar bodywork therapies, no oils or lotions are used and the client remains fully clothed. Because shiatsu is considered a preventative form of therapy, many people have treatments monthly to enhance health and general well-being.

▶ | PUT INTO PRACTICE

If you are considering trying shiatsu, seek out a qualified and experienced practitioner. Ask your health care provider for recommendations. You can perform a few simple shiatsu techniques on yourself, or with the help of a friend or partner, primarily to relieve muscle tension and stress. What follows is a simple shiatsu self-energizing routine called Do-In, which involves tapping, massaging, and pressing on different parts of your body; treatment from a shiatsu practitioner would likely include much more in the way of firm finger pressure applied to specific points. The Do-In is designed to improve and maintain general

physical health and mental well-being. There are many variations; this particular sequence takes about 15 minutes to complete.

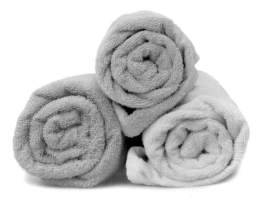

⚠ **CAUTION:** Not enough scientific evidence exists to confirm the effectiveness of shiatsu in managing any particular condition. Complementary or alternative therapies such as shiatsu should not be considered a substitute for conventional medical care. Consult your health care provider before having shiatsu treatments.

Tap Into Your Natural Energy

■ *Use Shiatsu Principles* Energize your own body even though traditionally shiatsu massage is provided by a trained therapist to another person. Here is a full-body routine you can try.

• In a quiet, well-ventilated room, stand on a yoga mat or carpeted surface. Have a pillow or thick towel handy for using later in the sequence. Breathe normally and try to keep your mind clear and free of thoughts that could make you feel stressed or tense.

• Begin by rubbing your hands together vigorously to stimulate the flow of ki in your body. Gently shake your arms and hands to relax them. One at a time, gently shake each of your legs and feet.

• Make loose fists with your hands. Keeping your wrists relaxed, begin tapping your head gently, starting at the top and moving around it in a counterclockwise direction. Cover your entire head, front, back, and sides. Then use the fingertips of both hands to massage your scalp, working from your forehead to the back of your neck.

- If you are pregnant, consult your health care provider before having any shiatsu treatment or performing any self-treatment.
- If you are undergoing chemotherapy or radiation, or have had a recent injury or surgery, talk to your health care provider before having shiatsu treatment.

• Place your hands on the sides of your face. Using the palms, slide your hands up and down the sides of your face, gently massaging your cheeks until the skin of the palms becomes warm. Immediately cup your warm palms over your eyes: Hold for 15 seconds (do not press on your eyeballs).

• Using your fingertips, apply gentle pressure to the skin overlying your upper and lower gums.

• Using your thumbs and index fingers, massage your ear lobes. Cup your right hand over your right ear and tap the back of the hand with the index and middle finger of your left hand three or four times. Repeat on the other side.

• Rotate your head gently to the right. Using a loose fist, tap gently on the left side of your neck with your left hand. Rotate your head to the left and tap gently on the right side of your neck with your right hand.

• With your right hand in a loose fist, reach over and tap all around your left shoulder. (Support the right elbow with your left hand.) Then switch sides, using your left hand in a loose fist to tap around your right shoulder.

• Straighten your left arm and hand. Using your right hand in a loose fist, gently tap the inside of the arm from the shoulder to the palm. Turn your left arm over and gently tap from the back of the hand up to the shoulder. Repeat the same procedure with your right arm extended, tapping with the left hand.

• Use your right thumb and index finger to massage the palm of your left hand, and then gently pull on and massage each finger and the thumb. Switch hands, using the thumb and index finger of your left hand to massage the palm and fingers and thumb of your right hand in the same way.

• Using loose fists, gently pound on your chest and across your rib cage. Open your hands, and with flat palms, pat your abdomen, moving in a clockwise direction. Bend forward slightly, and with loose fists, gently pound on your lower back and kidneys. Stand straight. Pound gently on your buttocks.

• Spread your feet slightly more than shoulder width apart, knees slightly bent. Tap with loose fists down the outside of each leg, hip to ankle. Tap up the inside, ankle to groin. Tap down the backs of your legs from your buttocks to your ankles, and finally tap up the fronts of your legs to your hips.

• Sit on the pillow or towel (you can also sit in a straight chair if that is more comfortable). Grab hold of one foot. Gently rotate, and massage the ankles. Press firmly around the heel and alongside the sole. Massage and gently pull on each toe. Using a loose fist, gently pound up, down, and across the bottom of your foot. Repeat the procedure on the other foot.

• Stand up with your feet shoulder width apart. Inhale deeply and raise your arms straight up. Exhale, placing your hands on the back of your head. Stroke downward along your neck. Place your hands on your upper back and stroke down your back, your buttocks and the backs of your legs, bending over gently in the process.

• Bring your hands around to the front of your ankles. Stroke up the fronts of your legs, up your abdomen and chest, letting your hands come to rest on your upper chest. Inhale, extending your arms outward, palms up. Exhale, bringing your arms gently down to your sides.

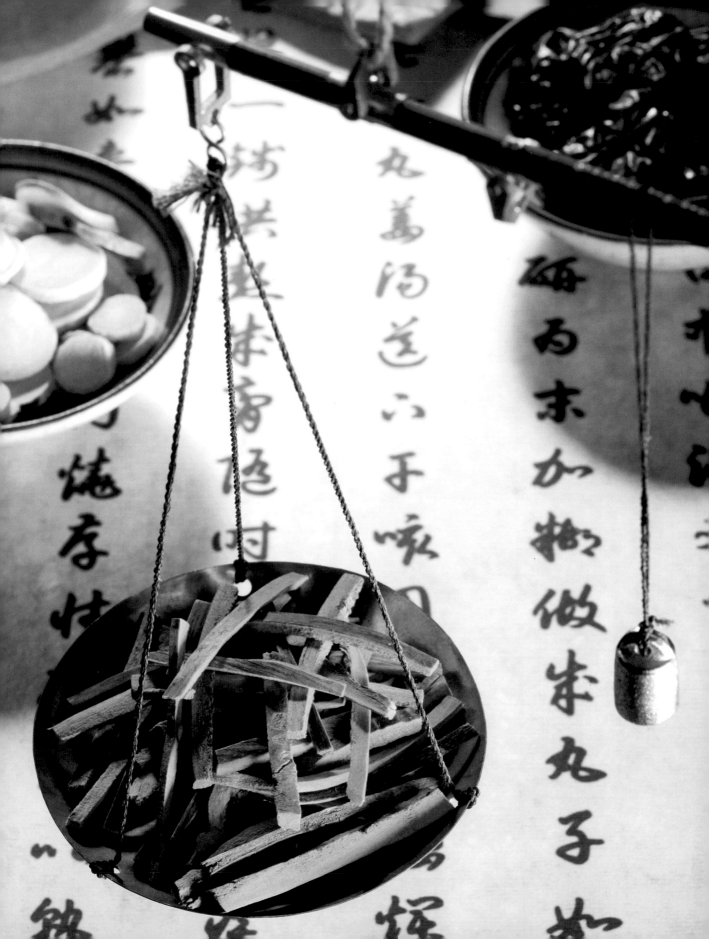

Traditional Chinese Medicine

7 MODERN PRACTICES FROM ANCIENT WAYS

Traditional Chinese medicine (TCM) is one of the world's oldest medical systems, with its origins reaching back at least several thousand years. It is a complex system of healing, and over the centuries, it has undergone a long and intricate development. Modern TCM represents a cumulative body of knowledge that has been assembled over time by practitioners using different philosophies, different medical approaches, and different cultural practices. This evolution continues even today. In many Chinese hospitals and clinics, TCM is practiced alongside, and often in combination with, Western medicine.

The TCM view of how the human body works, what causes illness, and how illness should be treated is much different from that of conventional Western medicine. In the West, health care providers typically view illness as something affecting a certain part of the body—a respiratory infection, heart problem, or an intestinal ailment. They work to treat that problem specifically, often in the most direct way possible—for instance, by surgically removing a cancerous tumor or using an antibiotic to treat infection. In TCM, illness is seen as a manifestation of imbalance in the whole person, not just one isolated part. According to this ancient healing tradition, the human body is a unified entity in which all the tissues, organs, and organ systems are utterly interdependent. TCM practitioners consider illness to be a sign of imbalance in the whole person. As a result, the goal in TCM is not to simply cure a disease or correct a problem, but to restore balance and harmony within a person and between the person and his or her environment.

▶ | THE BASICS

Practitioners and followers of TCM believe that a vital energy or life force called *qi* fills the universe and animates every living thing. They believe that qi travels through a person's body along a system of pathways called meridians. In a healthy individual, qi flows freely to every cell, tissue, and organ, without impediment. Blocks or imbalances in the circulation of qi result in illness. TCM practitioners use eight principles to diagnose a health problem and categorize its characteristics: cold/heat, interior/exterior, excess/deficiency, and yin/yang. These principles are also combined with the theory of five elements—fire, earth, metal, water, and wood—to help explain the relationship between a patient's physiology and an illness.

To illustrate the different approaches to illness in Western medicine and TCM, consider gout as an example. Western doctors would describe gout as a metabolic disorder brought on by an excess of uric acid in the bloodstream, which in turn causes crystals of uric acid salts to be deposited in the

HERBAL PRESCRIPTIONS IN TRADITIONAL CHINESE MEDICINE

In the West, we tend to use one herb at a time. In TCM and other herbal traditions, herbs are usually delivered in a prescription that can include from a few up to as many as a hundred herbs. A multivolume Chinese canon on herbal prescriptions collected from dozens of ancient Chinese herbals documents more than 14,000 prescriptions. A TCM prescription usually includes a "monarch" herb that "rules" the formula, with a "minister" herb to synergize the effect of the monarch herb. "Assistant" herbs are added to "supervise" the function of the main herbs. Finally a "guide" herb may be added to enhance the effectiveness or the flavor of the whole mix.

–Steven Foster
Herbalist and lecturer

joints, urinary tract, and soft tissues. These deposits lead to very painful bouts of arthritis and soft-tissue inflammation. From a TCM practitioner's viewpoint, however, the symptoms of gout (painful and hot joints, redness and swelling, and impaired movement) point to an obstruction of qi, due to a combined attack on the body's meridians (especially in the hands and feet) by wind, cold, and dampness that have led to a stagnation of the patient's vital energy.

▶ PUT INTO PRACTICE

To help restore the balance of qi in a sick person—and so treat illness by promoting a return to health—TCM practitioners use many different therapies. Each is designed to balance some aspect of the body, mind, or spirit, and restore the healthy flow of qi along the meridians that connect all the body's organ systems. Practitioners evaluate a patient's condition by carefully observing his or her appearance (especially the tongue), listening to and smelling parts of the body, touching and palpating various areas (including noting characteristics of the pulse), and asking detailed questions. Based on the

findings of these examinations, TCM practitioners develop a treatment for the patient that is highly individualized.

⚠ **CAUTION:** Never use TCM as a replacement for conventional medical care or as a reason to postpone seeing your health care provider about a medical problem, injury, or illness.

A Delicate Balance

■ *Use of Herbs* One of the most commonly used therapies in TCM is herbal medicine. The Chinese herbal pharmacopeia contains thousands of medicinal plants, as well as minerals and certain animal parts and products; each is classified by its perceived action in the human body. Depending on the illness or condition, different parts of medicinal plants may be used, ranging from leaves, flowers, and stems, to roots and seeds. Typically, herbal medicines are compounded according to ancient formulas, customized to a patient's condition, and often include multiple ingredients.

⚠ **CAUTION:** Licensed TCM practitioners are usually adamant that people should not use Chinese herbs and herbal formulations on their own. As in any medical system, proper diagnosis is essential for proper treatment. Many Chinese medicinal herb combinations can have side effects (just like Western medications) and they should only be used under the supervision and guidance of a trained TCM practitioner.

■ *Healing Through Acupuncture* An integral part of TCM, acupuncture is a therapy that aims to restore and maintain health by stimulating specific points along the meridians (acupoints) through which qi travels in the body. This is usually done by inserting fine (hair-thin), metallic needles into the skin at acupoints. The needles are usually left in place for 15 to 30 minutes. An acupuncturist may manipulate the needles—gently lifting, twisting, and rotating them—depending on the condition being treated. Uncomfortable as this might sound,

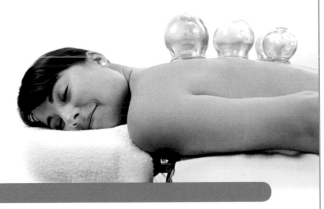

the experience is usually not painful. When the acupuncturist correctly locates an acupoint, a faint tingling feeling often follows. Numerous studies have been done on acupuncture: Many suggest that it can be useful for a wide variety of conditions. However, its effects are still not well understood, and much more scientific research is needed.

⚠ **CAUTION:** Acupuncture is considered safe as long as it is performed by an experienced practitioner using sterile needles. Acupuncture is not a do-it-yourself treatment.

- ***Adding Heat*** Another healing therapy often used in TCM is moxibustion. It involves burning a cone or stick of the herb mugwort (moxa) on or near the skin, often in conjunction with acupuncture. Indirect moxibustion, the most common form of this treatment used today, involves lighting a moxa stick and holding it close to acupoints on the body, typically until the skin at each point flushes from the heat. Alternatively, a needle is inserted into an acupoint and the end of the needle is wrapped in moxa, which is then ignited. The burning moxa heats the needle, and in turn, the skin and tissues around the acupoint. Moxibustion is believed to expel cold and help warm the meridians, which enhances the smooth flow of qi.
- ***Treating With Cupping*** Another TCM therapy, cupping shares some similarities with moxibustion. Heated glass cups are placed on the skin, typically over specific acupoints. As the cups cool, the air pressure inside decreases, causing the skin to be slightly "sucked up" into the cups, pulling on the tissue and drawing blood into the area under the cups.
- ***Qigong*** Qigong (see page 283) is a TCM mind-body therapy that involves exercise and meditation.
- ***Other Therapies*** Certain types of Chinese massage and special diets are other therapies often included as part of TCM treatments.
- ***What the Science Says*** Despite its popularity in China and Asia, and its use in the West, TCM has not been studied in depth in a systematic way. Most clinical studies have been carried out on acupuncture and its use in treating certain conditions. Many of these studies suggest acupuncture can be helpful for some things, such as pain, nausea, and vomiting, but more research is needed. Some herbs and herbal formulas used in TCM also appear to be beneficial for certain conditions, but again, more research needs to be done.

good to know: ABOUT TCM

- If you are considering TCM, consult your medical doctor before beginning any treatments.
- Learn about a potential TCM practitioner's qualifications before undergoing a treatment program. Many states require that acupuncturists pass exams and obtain licenses to practice, but some do not. Fewer states require certification to practice oriental medicine and Chinese herbal medicine.
- Although some Chinese herbal treatments may be safe, others may not. Some of the herbs in TCM herbal formulas can have powerful effects and may have serious side effects. Be aware that some herbal formulations may interact or interfere with prescription medications. There have also been reports of Chinese herbal products being contaminated with heavy metals, pharmaceuticals, pesticides, and various toxins or containing ingredients not listed on the label.

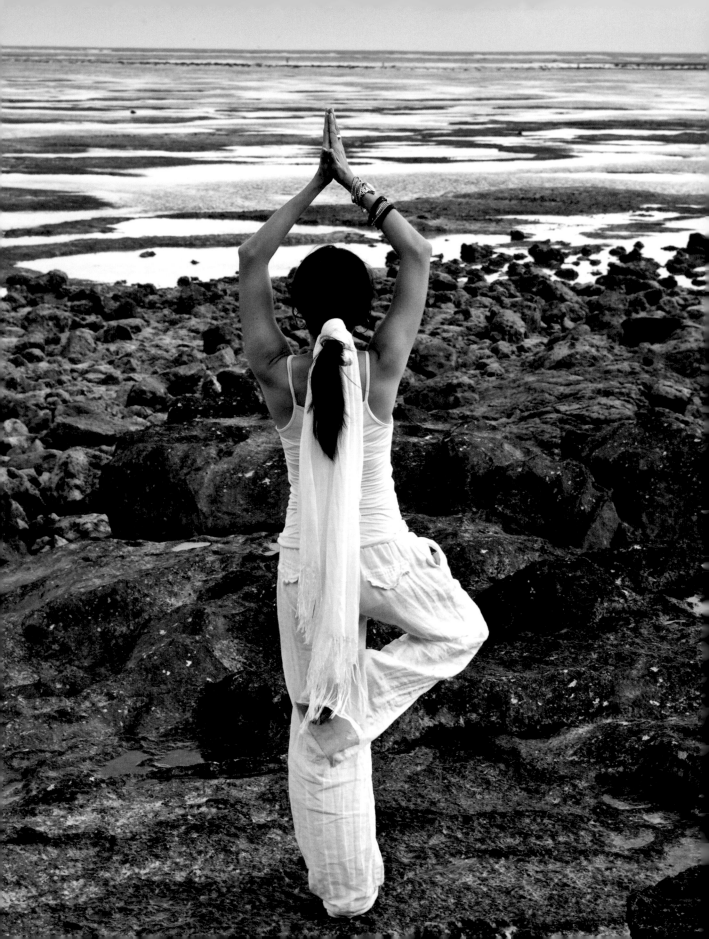

Yoga

8 WAYS TO STAY YOUNG & FLEXIBLE

I t's a common misconception that yoga—an ancient system of exercise, breathing, and meditation—is rooted in Hinduism, the predominant religious tradition of India. Archaeological evidence, though, indicates that yoga predates Hinduism by many centuries. Stone carvings that are at least 5,000 years old depicting people in various yoga positions have been unearthed in the Indus River Valley. One theory is that, as Hinduism evolved, it incorporated some of the practices and ideas of yoga, forging an association that continues to this day. Yoga itself, however, is not a religion; it's not associated with any creed or type of deity. Quite the contrary—the core of yoga philosophy is that all things come from within the individual.

The word "yoga" comes from the Sanskrit *yuj*, which means "to join or yoke together." The name may refer to the fundamental goal of yoga: to bring the body and the mind together in harmony. The earliest written record of yoga is the roughly 2,000-year-old *Yoga Sutras*, a text often credited to a scholar named Patanjali, who outlined what we think of today as "classical yoga." Patanjali divided yoga into eight basic parts, or limbs: (1) *yama* (moral behavior or ethics); (2) *niyama* (healthy habits or cleanliness); (3) *asana* (physical exercises or postures); (4) *pranayama* (controlled breathing techniques); (5) *pratyahara* (mental withdrawal from the senses); (6) *dharana* (concentration); (7) *dhyana* (meditation); and (8) *samadhi* (attainment of higher consciousness).

The techniques practiced within each limb have been passed down from teacher to student for thousands of years. It's not surprising that, over time, numerous schools of yoga have arisen, each incorporating the eight limbs to varying degrees. Among the most well known are Hatha, Raja, Jnana, Karma, Bhakti, and Tantra Yoga. Hatha yoga is the form most often practiced in the United States and Europe. It emphasizes physical movements (asanas) and breathing techniques (pranayama). Other yoga styles include Ashtanga, Bikram, Iyengar, Jivamukti, Kripalu, Kundalini, and Sivananda.

Yoga was hardly known in the United States until the 1960s, when a growing awareness of Eastern cultures sparked interest in this system of mind-body practice. Yoga's popularity has been on the rise ever since. Many research studies have demonstrated yoga's value in reducing stress, improving mood and feelings of well-being, lowering blood pressure and heart rate, improving muscle relaxation, strength, and flexibility, increasing lung capacity, countering anxiety and depression, and providing relief from insomnia.

Yoga is now recognized, even in the conventional medical community, as a valuable tool for promoting health—and perhaps even preventing or fighting disease. One recent study, for example, revealed that yoga may help suppress inflammation-inducing compounds that are thought to play a role in the development of cardiovascular disease, type-2 diabetes, and other conditions.

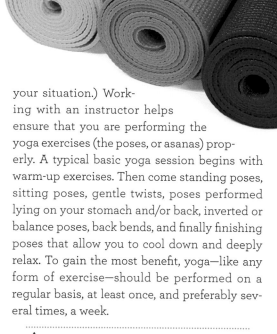

▶ | THE BASICS

Every style of Hatha Yoga (what you are most likely to encounter) centers around exercise, breathing, and to some extent, meditation. Yoga exercises are designed to promote relaxation, increase circulation to some of the body's important glandular systems, and improve overall muscle tone, strength, and balance. Breathing techniques are also fundamental to yoga practice, because the breath is considered the source of life. Controlling the breath, like controlling the body's position and movement, is considered a means to improve health and maintain function. Exercise and breathing, taken together, are an ideal preface to cultivating a quiet mind through meditation.

The best way to get acquainted with yoga is probably to take a beginning class from an experienced, qualified yoga instructor. (Ask specifically about the demands of the type of yoga being offered; tell the instructor about any physical limitations or health conditions you might have and ask whether the class is suitable for your situation.) Working with an instructor helps ensure that you are performing the yoga exercises (the poses, or asanas) properly. A typical basic yoga session begins with warm-up exercises. Then come standing poses, sitting poses, gentle twists, poses performed lying on your stomach and/or back, inverted or balance poses, back bends, and finally finishing poses that allow you to cool down and deeply relax. To gain the most benefit, yoga—like any form of exercise—should be performed on a regular basis, at least once, and preferably several times, a week.

⚠ **CAUTION:** Consult your health care provider before starting yoga. Yoga is generally considered safe in healthy people if practiced appropriately. However, people with certain medical conditions should not perform yoga or certain yoga poses. For instance, if you have spine or disk problems, glaucoma, a detached retina, high or low blood pressure, fragile blood vessels, risk of blood clots, severe osteoporosis, ear problems, or cervical spondylitis, you should not perform inverted yoga poses. Pregnant and menstruating women may want to avoid doing certain yoga poses as well. Never use yoga as a replacement for conventional medical care for any disease, condition, or illness.

JUST BREATHE

Breath awareness forms part of yoga practice. Ideally, your parasympathetic nervous system ("rest and digest")—rather than your sympathetic nervous system ("fight or flight")—governs your heart rate. Predominance of the parasympathetic system promotes a healthy variability in heart rate. During inhalation, the pulse rises subtly; during exhalation, the pulse slows. An overactive sympathetic nervous system elevates heart rate and blood pressure and blunts heart rate variability (HRV), raising the risk for cardiovascular disease.

Mindful breathing shifts you into "rest and digest" mode, restores HRV, lowers blood pressure, and reduces stress, anxiety, and depression. Try this: Lie on your back with one hand on your belly. Inhale to a slow count of four and notice how your hand lifts. Exhale to a slow count of four as your hand falls. Repeat.

–Linda B. White, M.D.
Educator and author

▶ | PUT INTO PRACTICE

Most people begin the practice of yoga by enrolling in a weekly class, where a trained teacher explains the poses and watches as you do them. As a very basic introduction to yoga, several simple and common yoga poses are presented. Consult your health care provider before attempting them. Move slowly and gently, breathing as directed. If any position causes pain, stop. Wear loose, unrestrictive clothing when performing yoga poses and stand and sit on a nonslippery surface; a rubbery yoga mat is ideal.

Joining Mind & Body

- **_Begin With Breathing_** Sit comfortably on a yoga mat or padded, carpeted floor. Cross your legs, placing your feet under your knees. Loosely clasp your hands around your knees, keeping your back straight and head erect. In this position (called Sukhasana) perform the Complete Breath, as described on page 268, five to ten times. You may close your eyes or keep them open.

- **_Do a Gentle, Reclining Twist_** Lie on your back with your knees bent. Have a pillow or thickly folded towel or blanket ready on either side of your body. Relax your neck, resting the back of your head on the floor. Extend your arms out about 90 degrees from your body. Shift your hips slightly to the left,

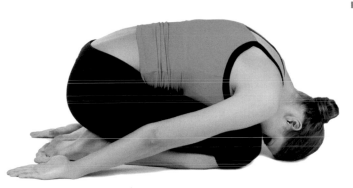

and let your knees fall gently to the right. Try to keep your shoulders in contact with the mat. If your knees can fall all the way to comfortably rest on the floor, fine. If not, push the pillow or other soft support beneath the knees so your legs can rest supported and be completely relaxed. Now turn your head to the left, away from your knees. Hold for five breaths, inhaling and exhaling through your nose. Bring your head back to center. Engage your core muscles and slowly bring your knees back up to the upright position. Shift your hips slightly to the right, and let your knees gently fall to the left. Support if needed, and turn your head slightly right, away from your knees. Hold for five breaths. Repeat two more times, if desired.

- **_Relax Forward_** This resting pose, called Child's Pose (Balasana), gives a slight forward stretch to the spine as well as the hips, thighs, and ankles. It is also very relaxing. Kneel and sit back on your feet with your heels pointing slightly outward and big toes just touching. Your knees should be separated about the width of your hips. (Note: If sitting like this is uncomfortable, place a folded towel between the backs of your thighs and your calves.) Lean forward, extending your arms forward

good to know: ABOUT YOGA

- Use a nonskid yoga mat; never work on a slippery surface.
- When performing the poses, or asanas, concentrate on your movements. Moving into and out of a pose is just as important as being in the pose.
- While performing yoga poses, you should be able to continue breathing in a slow, controlled fashion; in many respects, proper breathing is as, if not more, important than the physical pose.
- Yoga is not a competitive sport. If you are in a class situation, do not try to match what others are doing. Do only what you are safely able to do.
- Never force anything. There are alternative versions of every pose for different levels of ability (and flexibility). If a pose seems like it will be too difficult, ask your instructor to demonstrate an easier or gentler alternative.
- Never strain or continue to hold a yoga pose if it causes severe discomfort or pain; stop immediately.
- Investigate yoga props and get advice on how to use them. Props are any objects, such as foam blocks, bolsters, chairs, and benches, that help you perform yoga in a safer, more stable way with better posture.
- Keep your eyes open when doing poses, as closing them may cause you to lose your balance. (Closing eyes during resting or meditative poses, performed while sitting or lying on the floor, is fine.)

and alongside your head as far as is comfortable; let your forehead rest on the mat. While continuing to rest your forehead on the mat, bring your arms back around and to your sides, with your palms facing up. Hold this position for one to three minutes, and then return to the upright position.

⚠ **CAUTION:** Do not do this pose if you have knee problems or diarrhea.

■ *Improve Balance* This modified Tree Pose (Vrksasana) is good for strengthening the legs and improving balance and concentration. When you first try this pose, stand with your back close to (almost touching) a wall to keep yourself steady. Alternatively, stand near a stable chair that you can reach for at any time while doing the asana to maintain balance. Begin by standing with your feet about shoulder width apart. Exhale and bring the sole of your left foot to the inside of your right leg, as high as is comfortable, toes pointing down (your left sole might rest just above your right ankle, on your inner right calf, or if you are very flexible, on your inner right thigh; however, avoid placing your left foot against the inside of your right knee, as this could strain the knee joint). You will now be standing on your right leg only. Concentrate on maintaining your balance. (If you start to lose your balance, simply put your left foot back down, relax, and try again.) As you inhale, bring your arms up to extend out to the sides at shoulder height, palms facing up. Exhale and bring your palms together in front of your chest in a prayer position. Hold about 30 seconds, breathing normally, and concentrating on maintaining your balance.

On the next exhale, slowly bring your arms and left leg down. Relax for a moment, and then repeat the pose on the left side, bringing the right foot up and balancing on your left leg.

■ *Strengthen the Thighs, Straighten the Back* The Chair Pose (Utkatasana) helps strengthen the lower back and the muscles in your thighs. It looks deceptively easy, but isn't. Begin by standing with your feet about shoulder width apart, arms at your sides. Inhale and raise your arms as straight as possible over your head. Concentrate on lengthening your spine and keeping your chest full and open. As you exhale, bend your knees—keeping your lower back straight—and tip your upper body forward (arms still straight above your head) about 45 degrees. You will feel the tension in your thigh muscles as they contract to support you. Hold this position quietly, and breathe slowly and completely, allowing your breath to fill your belly as well as your chest. Focus on keeping your back straight and arms aligned with it, overhead. Continue holding, if possible, for at least two complete breaths, and then lower your arms and come back into an upright standing position.

■ *Arch Like a Snake* The Cobra Pose (Bhujangasana) can help to decrease stiffness in the lower back. Begin by lying on your stomach (on a yoga mat or carpeted surface) with your head resting on your lower arms. Raise your head slightly and focus on a point in the distance. Move your hands backward along the floor until they are slightly behind your shoulders; keep your arms close to your body. Engage the muscles in your lower back and arch your back slightly, raising the front half of your body up off the floor. Don't use your hands to support your weight; let your back muscles do the work. When you've reached the highest position you can comfortably attain (do not force yourself to go higher than is comfortable), tip your head back very slightly and hold this position, breathing slowing and evenly, all the while keeping your back muscles engaged. Try to keep your buttock muscles completely relaxed while doing the Cobra, as well as your arms; think of your arms as being there only for balance. Let the muscles of your lower back provide the power to maintain this position. Breathe slowly and evenly, keeping your eyes focused on a distant point ahead of you. Hold for two to three complete breaths, if possible. Then slowly let your upper body sink back toward the floor, sliding your hands and arms forward at the same time. When you are lying flat once again, rest your head on your arms and let your body relax. Concentrate on letting the muscles in your lower back release completely. Breathe normally several times. Repeat the pose once or twice more.

⚠ **CAUTION:** Be careful doing this exercise if you have had a lower back injury, such as a herniated disk. Some people with lower back pain find this exercise helpful, whereas others do not.

■ *Make Like a Corpse* This pose is a good one to end a yoga practice, or to relieve stress and deeply relax at any time. It is called the Corpse Pose, or Savasana. On a padded carpeted floor or a yoga mat, lie on your back with your legs shoulder width apart; let your feet naturally fall outward. Close your eyes and cover with an eye mask or a small clean cloth such as a folded washcloth. Let your arms lie naturally at your sides, with hands about 12 inches from your body. Roll your head gently to the left and then to the right, coming back to center. Adjust any

> ### *NAMASTE*—I BOW TO YOU
>
> Traditional yoga contains eight parts, or "limbs," in yoga parlance. Mainstream Americans practicing yoga as well as scientists researching its effects on the body have primarily focused on three of these limbs: the asanas (physical poses), breathing exercises, and meditation. Yoga classes often encompass all three. Studies show that a regular yoga routine can enhance well-being, sleep, and eating habits. The practice of yoga reduces feelings of stress, anxiety, and depression. It eases low back pain, headaches, arthritis, and the menopause transition. Strength, balance, and flexibility increase—physically and mentally. Unhealthy fat is lost. Cardiovascular disease and diabetes improve. The ideal yoga studio can cultivate gratitude, joy, compassion, kindness, and patience.
>
> **–Linda B. White, M.D.**
> *Educator and author*

part of your body until you feel completely at ease. Concentrate on letting your head, shoulders, back, pelvis, arms, hands, legs, and feet—every part of your body that is contacting the mat—sink into the ground. Take a deep breath, extending your abdomen and then filling your chest, and then release and breathe normally. Continue to concentrate on sinking into the ground and hold the pose, completely relaxed and breathing naturally, for several minutes. When you are ready to come out of the pose, open your eyes, bend your knees, and roll gently onto one side. Use your arms to help push yourself up into a sitting position, letting your head come up last.

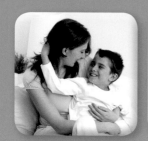
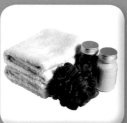
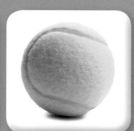
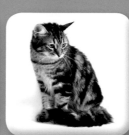
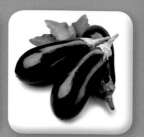

a healthy

lifestyle

Lifestyles

194 HINTS FROM THE WORLD'S HEALTHIEST

"You don't see many old men who are overweight and smoke," a wisecracker once noted. It turns out he was more accurate than funny. When writer and researcher Dan Buettner went on a mission looking for the secrets of the longest lived people in the world—those who live to 100 and beyond—he didn't run into any centenarians who were overweight and out of shape, with a cigarette in hand. What he found instead were healthy people with a zest for life.

Well-Known Secrets

In Buettner's best-selling book *The Blue Zones,* he chronicled the commonalities of people in regions of the world where people not only live long, they *thrive.* He found five mostly remote areas, where people by far outweigh the odds of living healthfully to the century mark and beyond. It's almost as if long life and happiness in these parts of the world are contagious. Could it be something in the water? That's what Buettner and his team of researchers from National Geographic wanted to find out when they went to talk to these people and investigate their lifestyle habits. As they documented their findings, it became clear that these centenarians share similar traits that contribute to a compelling whole: They practice healthy living.

As Buettner witnessed, healthy living is much more than feeding yourself well and getting enough exercise. It's also about positive thinking, a curiosity about the world, and an interest in other people. It's about having a purpose for living and the drive to reach that goal. It's about creating a personal environment, needing and enjoying others, and being surrounded by

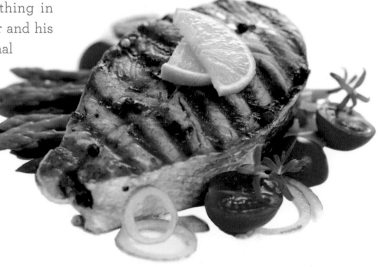

family and a happy and nurturing network of friends. It's about believing—in self, in others, and in spiritual pursuit.

Health and Happiness

In the world's cultures of longevity, health and happiness are interrelated. According to Buettner, who also wrote the book *Thrive,* which chronicles the lives of the world's happiest people, 50 percent of our natural predisposition for happiness, or the opposite, is genetic. The other half—which is 40 percent influenced by how we think and 10 percent ruled by our life's circumstances—is, for the most part, under our own control. That doesn't mean we can't rise above our genes. We can. So, if you have portraits of stern-looking ancestors hanging on your walls, don't fret. Happiness is a gift we can all attain.

Intuitively, we know we should lead a healthy lifestyle. The median life span for a child born in the United States today is 77.5, meaning half will die before that age and the other half will live longer. If you're 60 now, you can expect to spend another 21 years on this earth if you're a man and another 24 years if you're a woman. Of course, you want them to be productive years. You want to be happy and healthy until the day you die. But what about those centenarians Buettner encountered who were spry for decades beyond their natural life expectancy? Shouldn't we be reaching for those kinds of odds? Why not! There's nothing to lose and plenty to gain by practicing what science now knows is good for the body, mind, and soul. Let's take a look.

DOWNSHIFTING

The Danish Twin Studies, a population-based study of 2,872 twin pairs born from 1870 to 1900 in Denmark, established that genes dictate only about 20 percent of how long the average person lives—within certain biological limits. Lifestyle and overall health explain more about longevity. These aren't just more years; they are better, healthier years free of chronic diseases.

The secret to long-term health, as I see it, has less to do about diet—or even exercise—and more to do with the social and physical environment in which we live. The healthiest cultures live rewardingly inconvenient lives. They live in strong families that motivate them to make the effort to support loved ones. They know their life's purpose, actively pursue it, and have a ritual of "downshifting" each day. They experience the same stresses we all do—kids, health, finances—but manage stress through daily prayer, meditation, ancestor veneration, or citywide happy hours (like the Sardinians).

Sound too simple? Remember, simple doesn't mean easy. I don't recommend trying to change all these behaviors at once. Pick two or three to work on at a time. Research has shown that if you can sustain a behavioral change for six weeks, you should be able to sustain it for the rest of your life. As the world's centenarians have shown us, the rest of your life should be a long, long time.

Dan Buettner
Founder of Blue Zones, best-selling author, National Geographic fellow, and expert on longevity

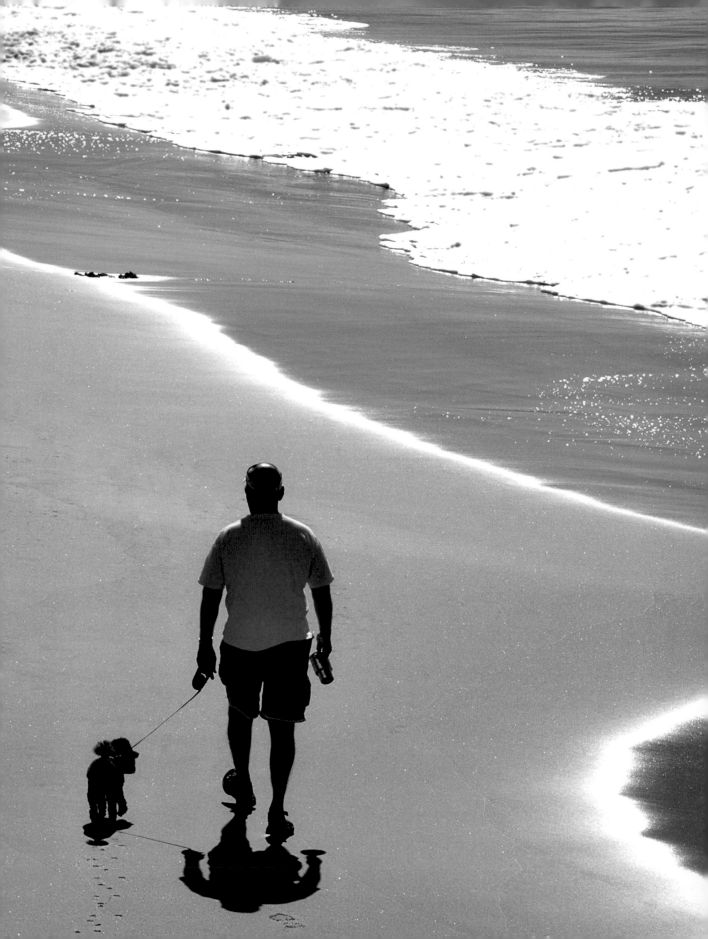

Banish the Blues

15 HABITS EN ROUTE TO HAPPINESS

How do you measure happiness? After all, what makes someone happy—say, having a house full of five-year-olds for the weekend—can make another person miserable. Despite the fact that scientists have been grappling with the concept of happiness for centuries and tons of data exist on happiness theories, there is no such thing as a happiness barometer. Happiness is a subjective phenomenon. However, there's one discovery that may surprise you: Despite the notion that we don't like getting older, studies show that we actually get happier as we age. The concept of happiness holds many surprises. So, let's take a look at some of these behaviors that stand between us and happiness and what we can do about them.

▶ | ANGER

Just how bad can a bad attitude be for your health and longevity? Really bad. Evidence suggests that the deleterious effects of anger's explosive fallout on the heart rank as high and possibly even higher than smoking.

When you feel rage, your body is going through a series of reactions that you cannot feel. When you overreact, so do your stress hormones—cortisol and epinephrine—which cause fatty acid levels in your blood to surge and also cause an increase in blood glucose levels. The process is called sludging and it can block off hundreds of tiny blood vessels for as long as 12 hours after a single outburst. This is how anger triggers a heart attack.

Anger is the antithesis of happiness. So if you're an angry sort, you can't find happiness—or even equilibrium—unless you learn to swallow hostility and smile.

Keep Your Cool

- **Learn to Be Appropriately Assertive** Your daughter-in-law sends your grandson to a sleepover ten minutes after you've just arrived for a visit after a long drive. Your mom has said you're starting to put on weight several times since you walked in the door. On top of it all, you're still boiling over the fact that your co-worker claimed credit for your great idea that has the whole company buzzing. There are times in all our lives when things can really get under our skin to the point we want to explode. Whether you shout it out or quietly seethe, both extremes are equally risky and affect your heart in a negative way. The best way to deal with situations that really get your goat is to take the middle ground. Get it out, but in an appropriately assertive way—calmly and politely. Here's how:
  - Don't accuse, insult, or use profanity.
  - Address the problem, not the person creating the problem.
  - Use "I" statements that acknowledge how you feel, rather than "you" statements.
  - Offer an appropriate solution.
- **Count to 10** Or even 100 if necessary. As the author Ambrose Bierce once said, "Speak when you are angry and you will make the best speech you'll ever regret."
- **Let Go of a Grudge** Holding a grudge is hard on your health. Studies show it creates personal stress equal to a major event, such as a death in the family. It also is bad for the psyche and can numb you into unhappiness. And what's the point? The person it is affecting the most is you. There's no grudge worth dying over.

- **Learn to Forgive** Forgiveness doesn't mean you have to forget. Forgive for your own sake, if not for the sake of others. It releases stress and gives you a feeling of relief.
- **Learn to Laugh at Yourself** Don't get angry with yourself if something goes wrong or you do something stupid. Admitting and accepting your faults adjusts your perspective on life.
- **Keep Tabs on Your Hot Buttons** Many people spend so much time being angry they don't pay attention to what's pushing their buttons. People often tend to fire their anger in the wrong direction. For example, yelling at the cashier because the checkout line is too long and slow isn't going to get you anywhere, but it will make you look like a jerk. Remember, count to 10 and think before you react.
- **Surprise Them With Kindness** If you're the recipient of anger, surprise your assailer with kindness. The cashier who responds to the impatient customer, "Have a nice day, sir," said without anger, not only deflects an angry reaction but will likely get a lot of smiles from others in line. Everyone benefits.

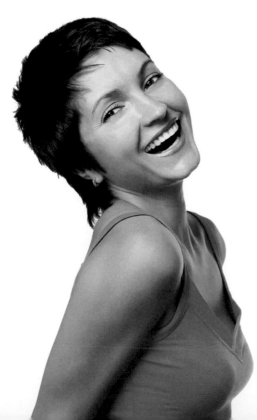

▶ | THE BLUES

There are good days and bad days, good times and bad times. When the bad start to outnumber the good, it can get to you. Smiles turn into frowns. The slight skip in a walk turns into a shuffle. Getting the blues can make your whole life feel like a bad hair day. We can't be perky all of the time, but we can be perky some of the time! There are plenty of ways to banish the blues. These are among the techniques that work.

WHEN TO CALL THE DR.: Getting the blues is a normal feeling we all experience from time to time, but true depression is not. Depression is a mood disturbance characterized by profound sadness and despair. It affects overall physiologic functioning: Appetite can increase or decrease. Weight may go up or own. Sleep is disturbed. Depression involves fatigue, difficulty concentrating and making decisions, guilt, and more. It's a condition that should be treated with professional counseling and medications. Anyone suffering from depression should seek medical intervention.

Picker-Uppers

- **Fill Your Life With Happiness** When you occupy your mind with happy thoughts and activities, you don't have time to think about your troubles. Don't sit and brood. Do something you love. Go to an art show, go shopping, grab a book, go to the beach, or attend a sporting event. Whatever you do for pleasure when you're happy becomes even more important to do when you're blue.
- **Laugh a Lot** When was the last time you had a good belly laugh? If you can't remember, then you're probably taking life too seriously. Laughter melts tension, which lifts your spirits. If you can't find something to laugh at, seek out funny people who can make you laugh.
- **Watch a Funny Movie** Research shows that watching a funny movie is therapeutic.

Researchers proved this when they observed blood flow in people exposed to comedy versus drama. When study participants watched 15 minutes of the comedy, *Kingpin*, blood flow to the heart increased 22 percent. After 15 minutes of exposure to the dramatic movie, *Saving Private Ryan*, blood flow decreased by 35 percent.

- *Move Your Body* Feeling blue? Take a walk. Go for a run. Jump on your bike and ride around the block. Even just getting up from your desk and walking for five or ten minutes—inside the office building or around the block—can make a major difference in the way you feel and the energy level you bring with you when you return to work. Numerous studies have found that exercise is a powerful mood elevator.

- *Check Out of the Bar* Although alcohol can initially lift spirits, drinking too much—that is, more than two drinks a day—is a depressant. If alcohol's effect brings on the blues in you, don't drink.

- *Think Positive* Check your inner monologue and truly listen to what it's saying. If it's filled with a lot of negatives—I can't, I'm just not lucky, this always happens to me—make a concerted effort to change your attitude, even if it requires seeing a counselor. Happy people are positive people.

- *Let the Sun Shine In* Many of us feel happier after spending time in the sun. One reason may be that, when exposed to the sun's ultraviolet light, our skin manufactures vitamin D. Tissues throughout the body, including in the brain, have receptors for this vitamin. Lab studies suggest vitamin D may protect nerve cells and regulate brain chemicals involved in mood. During the fall and winter, however, in higher latitudes (above the 37th parallel or about the level of Santa Cruz, California), the sun's intensity falls below the threshold to produce vitamin D in us. Furthermore, few foods naturally contain this vitamin. Not surprisingly, insufficiency of this important vitamin is common. Researchers speculate that troughs in vitamin D might explain "winter blues," or seasonal affective disorder (SAD). Vitamin D has many other clearly established benefits: it helps maintain strong bones and muscles and reduces the risk of infections, heart disease, diabetes, some cancers, multiple sclerosis, allergies, and asthma. So, by all means, go outside.

BLUES BATH

Aromatherapists use these essential oils to help lift mild cases of depression:

3 drops lavender essential oil
3 drops ylang-ylang essential oil
3 drops geranium essential oil
3 drops basil essential oil
¼ cup bath oil

Stir the essential oils into your regular bath oil and swirl into warm bath water. Get in and soak.

good to know: ABOUT THE BLUES

One of the hallmarks of depression is negative thinking. Everything seems hopeless and pointless. People feel guilty and ashamed of their condition. If that weren't misery enough, anxiety often accompanies depression. Meditation has been found to work for many people. Cognitive behavioral therapy can gradually improve habits of thought and action. This psychic malaise feels terrible, and it can have physiological sources as well. Fortunately, treatments do exist. If symptoms of anxiety or depression just won't go away, though, call a health care professional for help. You deserve to get better.

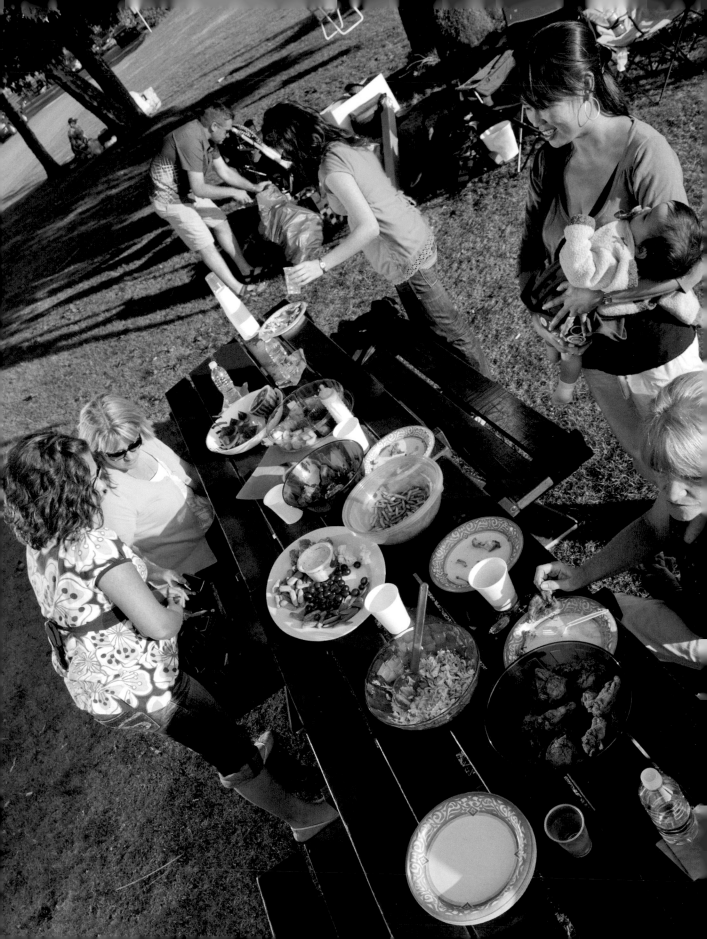

Build Healthy Social Networks

18 PEOPLE-FRIENDLY CHOICES

What's one of the secrets to happiness? Being around happy people. What makes people happy? Being positive about life, doing the things they love, and having a sense of purpose and a goal. What's the payoff? Better health and a better prospect for a longer life. When Dan Buettner was scouring the world for the longest lived and happiest people, one commonality he found among them all was their joie de vivre—their joy for life. They love to be around people and they make choices that help encourage socializing.

▶ | SOCIALIZE

Good friendships can last a lifetime and play a major role in your own love of life. Surrounding yourself with the right people, and arranging your life to spend as much time as possible with them, is an important part of a healthy lifestyle. Here are some ways to help you create healthy social bonds.

Connect With the World

- **Join a Club or Social Group** One study found that joining a social group in which you actively participate, even if only on a monthly basis, produces the same degree of happiness as doubling your income. Think about your interests and talents and identify an organization you can join that will nurture them. Join a yoga class or an exercise class. Regular attendance creates an opportunity for a sense of community. And exercise alone acts as an antidepressant.
- **Keep It Casual** You don't have to become a dues-paying member of a formal club to expand your network of friends. Friendships develop at work, at the gym, in the neighborhood, and at church. All it takes is a little effort. Having friends whom you care about and who care about you will make the world seem a whole lot better.

- **Gather Around the Table** When researchers divided the day into segments to find out which is the happiest time of day, dinnertime came in number one. The reason: It is the time of day when you can relax and interact with family and friends. The unhappiest time of day? Commuting alone to work or school.
- **Set Out the Wine Glasses** Wine is well known for the benefits it bestows on the heart but there is another, lesser known reason to raise a glass and say *Cheers*. Drinking just one glass of wine increases the happiness-inducing chemical dopamine in the brain. Enjoying that glass with friends will add to the cheer. (According to Buettner in *The Blue Zones*, the key to drinking wine "effectively" is drinking the same amount consistently and in moderation. More important, however, drinking a glass of wine socially, and/

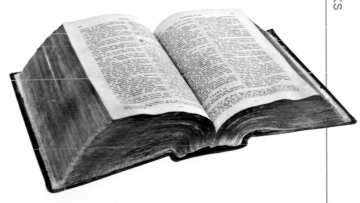

or with a meal helps create an "event, and thus makes it more likely you'll eat more slowly." Also, Buettner recommends taking it easy: "A serving or two per day of red wine is the most you need to drink to take advantage of its health benefits. Overdoing it negates any benefits you might enjoy," and can do harm to your liver, brain, and other organs.)

- ***Find Religion*** Or at least *your own* definition of religion, faith, or spirituality. According to Ed Diener, author of the book *Happiness,* it's religion's *lessons* that lead to happiness, including acting morally and selflessly and having a sense of purpose. Churchgoers have social support. Population studies show that churchgoers—that is, those who attend services at least once a week—live an average of 14 years longer than people who don't go to church.

- ***Help a Friend in Need*** That's what friends are for. When you offer your help, be specific about what you can do. A *Let me know if I can be of help* will only elicit a *Thank you,* but the offer of a specific service—*I can babysit for you on the weekend while you're caring for your sick mother*—is more likely to find a taker. By the same token, accept the help of your friends in your own time of need.

▶ REDEFINE FAMILY

Whether it's the cousins you haven't seen since childhood, the neighbors you keep meaning to invite for dinner, or the fellow volunteers at your town's weekly soup kitchen, making new connections and making a commitment to keep them for a long time will go a long way toward your happiness quotient. Be there for others, and others will be there for you. Even just knowing that they are there when you need them can improve your worldview.

Opening & Closing the Circle

- ***Practice Tolerance*** People who live in happy environments are tolerant of other races and lifestyles.
- ***Consider Everyone Social Equals*** Accumulating the most material possessions does not a winner make. Build a social network of people who accept you for who you are, not what you have.
- ***Learn How to Communicate*** Open and honest communication is at the heart of every lasting relationship. This means listening, even if what you are being told is not that important or interesting to you. It means agreeing to respect each person's differences. It means reminding rather than nagging and suggesting rather than complaining.
- ***Put Family First*** Tending to family is the epitome of social networking. People in these cultures tend to marry, have children, and build their lives around family life. In Okinawa, a sense of family transcends everything else. Older Okinawans begin their day by honoring their ancestors' memories. Picnic tables are set up at gravesites so families can celebrate Sunday dinner with their deceased relatives. In these cultures, nursing homes are unheard of. Rather, the young take care of the old and consider it a privilege and duty.

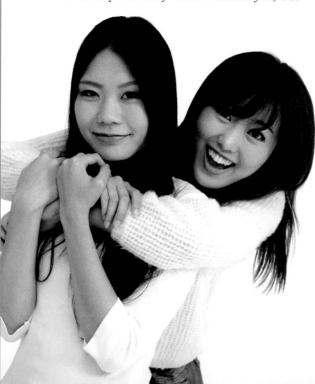

- *Extend Your Family* In the world's happiest nations, family is deemed the center of life. This doesn't mean you have to miss out if you have little or no family. Remember, you can pick your friends, but you can't pick your relatives. Draw those you love into your closest circle and treat them as if they were kin.

▶ | SHARE THE JOY

Happiness is contagious. One study of a small community of 12,000 people in Massachusetts found that the happiest people had the largest network of friends. As their social circle got bigger, they got happier. Research shows that behavior patterns are spread partly through subconscious social signals we pick up from the people with whom we share our space.

The World Smiles With You

- *Laugh a Lot* People who live in Mexico seemingly do not have a lot to laugh about when you consider the country's poverty and crime problems. Nevertheless, Mexicans are considered to be among the happiest people in the world. One of their secrets? Laughter. Mexicans have an amazing ability to laugh even in the face of hardship. It helps make dealing with strife more tolerable. Laughter produces an insulin-like chemical that acts like a mood enhancer, as an antidepressant and anxiety reducer. So, next time you don't think there's anything worth being happy about, try cracking a smile.
- *Find Happiness at Happy Hour* Socializing after work has been found to be one of the most satisfying activities to enjoy on a daily basis. If your fellow workers have a favorite after-work hangout, join in. If they don't socialize, send out an invitation and start a new tradition.
- *Revel in Good Conversation* Research shows that we're likely to get more satisfaction from friends with whom we can have meaningful conversations. Such conversations, researchers speculate, help us find more meaning in a chaotic world.
- *Tell a Joke or Two* Researchers at California State University studied the link between humor and satisfaction in life by introducing a happiness and humor program, including joke telling, to a group of senior citizens. They found it significantly increased self-reported life satisfaction.
- *Develop Your People Skills* Learning how to listen constructively, build consensus, and feel compassion for others are but a few of the people skills that will help you build and maintain a social network. Remembering people's birthdays, asking people about themselves, or asking after someone's ill spouse goes a long way in bonding relationships. And here's another one many Americans have a hard time conforming to: Let others finish their sentences before chiming in with your own thoughts and ideas.
- *Get Rid of Toxic Friends* One analysis found that every positive friendship adds 7 percent to your happiness quotient, but negative people or people who have a negative influence on your life drain it by 9 percent.
- *Count Your Blessings* According to Buettner's findings, 90 percent of happiness is the pursuit of contentment. The more you can take the focus off yourself and your problems, the happier you will be.

good to know: ABOUT HAPPINESS

- The measurement of well-being is a combination of how people perceive their personal happiness, fulfillment, life satisfaction, and peace.
- The happiest profession? Teaching. Teachers tend to view life more positively, are more optimistic, and lead a healthier lifestyle.

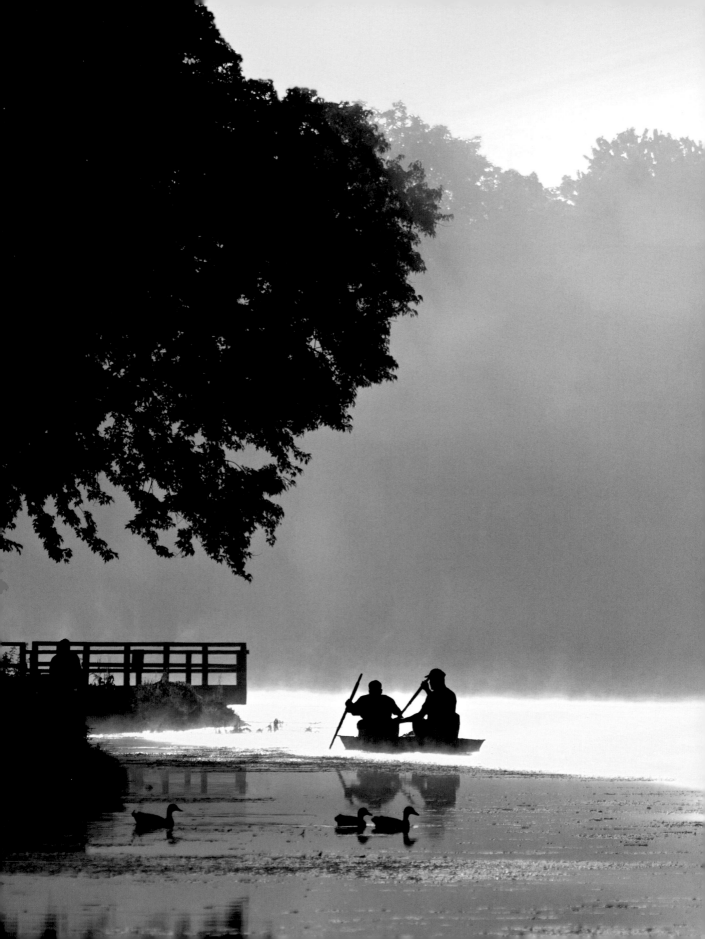

Build Relaxation & Ritual Into Your Day

9 WAYS TO CUSTOMIZE YOUR DAYS

Relaxation is something we all desire, yet few of us know how to experience. Modern life is just too hectic. We get strung out, stressed, and overwhelmed. Some people don't know how to relax, and for good reason. The stress response is automatic—it just happens—but the relaxation response is not. We have to learn it. Almost any American knows what stress is like, but for many of us *relaxation* is a foreign word. Conversely, most of the people who live in the cultures of longevity and happiness have a hard time even grasping the concept of stress. Multitasking is more of an American phenomenon than a universal concept.

Too often, we attempt to multitask and may even think we're successful. Science shows the brain actually shifts attention rapidly from one task to another. As a result, we may miss a chance to fully appreciate any one activity. To live life to its fullest, we need to experience it by savoring it moment to moment. At the very least, you should take the time to look out the window. The following are some ways to slow down and stop moving so fast.

▶ | STRESS

Stress happens when something sudden, unexpected, or unknown steps into your life. When one of those significant changes occurs, your brain activates the stress response. The change can be good or bad: A car runs the red light as you step into the crosswalk, or your beloved proposes marriage. In a reflexive action, the fight-or-flight nervous system kicks into high gear and stress hormones like epinephrine (adrenaline) flood your bloodstream. Your heart races, muscles tense, and blood pressure surges. If the challenge is physical, your body's heroic response can save your life. If the challenge is psychological, this response can be harmful. Fortunately, higher brain areas can reassess the situation and decide to call off the stress response.

Some stress is good, like the kind you feel when you are heel to toe against a competitor in a road race, or nearing the end of a deadline on an exciting project, or you're racing to get to a meeting. This type of stress comes and goes. It's also exhilarating. Most dangerous to your health is the kind of relentless stress that frays the nerves and makes knots in the stomach, caused by anxiety or constant worry, such as the day-to-day fear of losing your job, or the inability to pay your bills, or the struggle in a pursuit that is just not working.

Relaxation is the flip side of stress. We can't avoid stress, but we can manage it. When you know how to handle stress and learn how to relax, you achieve the ultimate—balance. It's something we all talk about, but few of us rarely achieve. There are many natural and enjoyable ways to get stress under control without resorting to prescription medications and their unpleasant side effects.

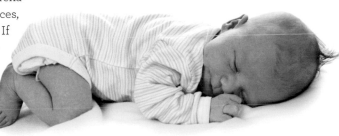

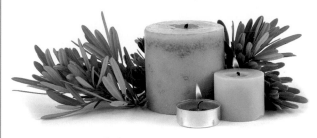

Better Than Counting to 10

■ *Breathe Like a Baby* The first breath we took as a baby came through the diaphragm, drawing in a chest full of oxygen. Somewhere along the growing path, diaphragmatic breathing, or belly breathing, converged into breathing through the chest. Many stress experts believe belly breathing is best because it allows us to take in more air, so we don't have to inhale as frequently to get oxygen. As a result, breathing slows, heart rate goes down, and we relax. Relearning how to belly breathe takes a little practice. Here's how to go about it: Lie flat on the floor and place one hand on your stomach just below the rib cage and the other on your chest. Inhale and then exhale. Both hands should rise with inhalation and fall with exhalation. A full breath will bring air all the way into your lungs from bottom to top.

■ *Relax Progressively* This relaxation ritual can be addictive! It is easy to do and can be done just about anywhere. Just be careful where and when you do it, as it might make you fall asleep. Find a comfortable place to lie down and stretch out. Close your eyes and give yourself a moment or two to get still and relaxed. Then, focus your mind on your breathing and take a few deep, slow, and even breaths. Notice where you feel tight and where you feel tense. Starting with your feet, release your tense muscles as you exhale,

BREATH: A RITUAL FOR WHOLENESS

When your breathing is slow and calm, tension simply fades away. Your heart rate slows, blood pressure lowers, digestion is enhanced, and muscles relax. A daily breathing ritual will improve your health and take only a few minutes of your time:

• Breathe in slowly and quietly through the nose for the count of four, letting your belly expand, while your chest stays soft and relaxed.
• Hold your breath for the count of seven.
• Open your mouth and exhale audibly and completely for the count of eight.
• Repeat this one-breath cycle three more times for a total of four breaths.
• Repeat two to three times a day.

–Tieraona Low Dog, M.D.
Author and integrative medicine expert

gradually moving up your body until you reach the top of your head. When you're finished, stay put for a few minutes longer.

▶ | BALANCE

Driving with a coffee cup in one hand, the other on the steering wheel, and chatting on the cell phone. Talking to your spouse about dinner while paging through your emails. Eating at your desk while finishing up a report. Correcting test papers on your kitchen counter while waiting for the oven to heat up. Doing two or more things at once, what we boastfully call multitasking, might sound like a good idea, but most experts agree that it's not. Instead, it creates stress, the kind that's not good for your health. Further, the brain can't actually multitask; it merely shifts tasks quickly.

Simplify, Simplify

■ *Don't Multitask, Unitask* You can't savor life when you're not focused on what you're doing. You'll appreciate your day more and probably even perform

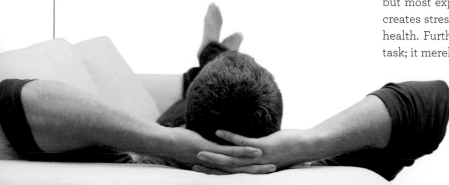

better by slowing down and doing one thing at a time.

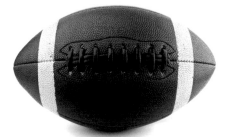

- **Honor Your Workweek** People who work long hours have less time for social activities, interaction with friends, exercise, hobbies, and culture. There's no room in your vocabulary for workaholic. The American full-time workweek ranges from 35 to 40 hours. Stick with it.

- **Take the Time Off You Deserve** Some people take great pride in "never taking a day off from work." Yet, vacations lower stress, allow time to pursue interests, and leave us reenergized as we return to the job. A study conducted in the nation of Denmark found that people are most satisfied with an average of six weeks of vacation a year. The average American takes 8 to 16 days a year!

- **Practice Delegation** This applies to both work and home. Bosses who feel no one else can do a task as well as they can are delusional. In *Thrive*, Buettner lists delegating responsibility as one of the key traits of an ideal boss. At home, Mom shouldn't be expected—and shouldn't feel the need—to do all the chores.

- **Find a Special Relaxation Ritual** Be it girls' night out, Monday night football with the

boys, or a couple's weekend rendezvous, people who create structures in their lives that allow relaxation and enjoyment are happier. They deal better with stress, make more rational decisions, and tend to be more attentive at home or work.

- **Learn to Be Mindful** Mindfulness is a state of mind or type of meditation that helps us get better in touch with life by seeing it with more deliberation and clarity. It is simply the ability to pause and deflect distracting thoughts, feelings, and sensations by concentrating on one thought or thing to the exclusion of everything else. In essence, it's the ability to experience the moment. Though it sounds simple, it takes a lot of practice to achieve. But work at it. Studies show the results are profound. People who are mindful are less reactive, more objective, better able to cope when a situation gets out of control, and make more skillful choices when challenged. Learning to be mindful also improves overall health, sharpens the mind, and enhances happiness.

 WHEN TO CALL THE DR.: We all experience stress, but anxiety is an emotion of a different dimension. It's a feeling of uncertainty or impending doom that can seem at times to come from nowhere. It also has certain characteristics, including sweating, shaking, a pounding heart, and visible distress. When anxiety interferes with life, it means you have an anxiety disorder that requires medical attention.

good to know: ABOUT STRESS & BALANCE

- People who respond poorly to stress are more likely to develop high blood pressure than those who know how to go with the flow. In fact, the link is so strong that researchers say they can predict, among young people, who is likely to develop high blood pressure by the age of 40 simply by observing their reactions to stressful situations.

- Mandatory breaks are required by law for a reason. Take at least a 30-minute break during the workday. Better yet, take an hour.

- Don't spend your vacation time doing a major chore such as painting the siding or just hanging around the house. Research also shows that part of the pleasure of a vacation is planning it.

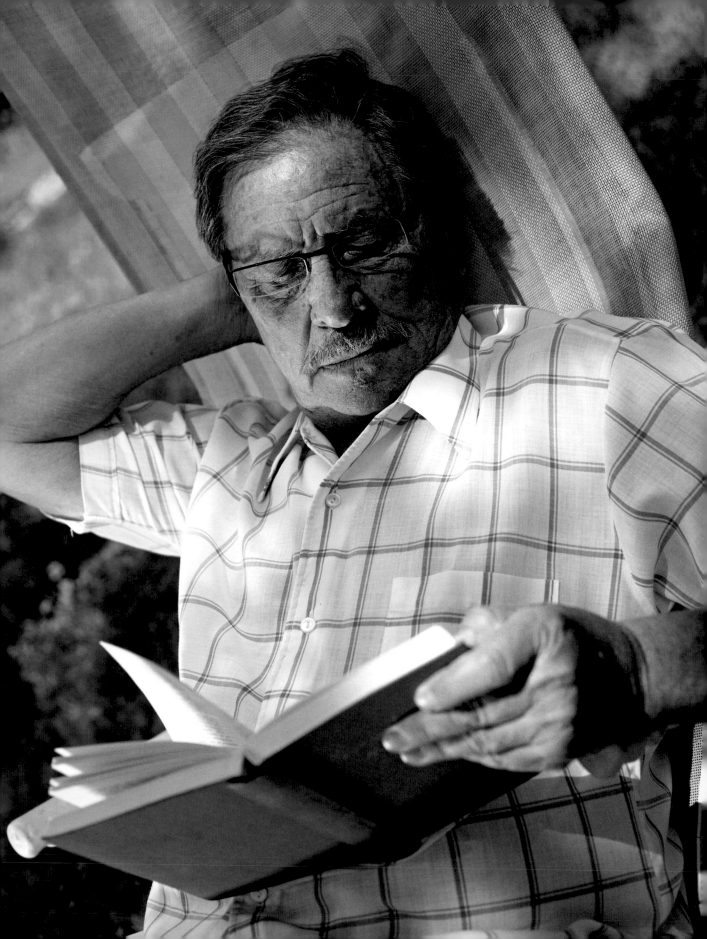

Create a Quiet Space

14 APPROACHES TO YOUR COMFORT ZONE

Several years ago, a major household appliance company conducted a survey in which mothers were asked to rate six responsibilities according to the order of importance in their lives. In order of importance, self came in dead last, behind kids, home, career, the family pet, and the spouse. Many people, but women in particular, tend to put everybody and everything ahead of themselves. This may be good some of the time, but it definitely isn't good all of the time. Even people who understand the importance of eating healthfully and exercising regularly are surprised to find out that tending to others and other things to the exclusion of self is a blueprint for unhappiness and possibly a heart attack.

Finding and taking the time to do something for yourself alone may sound selfish to many, especially busy mothers who cater to children, a spouse, house, and a job. Consider that for all the love, care, and attention you give to others, you ought to be finding a way to give back to yourself. Creating a time and space for quiet is one way to do it. You owe it to yourself—and to those you love and interact with on a regular basis—to be good to yourself.

▶ | FIND A SPACE

A quiet space doesn't have to be a room of your own, such as an office or a "man cave." Finding space can be any actual place or an activity you like, as long as it is something special to *you,* be it a bath, a solitary walk in the woods or on the beach, or a ticket for one to a movie or spa.

Give Yourself A Break
- *Pamper Yourself With Solitary Pleasures* Resolve to reserve some time in every day— workdays and weekends—in which you allow yourself an activity you have chosen simply for your own enjoyment. Soothe your psyche every day with some little pleasure that makes you feel good, be it a manicure, a drive in the country, a massage, or reading a book.
- *Set Aside Time to Enjoy What Means Most to You* Set aside a day, if possible, or a few

hours during the weekend to slow down and put life in perspective. For example, Seventh-day Adventists create a "sanctuary of time" on their Saturday Sabbath in which they focus on God, their families, and nature. No work takes place. Kids aren't out playing or doing homework. The result is a greater sense of well-being, says Buettner in *The Blue Zones.* And a richer life.
- *Find Your Sanctuary* You can't find a place more quiet and, in most instances, more beautiful than a place of worship. Healthy centenarians have faith, says Buettner, and people of faith tend to live longer. Studies show that people who have a spiritual bond have lower rates of heart disease, depression, stress, and suicide, and have a stronger immune system.
- *Connect With Your Surroundings* If you don't take the time to chill out and smell the roses, you are missing out on one of life's biggest pleasures. Centenarians who live in the cultures of longevity identify with their surroundings. They love their land and spend hours in their gardens. They have their

favorite time of the day, their favorite chair, and their favorite place to be. They feel snug in their comfort zone. Given the option, most would not want to live anywhere else, even if it meant a richer style of living.

▶ | TAKE THE TIME

Quiet time. The words alone sound soothing, solitary, and peaceful. So, why aren't you finding it? Because you're not making it happen. Words like *mellow, calming,* and *slow* are foreign in a life governed by to-do lists that are too long and superstores beckoning you 24/7. If "my time" is not at the top of your to-do list, your first step is to make a correction and write it in ink.

Create Sanctuary

- *Have a Room of Your Own* If there is a room in your home that is seldom used, make it your room. Decorate it to please yourself and fill it with the things you love. Let others know that if they are using the room when you're not around, you expect them to leave it as they found it.

- *Indulge in an Aromatic Soak* In today's fast-paced world, we rush to fit in a fast shower in the morning. A soothing bath at night is not on the program! A long meditative soak, however, is a great way to relax, unwind, and spend some peaceful time alone. In addition to a tub, all that is required are the right water temperature and some soothing essential oils. The water should be warm

but not hot—somewhere between 92°F and 100°F is ideal. Add a few drops of chamomile, lemon verbena, lavender, or rose essential oils. Before stepping into the bath, disperse the essential oils with one hand (or they can irritate sensitive mucous membranes). Light a candle, lower the lights, and step in. (See "Soak Away Pain" in the rosemary section and "Soak Away Stress" in the lavender section of Chapter 2.)

- *Spend Time Alone With Others* Explore antique shops with your best friend, enjoy a girls' night out, play poker with the sisters on the lane, or attend a retreat with old school buddies. There's no rule dictating that a quiet space requires solitude. If it feels as good or even better than a good massage, then go for it.

- *Put Out the "Do Not Disturb" Message* If it's a space you want as your own, or time of day you need to yourself, let those in your immediate life know about it. Be polite, but firm. Let them know that this is your time and space and you are not to be disturbed. It's nonnegotiable.

▶ | INNER SPACE

As selfless and altruistic as it sounds, giving all to everyone and nothing to yourself can lead to your own undoing. People are most content with life when they treat others well *in addition* to themselves. Taking time for yourself—creating your own kind of solitude—cannot be understated. The following are a few suggestions on how to go about it.

Look Inward for Quiet

- *Put Your Mind in a Quiet Place* Visualization is a wonderful place to go when life around you suddenly gets to be too much. Anyone who loves to daydream knows how to do it already! If possible, go to a quiet place where you can sit or lie down and relax. Close your eyes, and through your mind's eye, picture an idyllic spot or a place that you'd love to be. As the picture comes into

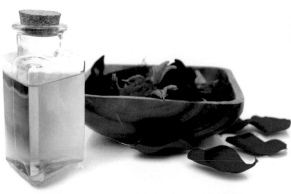

A HEALTHY QUIET PLACE

Ensuring that the world around you is as natural as possible, even in the 21st century, offers a life of transformation and renewal in more ways than just having a healthier body. The healing of your outer world works deeply for body, mind, and spirit. You feel fully at home.

Our sixth sense, or intuition, is keenly aware of when we are in balance with our surroundings. We know when we are breathing fresh, clean air, when we drink water that is as sweet as sugar, and when our surroundings feel healing. We know deep down inside what feels right and true—something sings inside of us.

Listen to your intuition about your surroundings as that is your everyday guide and will help you know what to change in the world around you. A plant here, a picture there, perhaps?

–Annie B. Bond
Author and eco-friendly living expert

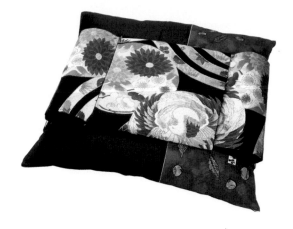

your head, put your other senses to work. If it's the beach, listen for the waves lapping the shore and the plovers chirping in the sand. Feel the warmth of the sun caress your body and the sea mist brush your face. Hold the thought as long as possible, open your eyes, and release.

■ *Meditate* Learn how to slow down, appreciate life around you, and excise stress by learning how to meditate. Create a space in your home that is quiet, neither too hot nor too cold, not too bright, and with a door to snuff out noise and other distractions. Furnish it with a meditation cushion. Establish a meditation schedule (some people prefer first thing after rising). Start out with 10 minutes a day and work up to 30 minutes.

■ *Let Music Quiet Your Mind* Hundreds of studies show that music is a powerful healer. Music has a very long list of benefits that can help lower blood pressure, boost immunity, ease muscle tension, and reduce pain and stress. Music accentuates your quiet time by activating the relaxation response, a benefit that will last long after the music stops.

■ *Set a Time as Sacred* Decide on a time when, every day, you will take 5, 10, or 15 minutes to find a quiet space and be by yourself. If you live with others—roommates or family members—let them know your plan and ask their help in respecting your practice.

■ *Find a Quiet Space Outdoors* A long walk out-of-doors could be the best way to find private space and inner quiet. If you live in the city, it might mean a walk in the park, where you will find many fellow seekers after quiet and solitude.

■ *Find Your Favorite Sounds of Silence* Quiet does not have to mean silence. It can be music, or city street noise, or the rush of water in a fountain or a mountain stream. Quiet is a state of mind—calm and paying inward attention rather than noticing distractions around you. Some people in busy offices even purchase white noise machines, which generate a fuzzy static that drowns out other people's conversations.

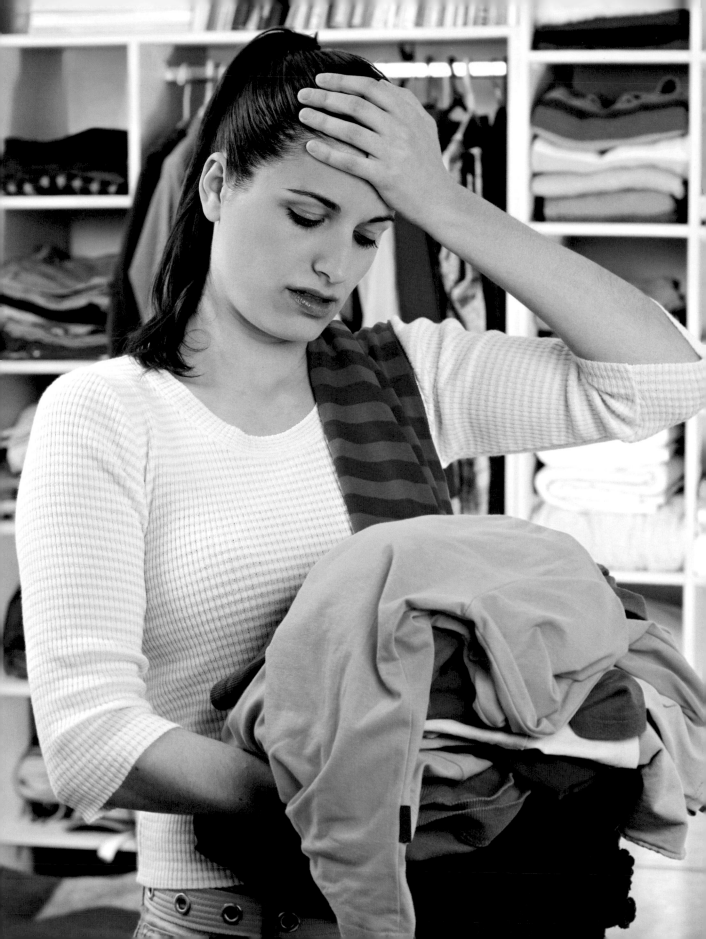

Cut Clutter

13 WAYS TO CLEAN UP YOUR ACT

Reality television shows about hoarding may be good entertainment, but hoarding as a lifestyle is nothing to laugh about. In addition to the all-too-obvious intrusion it makes on life, hoarding can turn into a genuine psychological condition. Fortunately, compulsive hoarding—what doctors call hoarding disorder—is rare. Nevertheless, millions of Americans have an inexplicable attachment to their goods that creates needless stress and makes managing life difficult. Closets, and in some instances, "empty" rooms all over the country are filled floor to ceiling with goods that haven't been seen or used in years, including clothes owners wouldn't even wear to a Halloween party. As kids move out and move on, parents far too often remove the beds and dressers and eventually replace the memories with useless and mostly worthless "relics" that end up on a garbage heap as soon as the estate is settled.

▶ PILED UP

Collecting something of value is one thing, but collecting junk with no intrinsic value is something else. For at least one segment of society, however, clutter is its bread and butter. The storage unit business is a big and burgeoning industry. An estimated one in ten American households has so much stuff they have to rent a storage locker to hang on to it. It's not uncommon for people who have one storage unit to move on to more storage units.

Too Much of a Good Thing?

- *If It's Worth Something, Sell It* Just because you paid $2,000 for a mink coat is no reason to take it with you to your retirement home in Florida. If you have something of value, sell it online or take it to a consignment shop. Recovering a portion of the cost will help lessen the psychological stink of getting rid of something expensive.
- *Apply the One-Year Rule* If you haven't used it or worn it in a year, then you really

don't need it. Give it the old heave-ho—don't even hesitate!

- *Stay Away From Yard Sales* If you have a penchant for buying something for no other reason than it being "a bargain," then avoid cruising yard sales and secondhand stores. The only yard sale you belong at is your own. Adopt the attitude, "someone's junk is not someone else's treasure"—at least not yours.
- *Give It to Charity* Sometimes it is painful to part with something. Downsizing, for example, can create a lot of anxiety when you're looking at furniture that is too big to fit into your smaller home. Donating belongings to a charitable foundation can help make the separation less painful. There is comfort in knowing someone less fortunate can enjoy what you can no longer use.

▶ LETTING GO

Health experts are hard-pressed to find a good explanation as to why many of us have an attachment for something we know deep down we have no use for and will probably never

CLEAN AS YOU GO

Cook with a plan, make every movement mindful and purposeful, and never let anything sit dirty. Be mindful that the preparation is as much a part of the meal as the final product. The best reward after a delicious meal is a kitchen that is already clean! Thomas Jefferson said it best: "Never put off for tomorrow what you can do today." This works as well in your office as in your kitchen—an uncluttered environment helps to keep your mind clutter free. Organized environments reduce anxiety and lead to more productive work.

–Barton Seaver
Chef and sustainable food expert

need again. Some fear they might need something someday—for example, the still unused electric juicer you got for a wedding present 20 years ago—and hold onto it "just in case." Some can't stand to part with something because it "cost a lot of money" even though it is a reminder of a spending mistake. Parents hate to throw out their kids' old toys and trophies for "sentimental reasons." Crates of old family photos collect dust and mildew in the basement because "they're family," even if you can't name or recognize most of the people.

Attachments Included

- ***Let Go of History*** Many people feel obligated to hang on to old photographs and objects for sentimental reasons or to keep family history alive. Where are these items now? If they're hidden away somewhere and haven't been

looked at in years, where's the sentiment? Truly meaningful possessions are kept in a prominent place.

- ***If You Don't Want to Display It, Don't Keep It*** A good way to assess the true personal worth of something is to ask yourself, Would I put this in my living room? If not, sell it or chuck it. You won't be insulting the memory of dear old grandma by getting rid of her old china figurines.

- ***If the Kids Might Want It Someday, Give It to Them Now*** Those old sports trophies and roller skates may be sentimental to you, but do they have the same appeal to their rightful owners, your kids? Ask them. Pass them on if they want them. Otherwise, you know what you should do.

▶ | MAKING SPACE

There is no rationale for living among clutter, especially if you're spending money every month to store it. Decluttered living, say specialists, is less stress-driven and more focused. It also cuts down on needless dust, mildew, and other allergens. The following are some principles to live

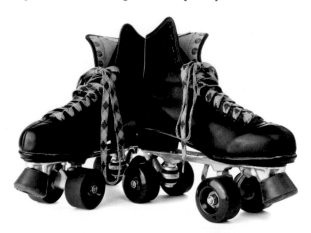

good to know: ABOUT HOARDING

Estimates say hoarding disorder, or compulsive hoarding, is a problem in anywhere from 2 to 5 percent of American households. The Mayo Clinic defines compulsive hoarding as the accumulation of items for which there is no use or space to the point of making living conditions unsafe and unsanitary. Frequently, stockpiles get so vast they spill into the outdoors. Some people even hoard animals—the proverbial "cat lady" is the perfect example—and it is not uncommon for some people to have 100 or more animals. Ironically, hoarders often do not recognize the problem they are creating.

by so you don't turn your neighborhood into the next backdrop for a reality show.

Clean Out the Closets

- **Adopt the One-In, One-Out Rule** One woman we know tells the story of her mother who always complained of having nothing to wear, even though she had three closets bulging with clothing and a spare bedroom full of dress shop clothes racks. When her daughter went through the belongings after her mother passed away, she lamented, "Mom was right, she didn't have anything to wear. She just never threw anything out." This won't happen if you adopt the one-in, one-out rule. If you buy a new sweater, get rid of one. When new monthly or weekly magazines arrive, discard the old ones. Recycle newspapers daily.

- **Cut Noise Clutter** Rid your home of as many noisemakers as possible. This would include television, radio, and Internet. Ideally, electronic devices should be placed in one central location.

▶ | CLUTTER-PROOF

If your quarters are feeling a little tight—not to mention messy—the time to do something about it is right now. Go out and buy a bunch of garbage bags and grab pencil and paper. It's time to take inventory. With every effort to clutter-proof your space you'll literally be sweeping stress out of your life.

Clean Up That Mess

- **Tackle the Mess One Room at a Time** Fight the urge to put out all the fires at once. Start in one room and work it section by section. Start with the big picture—the stuff you see around you—and move inward to closets, cabinets, and drawers. Stay focused until you are completely satisfied that everything in the room now serves a function and purpose. Don't move on to another room until you're satisfied.

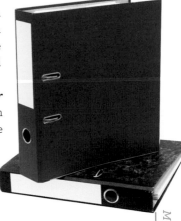

- **Divide and Conquer** As you go through each room, singling out the things you don't really need, sort your stuff into groups: (1) No one will want this; it goes into the trash. (2) Someone might want this; it goes out for donation. (3) This is really valuable, but I don't need it; consider putting it up for sale. Have a box or bag ready for each category, and once you have filled them, don't let them sit around. Throw out the trash today. Carry items to charity tomorrow. And if you don't get around to selling the valuables in a week's time, donate them to charity too.

> ⚕ **WHEN TO CALL THE DR.:** If you or a loved one illustrates signs of excessive hoarding, talk with a doctor or mental health agency. Some communities have agencies set up to help with hoarding households. Check with your local government for resources in your area.

- **Say Goodbye to a Good Book** One of the biggest (and heaviest) stockpiles in many households is books. People like to hang on to old books because they liked them. The better question is this: Are you ever going to read it again? If you can't say "yes" with certainty, then say goodbye ol' buddy.

- **Go Digital** As go books, so go newspapers and magazines. Unread print materials take up valuable space. These days so many past periodicals can be read either online or in the library, so if there is an article in there somewhere that you really ought to read, it won't disappear if you take your own copies to the recycling center.

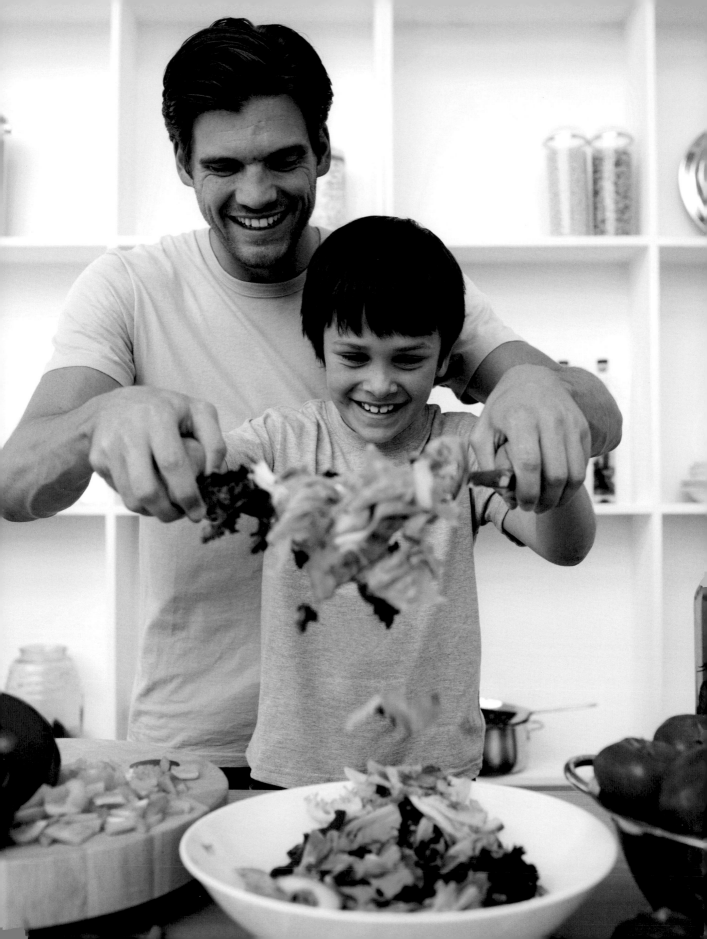

Eat Less

21 TIPS TO SLIM DOWN YOUR DIET

By all evidence, Americans have the worst dietary habits in the world. The proof can be found in the declining health and expanding girth of people from Asia and other parts of the world who immigrate to the United States and adopt American customs and eating habits. As a nation, we are fatter than ever, so fat that the Centers for Disease Control calls it an epidemic. Recent statistics show that 73 percent of men and women between ages 45 and 64 are overweight or obese. Time to learn from those who happily eat less.

▶ | EATING STYLES

People in the cultures of longevity enjoy eating as much as everybody else, but their eating habits are a stark contrast to American customs. Fast food chains are uncommon in these cultures, where many centenarians never even heard of a Big Mac, let alone tasted one. When Dan Buettner was doing his research for *The Blue Zones,* one commonality he found among all the centenarians he met was that they all maintained a healthy weight all their lives. In addition to their active lifestyles, much of the credit goes to their style of eating: They thrive on a diet of whole foods and very little meat. Plus, they follow many of the following healthy eating practices.

Believe Your Belly

- *Know the Difference Between Filled and Full* In Okinawa, a nation of one of the world's longest lived populations, you can frequently hear people intone *hara hachi bu* before starting a meal. It's a reminder to stop eating when hunger is sated, which is 80 percent of the way to feeling full. Some experts suspect this is a major key to longevity. It's a strategy that has been proven in animal studies and anecdotally in humans. Experts believe that caloric restriction somehow helps curtail the cellular damage caused by free radicals, which have a corrosive effect on the body like rust on an aging car.

- *Eat Mindfully* There's a big calorie gap between an American who says "I'm full" and an Okinawan who says "I'm no longer hungry." There are several reasons for this. One is the supersizing of American meals and menus. Another is the ritual of eating while doing something else, such as watching TV, reading the paper, playing games on a smart phone, or eating on the run. However, when you eat mindfully—that is, when you pay attention to what you're eating by purposefully savoring each bit and chewing slowly—you connect to the physical act of eating and you'll be more mentally in touch with your satiety level.

- *Eat a Little a Lot* If a larger meal earlier in the day doesn't fit your lifestyle, many weight loss experts recommend eating small meals more often, up to as many as six a day. This doesn't mean you should be adding calories to your day; rather, you should distribute differently. Eating smaller meals helps keep insulin levels normal and discourages fat storage.

- *Never Eat Standing Up* Consider the candy dish you mindlessly reach for when walking by the reception desk, the people luring you to try a taste of this or that when you're cruising the aisles of the supermarket or craft fair, the trays that pass by at cocktail parties. Without really realizing it, we take in a lot of calories when we're not sitting and eating. One strategy that helps many people lose weight and maintain a healthy weight is never to eat standing up.

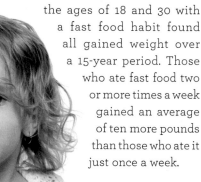

▶ | FAMILY MATTERS

More alarming than adult obesity is the growing rate of overweight children, even toddlers. Statistics show that nearly 40 percent of young Americans between the ages of 2 and 19 are overweight or obese. This does not bode well for their future health or their longevity. Studies show that 70 percent of overweight children are destined to become overweight adults. This means they are at a greater risk of adopting life-threatening adult diseases at a younger age. Type-2 diabetes used to be uncommon in children, but doctors are now diagnosing type-2 diabetes, what used to be called adult-onset diabetes, and heart disease in children. One study of 343 extremely obese kids, conducted at Cincinnati Children's Hospital Medical Center, found they were all already showing signs of a thickened heart. Their average age was only 12. If obesity continues to grow at its current rate, the life span of future generations is going to go down instead of up for the first time in our nation's history.

Make It a Family Affair

■ *Go Meatless Three Days a Week* Studies show that, on average, vegetarians are slimmer, have lower blood pressure, better cholesterol levels, lower rates of certain types of cancer, are less likely to develop diabetes, and have a lower risk of heart attack and stroke than omnivores. To garner similar benefits, nutritionists recommend going vegetarian at least three days a week. Eat a veggie burger instead of a beef

or turkey burger. Eat spaghetti with pesto instead of meat sauce. Eat meatless chili and vegetable spring rolls. Frequent ethnic restaurants, such as Thai and Indian, which are known for offering memorable flavor-inspired meatless meals. You can work up to it by starting out eating meatless one day a week and working your way up.

■ *Eat Your Big Meal Early* When you eat, blood goes to the stomach to aid digestion, which requires a larger supply of blood. This means insulin has to work harder, which also makes the heart work harder. In the cultures of longevity, the biggest meal of the day is eaten in the first half of the day and the smallest, and last, meal of the day is eaten in late afternoon and early evening. If this is a style of eating you can fit into your lifestyle, it is worth a try.

■ *Drive by the Drive-Through* Supersize portions and all-you-can-eat chains are major contributors to our obesity epidemic. Add to that the bounty of studies linking a fast food habit to a host of diseases, and the evidence is pretty convincing. For the record, here's another example: One study that followed 3,000 young women between the ages of 18 and 30 with a fast food habit found all gained weight over a 15-year period. Those who ate fast food two or more times a week gained an average of ten more pounds than those who ate it just once a week.

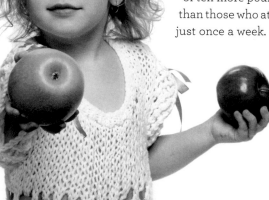

- **Shop at Safe Places** You can be easy on yourself and save a lot of aggravation by shopping at whole food markets and health food stores. Buying all natural all the time may mean spending more, but it may also mean spending more active years later in life.

▶ | BEST CHOICES

Garden vegetables, fruits, and whole grains are the cornerstone of all longevity diets, says Buettner. People in the cultures of longevity typically eat meat only a few times a month. In some regions, it is only consumed during times of celebration. Although these people wouldn't call themselves vegetarians, they mostly depend on what they grow themselves, most of which comes from plants.

Be a Picky Eater

- **Go for an Abundance of Color** Antioxidants, even more than vitamins and minerals, are believed to be the powerhouse of our food supply. They chase and annihilate free radicals that accumulate in the body and damage cells. A major source of antioxidants is phytonutrients, nutrients that come from plants, which are found in vegetables, fruits, grains, herbs, and spices. There are literally thousands of varieties of phytonutrients. A general rule of thumb is: The more colorful, the richer the phytonutrient content. (See Rainbow Veggies, pages 183–185.) Blue-purple fruits are packed with a particular type of potent antioxidant chemical. But pale and colorless foods like garlic, onions, ginkgo, green tea, and soybeans are also rich in antioxidants.

- **Substitute Soy Protein for Animal Protein** Soy is an excellent substitute for meat because it comes in many varieties. It is an almost complete protein, meaning it contains most of the essential amino acids necessary to build healthy cells—a rarity in the plant world. Add soy to soup, smoothies, and breads. The star soy is tofu because it has the ability to change in taste depending on the other ingredients it mingles with in a dish. Because tofu is minimally processed, it makes an ideal substitute for meat in many dishes.

- **Become Fat Savvy** Dietary fat has been a known villain for decades but studies now show conclusively that the real troublemaker is a specific type of fat—saturated fat, which is found only in animal products, such as red meats, poultry skin, cheese, and milk products. Good fats are polyunsaturated and monounsaturated fats, the kind found in plant oils, nuts, and avocados. Nutritionists say it's best to keep saturated fat intake at no more than 10 percent of calories and total fat around 30 percent. The really bad fats are the trans fats. (See Nuts and Olive Oil & Avocado, pages 167–169 and 171–173.)

- **Get Trans Fats out of the House** Trans fats, the man-made artificial substance synonymous with convenience foods, are arguably the most dangerous substance in the American food supply. Activists argue that banning trans fats could prevent 30,000 to 100,000 deaths from heart attacks alone and would help put the brakes on obesity. The evidence against trans fats is so overwhelming that the Food and Drug Administration and the American Heart Association have declared there is "no safe level" for human consumption. The easiest way to avoid trans fats is to stay away from processed, packaged, and other convenience foods.

- **Beware of Packaging** If you're going to buy commercial products, read the labels carefully. The words "hydrogenated" or "partially hydrogenated" are other names for trans fats.

■ *Challenge Trans Fat–Free Labels* A manufacturer is allowed by law to claim a product is free of trans fat as long as the content is under a half gram per serving, not per package. And there is no law that regulates what constitutes a serving. You can, however, figure out how much trans fat is in your products by doing the math: Check the nutrition label for the total grams of fat. Then add up the grams of the individual types of fats listed. Subtract the total of the individual fats from the amount of total grams listed on the label. If the total amounts to 12 grams, but you can only count 10, then you know the other unmentionable grams of fat are trans fats.

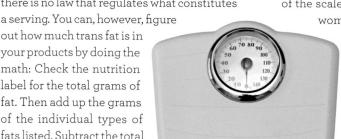

▶ | WATCH & WEIGHT

Here's a bit of irony: At any one time, nearly half of all Americans are on some kind of diet, yet as a nation we're eating more than ever before. Statistics show that we're taking in an average of 530 more calories a day than the typical American ate in the 1970s. With overeating all around us, what's the best way to start toward more healthful eating habits? First of all, consider alternative ways to assess your own body weight and condition.

Scales Plus

■ *Keep Tabs on Your BMI* BMI—body mass index— measures body weight in relationship to height and is the formula scientists and doctors use to determine the effect of body weight on disease risk. A normal BMI ranges from 19 to 24.9. Aim to stay on the lower end of the scale. This is especially important for women, as the BMI does not differentiate between male and female. A BMI of 25 to 29.9 means you're overweight; above 30 indicates obesity. BMI charts are readily available at your doctor's office and online.

■ *Watch Your Waist* Numerous studies have convinced health experts that abdominal fat is a better indicator of heart disease risk than BMI. It's the apple shape rather than the pear shape, or the pot belly rather than the big bottom. Both men and women can be apple-shaped. A woman's risk gets greater after menopause, when waists tend to thicken.

■ *Put Your Hands on Your Hips* You can figure out if your waist is putting you at risk by measuring your waist-to-hip ratio. Figuring it out is simple math. Measure your waist just above the navel. No sucking in your gut! Measure your hips at their widest. Then, divide your waist measurement by your hip measurement. The safe cutoff ratio is 0.8. Higher than that? Consider reducing your waist by reducing your weight.

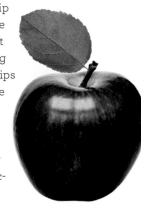

---

good to know: ABOUT FOOD CHOICES

— Yo-yo dieting isn't good for you. A long-term study at the University of Michigan found that women whose weight fluctuated five times in one year had lower-than-average blood flow to the heart, a precursor to heart disease.

— Soy is rich in phytoestrogen, a plant compound akin to the female hormone estrogen. Many nutritionists believe that eating too much soy can cause hormone imbalances, particularly among postmenopausal women. Because of this, the Food and Drug Administration recommends eating no more than 25 grams of soy protein a day.

— Some people make the mistake of reducing fat (which has health benefits and curbs appetite) and increasing carb intake. An excess of calories in any form leads to accumulation of body fat, and a balanced diet in moderation is the best approach.

WINTER BEAN & ROOT VEGETABLE CASSEROLE

Here's a tasty and healthful way to go vegetarian:

2 tablespoons olive oil
8 cloves garlic, peeled
1 teaspoon black mustard seeds
1 large turnip, peeled and cut into large chunks
4 small red-skinned potatoes, quartered
1 15½-ounce can garbanzo beans, drained
2 cups vegetable stock
½ cup chopped parsley
Salt and pepper to taste

8 large shallots, peeled and cut in half
1 teaspoon fennel seeds
4 large carrots, peeled and cut into large chunks
1 parsnip, peeled and cut into large chunks
2 15½-ounce cans of great northern beans, drained
1 14½-ounce can crushed tomatoes
2 bay leaves
2 cups croutons

Heat the olive oil in a large Dutch oven and add the shallots and garlic. Sauté three minutes and add the fennel and mustard seeds. Sauté until the seeds release their flavor and the mustard seeds start to pop. Add the vegetables, beans, tomatoes, stock, and bay leaves. Bring to a low boil, season to taste, and reduce the heat. Simmer, covered, for one hour or until the vegetables are tender. Remove bay leaves. Serve topped with croutons and parsley. Serves four.

▶ CALIBRATE INTAKE

Dieting through deprivation isn't natural and can be self defeating. Dieting is so difficult because the body is built to naturally protect itself from starvation. When the body senses a decrease in energy—that is, calories—metabolism slows. Even more insidious is the fact that when diets fail and weight creeps back, your fat cells fill up with more fat. One big problem is that when you curtail calories and lose weight, hormones that regulate appetite/hunger become deranged and you feel hungrier. And the hormonal shifts can last for many months.

Diet Is a Four-Letter Word

- *Eat From Nature's Supply* Fruits, vegetables, and grains that grow in the ground and on vines, stalks, and trees contain the essential vitamins, minerals, and antioxidants we need to sustain good health. Most of Mother Nature's foods are low in fat and high in complex carbohydrates, the body's main fuel source.

- *Don't Ban Carbohydrates* The popularity of low-carbohydrate diets is a detriment to good health. Many health organizations, including the American Obesity Association, the American Heart Association, and the American Institute for Cancer Research have come down hard on low-carb diets. This is because studies show that complex carbohydrates—vegetables, fruits, beans, and whole grains—reduce the incidence of heart disease, cancer, stroke, diabetes, and many other health problems. Conversely, high-fat, high-protein diets have been linked to causing many of the same problems. One study of 29,000 older women found that those who consumed the highest intake of protein from red meat and dairy products, such as butter and cheese, had a 40 percent higher risk of dying from heart disease within a 15-year period than others.

- *Don't Be a "Simple"-ton* The kind of carbohydrates you want to and should avoid are simple carbohydrates, fast-acting nutrients that rush into the bloodstream, causing insulin and blood sugar to go into a frenzy. (Complex carbohydrates work just the opposite.) Tip: Simple carbohydrates are easy to spot because they are mostly white—sugar, flour, rice, and so on.

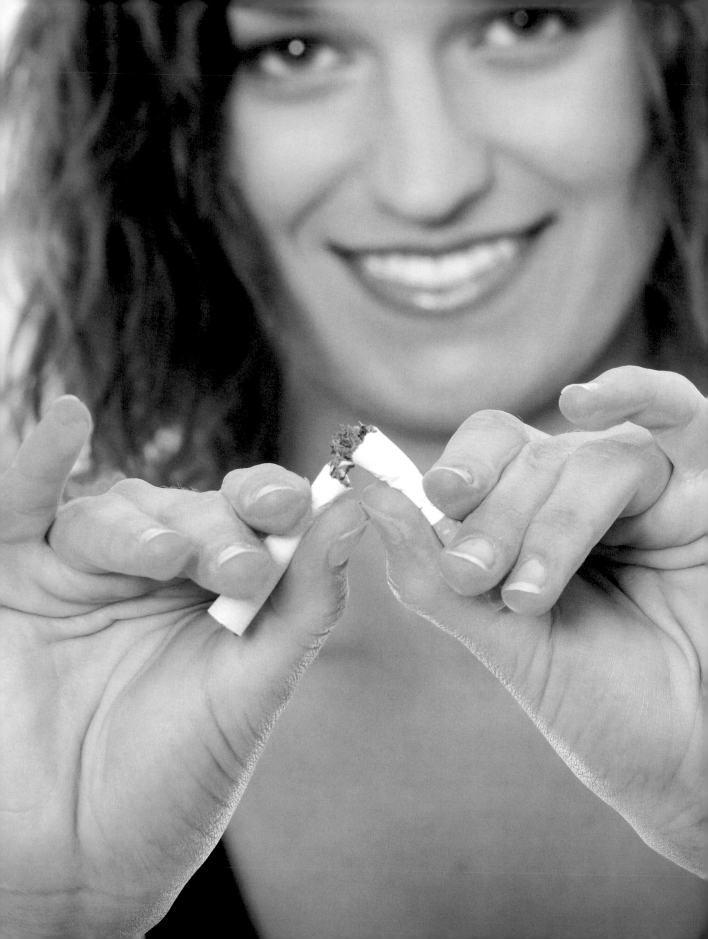

End Nicotine Dependency

10 WAYS TO KICK THE HABIT

The message has been front and center for a half century: Smoking is bad for your health. In fact, most authorities consider it to be the most dangerous lifestyle habit anyone could ever adopt. If in doubt, consider these indisputable facts: Tobacco—whether you smoke it or chew it—is the number one cause of premature death throughout the world. It is associated with 13 different types of cancer and linked to 80 percent of all cancer deaths worldwide. It is also dangerous to your heart. Statistics show that 50 percent of all nonfatal heart attacks could be avoided if people would just stop smoking. If you've had a heart attack and continue to smoke, well, it is akin to playing Russian roulette.

▶ | LONG-TERM LOSSES

Smoking is extremely hard on the body. It makes the heart beat faster. It causes arteries to constrict, which slows blood flow. It's a risk factor for high blood pressure. Studies show smoking can lower levels of good HDL cholesterol and raise levels of bad LDL cholesterol. It increases the risk of hip fractures and osteoporosis later in life, especially for women.

Hamper the Habit

- *Make Your Reason Your Mantra* People who smoke and want to quit have personal reasons to do so—their health, their family, or just the desire to breathe better. Write down your reasons and post them in a place where you can see them, so they become your mantra. For example, post them as your wallpaper on your computer or mobile phone, make them into a bookmark for the novel you are reading, put them on your refrigerator, or put them in your wallet so you see them when you're tempted to buy a pack of cigarettes.
- *Use Visualization* Anecdotal evidence suggests visualization can help. One person who smoked three packs a day for 20 years recognized that the act of lighting up was his habit more than the smoking after he noticed many virtually untouched cigarettes burning out in the ashtray. When he got the desire for a cigarette, he visualized a rolled-up $10 bill burning. Another recalls going cold turkey one morning while walking on a beach after a night of smoking and still feeling nicotine fumes every time she tried to take a deep breath of sea air. Whenever she got a craving for a cigarette, she visualized the same beach scene and unsavory feeling in her lungs.
- *Face the Reality* As you try to stop smoking, recognizing the nasty aspects of the habit may serve as incentive. One smoking cessation technique is to find a large glass jar with a screw-on top and place every cigarette butt into it during the period of time you are trying to cut back

on smoking. Over time, the accumulation of sight and smell may help to dissuade you from further smoking.

- **Enlist the Help of Others** Studies show that combination therapy—medication plus counseling—can dramatically increase the likelihood of beating the habit. This can include one-on-one counseling with a health care professional, a support group, or telephone counseling with a trained supporter, who is either a health care professional or a former smoker.

▶ BAD HABIT

Though smoking has declined by more than 65 percent since it was deemed dangerous to health in the 1960s, an estimated 25 percent of Americans still smoke. Further, according to the World Health Organization (WHO), an estimated 1.3 billion people smoke worldwide. Surveys conducted by WHO and other organizations estimate that 70 percent of smokers would like to kick the habit but can't.

Addictions are hard to break, and smoking is one of the toughest. For reasons doctors don't fully understand, smoking is a tougher addiction to break for women than for men, even though they smoke less, inhale less deeply, and don't take it up at as early an age as men do. One theory is that women smoke for emotional reasons—to ease tension, combat stress, and as a

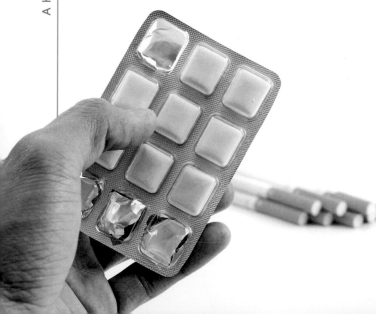

diversion from food. All are triggers that are difficult to overcome.

So, how's this for encouragement: It's never too late to stop. If you stop now, you can reverse the damage already done to your heart by half. In 15 years, you can lower your risk of heart disease to that of a nonsmoker. Additionally, cancer risk starts to decline the moment you take your last puff. Relative risk declines after five years and gradually continues to go down thereafter. Skin experts say that smokers who quit will be able to see a difference in their appearance after two months, the amount of time it takes for the skin to replenish itself twice. Skin will likely look less sallow, though wrinkles are probably not going to vanish.

Admit the Addiction

- **Try Going Cold Turkey** For some people it works, but for most it doesn't. Statistics on the success rate of going cold turkey are as low as 10 percent. It can work, however, when motivation is strong.
- **Get Some Over-the-Counter Therapy** Of all the pharmaceuticals available to stop nicotine addiction, including prescription drugs, studies have found the most effective is over-the-counter nicotine replacement therapy, which is packaged as a gum, lozenge, patch, or an inhaler. It works by helping relieve uncomfortable symptoms of withdrawal. One study found it was almost twice as successful as a placebo. Generally, it takes 8 to 12 weeks to work.
- **Avoid Weak Spots** Self-help organizations such as Alcoholics Anonymous counsel people to avoid people, places, and situations that are associated with their addiction. For example, if you smoke after meals, immediately get up after eating and go for a walk in the fresh air. It will get your senses in touch with the total opposite of a cigarette—fresh air.

▶ | SMOKE-FREE

And, here's another motivator. Nonsmokers seem to be happier people. San Luis Obispo, California, named the nation's healthiest and happiest city in America in the book *Thrive*, was the first city to enact antismoking legislation in bars. Today, you can't light up in public anywhere in the city. (Of course, there are other reasons for its happiness quotient: It's a college town, in a beautiful setting, and a fairly affluent area. Those are a few of the other factors that help make it a healthy, happy place.)

Trade Smoke for Smiles

- **Substitute a Healthy Habit** Fill the void of all the time you spent smoking with a healthy pursuit, such as exercise, knitting, gardening, doing a crossword puzzle, or any other pleasure that keeps your mind focused and your hands busy. Eventually, the new habit will replace the old.

- **Don't Swap One Bad Habit for Another** Some smokers rationalize that puffing on a pipe or a cigar does not carry the same health risks as smoking cigarettes, but this

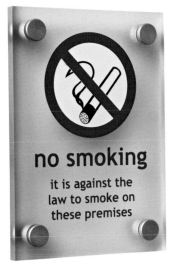

no smoking
it is against the law to smoke on these premises

is a misconception. In fact, WHO reports higher rates of lung cancer among people who switched from cigarettes to cigars or a pipe than in people who smoke cigars or a pipe exclusively. One study found that, compared to nonsmokers, the risk of lung cancer increased five- to sixfold in men who switched from cigarettes to another form of nicotine.

- **Manage Stress** Withdrawal from nicotine dependency is, by definition, stressful. It undermines efforts to quit and raises the risk of relapse. Stress-management techniques seem to improve success. For instance, research shows that walking, aerobic exercise, yoga, and meditation (see page 279) help combat withdrawal symptoms. One study found mindful attention a way to help relieve cigarette cravings: To do it, assume a relaxed position and focus on breathing slowly and deeply. With each breath, mentally scan a part of your body—feet, calves, thighs, torso, shoulders, arms, hands, neck, head—relaxing those muscles with each exhalation. Finish by focusing on the breath itself as it fills the body.

---

good to know: ABOUT SMOKING

- The habit of smoking has great impact not only on your heart, lungs, and internal systems but also on your outward appearance. Smoking yellows teeth, dulls hair, and gives the skin a sallow appearance.

- Smoking is one of the major causes of premature wrinkles—a not-so-attractive look that goes by the moniker "smoker's face." Research at the University of California, San Francisco, found that smokers are two to three times more likely to develop premature wrinkles than nonsmokers. This is because smoking causes skin fibers to lose their elasticity. Nicotine narrows blood vessels, preventing oxygen-rich blood from reaching the tiny capillaries in the top layers of the skin, making the skin appear dull, lifeless, and leathery.

- If you're a former smoker or a nonsmoker, be proactive about getting smoking bans in your community. Nearly half of all Americans who don't smoke are regularly exposed to secondhand smoke. According to the American Cancer Society, secondhand smoke kills an estimated 53,000 nonsmokers a year, and 10 to 15 percent of lung cancer in people who have never smoked is attributed to secondhand smoke.

- Smoking bans are working. Three months after New York City implemented a citywide smoking ban in July 2003, smoking-related symptoms among hospital industry workers dropped 88 percent.

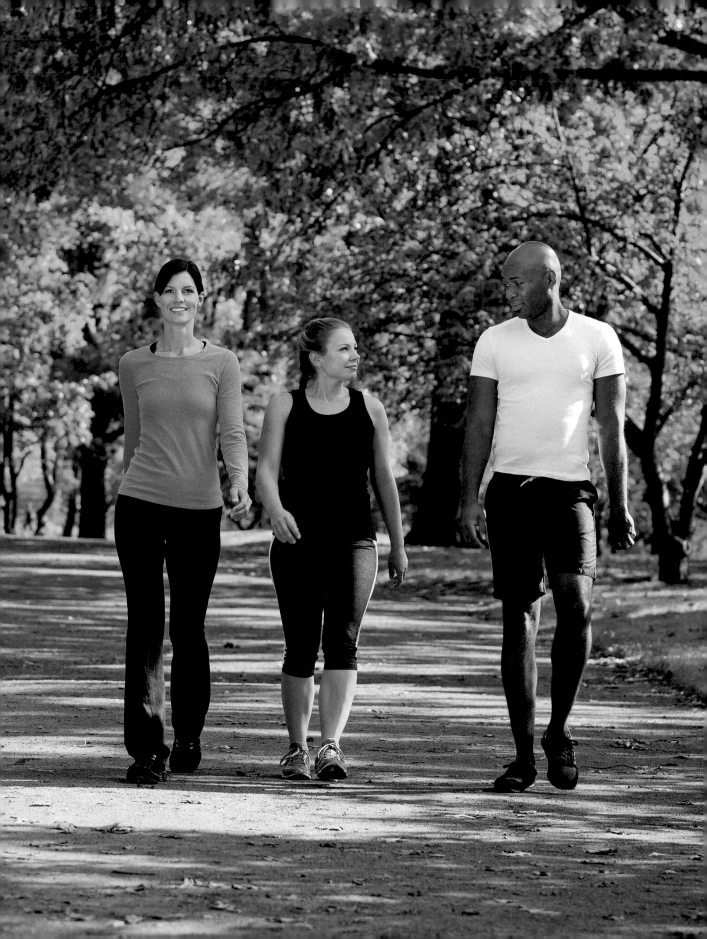

Exercise Regularly

24 SURE MOVES TO A MORE ACTIVE LIFE

I f doctors were asked to choose their prescription for health and longevity for their patients, given the choice between moving the body more and eating less, it's a good bet that the majority of them would say "exercise." That's because leading a physically active lifestyle can go a long way toward avoiding a lot of problems associated with a diminished quality of life. And while physical activity might mean for some a daily visit to the gym for a workout, there are plenty of other ways to put movement and activity into your routine. Get away from the desk, get off the sofa, get out of the car—you will feel better and live longer.

▶ | GET MOVING

The consequences of a sedentary lifestyle are major and contribute to the two leading causes of death in the United States and throughout the industrialized world—heart disease and cancer. Sitting in a chair all day is just as bad for the heart as smoking, high cholesterol, or high blood pressure, says the American Heart Association. One study at the University of Florida College of Medicine in Gainesville concluded that inactivity in women puts them at an even greater risk for heart attack than does obesity.

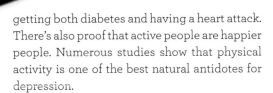

On the other hand, regular exercise is well known to help keep the heart healthy. Studies show that people who get the most physical exercise have the lowest risk of a heart attack. One study at Northwestern University in Chicago, involving 4,400 men and women, found that as levels of fitness rose, risk factors for heart disease dropped.

A sedentary lifestyle is also a risk factor for certain types of cancer. Studies have found inactivity increases the risk of breast, colorectal, endometrial, and prostate cancers. Conversely, numerous studies show that as physical activity increases, the risk of getting some cancers drops.

Inactivity increases the odds that you'll get diabetes. It is the leading risk factor in a combination of symptoms that compose metabolic syndrome, a condition that raises the chances of getting both diabetes and having a heart attack. There's also proof that active people are happier people. Numerous studies show that physical activity is one of the best natural antidotes for depression.

Make Your First Moves

- ***Don't Let Time Be Your Excuse*** "I don't have the time" is the refrain of millions of Americans. Sports medicine doctors say that's nonsense. If you can't find a half hour or an hour at a time to devote to exercise, then break it up into 10-minute sessions. One study at Southwest Missouri State University found that three 10-minute bursts of energy can be just as effective as a 30-minute workout. This could be a 10-minute walk over your lunch break, climbing up and down the stairs during commercial breaks when you're watching TV, or 10 minutes riding a bicycle after dinner.
- ***Find Your Own Niche*** If you're going to stick with an exercise, it has to be something you like. You don't need to be a runner or go to a gym to get in shape.

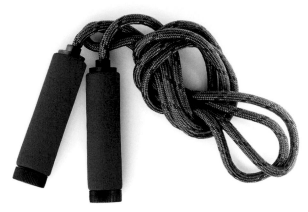

- *Find a Buddy* It's harder to give in to excuses when two or more people are in it together. If you're going to go for the buddy system, however, choose people on the same fitness and stamina level as you are. Nothing is more deflating than petering out when everyone else is still raring to go.

▶ | CHANGING HABITS

As a nation, America is far too inactive. According to recent national statistics, 56 percent of Americans—60.1 percent of women and 50.3 percent of men—report getting no vigorous exercise that involves working up a sweat and getting the heart pumping. And, 35 percent of women and 30 percent of men report spending no time at all in leisure-time activity that involves working the body moderately or even a little bit. Doctors and scientists dedicated to protecting the health of Americans find these statistics grim, and for good reason. Your level of physical fitness determines if your heart will be strong enough to help you live an active, independent life in your later years.

In Dan Buettner's investigations, the one thing all centenarians he interviewed had in common was a lifetime of activities that kept them on the move. We're not talking marathoners and gym jockeys. We're talking about people who keep up habits they adopted long before the world got so computerized. Daily activity is a part of their routine. They walk to the market every day and prefer riding a bicycle to driving a car. They love working their gardens and land. They spend a lifetime making a living that does not involve sitting behind a desk all day.

Exercise at Any Age

- *Don't Let Age Be an Excuse* Starting a regular exercise program, even in midlife, helps improve quality of life as you age, according to researchers in London who followed the exercise habits of 6,398 people ages 39 to 63. They found that those who exercised moderately for 2½ hours a week or strenuously for 1½ hours a week, including those with chronic health problems, were fit enough to maintain an independent lifestyle into old age.
- *Get Into Balance With Yoga* As you age, maintaining good balance is importance, as accidents are the fifth leading cause of death in the United States, and one in three Americans over age 65 falls each year, resulting in death or injury. When done properly, yoga is excellent for helping to maintain and increase balance. It also increases flexibility and strengthens muscle groups.
- *Work Out With Weights* Resistance training actually gets more important as you get older. It strengthens and firms muscles and lubricates joints. If you can't join a gym, invest in hand weights. You can use them anytime and almost anywhere, even while watching television.

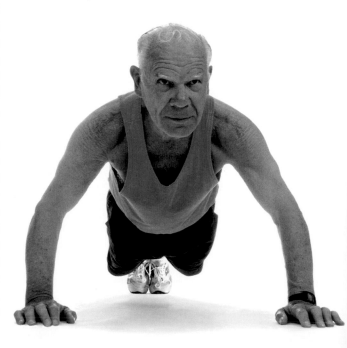

- **Get Your Kids Moving** Kids just aren't as active as they used to be—and there's plenty of evidence to prove it, the most obvious being the startling rise in obesity among young children and teens. Kids aren't all that active after school, either. Recent statistics show that only 45 percent of boys and 27 percent of girls report engaging in physical activity for at least an hour five days a week. So, make exercise a family affair. Walk, hike, and bike as a family. Organize family sports, such as tennis, badminton, or swimming.

- **After-School Action** At one time, parents could depend on school to get their kids physically active, but not anymore. In many public schools today, recess and physical education are the exception rather than the rule. National statistics show that only 33 percent of American students in kindergarten through 12th grade attend daily physical education classes. Fewer than 50 percent of teens between the ages of 14 and 17 meet the physical education requirements of the National Association for Sport and Physical Education.

- **Encourage Sports** Because of budgetary cutbacks in many schools, it is becoming increasingly important for parents to make sure their kids get involved in organized sports. Most communities offer programs independent of schools that can teach children skills and give them a sense of self-worth.

WHEN TO CALL THE DR.: If you are out of shape, are age 50 or older, or you are being treated for a chronic health condition no matter what your age, consult with your doctor before starting any exercise program.

▶ | WALK

Think of walking as a savings plan for your old age. The more you put into it, the more freedom you'll have to enjoy life in your later years. Make a daily deposit and you'll be vested in no time. Walking offers other major benefits. It is easy, cheap, and enjoyable—factors that give walking the lowest dropout rate of any form of exercise. Walking can also boost your energy, help you lose a few pounds, perk up your mood, and cut your risk of a heart attack by *half*.

The Word on Walking

- **Put Aside a Half Hour a Day** The American College of Sports Medicine and the Centers for Disease Control and Prevention say that all it takes is 30 minutes a day of moderately intense heart-pumping walking—what's called "cardio" in the gym—to elevate heart and breathing rates. For the typical person, this means walking at a brisk pace of three to four miles an hour, or about two miles in a half hour. If you can speak, but not comfortably carry on a conversation, you're doing cardio. If you're huffing and puffing so much you can't speak, you're going too fast. If you're walking along and can easily carry on a conversation, you're going too slow.

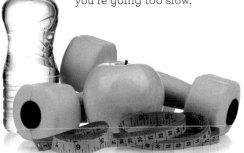

good to know: ABOUT EXERCISE

Give It Time If you are out of shape, exerting yourself the first few times can feel pretty lousy. However, experts urge you to stick with it. Totally sedentary folks will be able to feel the difference within a week or two. And if you're starting again after a long time off, you'll feel yourself come back even faster.

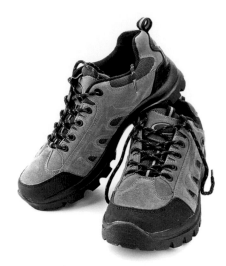

- **Join the 10,000 Steps Club** It's the largest walking club in America. The 10,000 Steps Program is a federally funded endeavor sponsored by Shape Up America! to help Americans get fit. Anyone can join and all it costs is the price of a pedometer. In case you're wondering, 10,000 steps is the equivalent of approximately five miles and it keeps you in motion for about 2 to 2½ hours a day. The sponsors of the program say most Americans can't go nearly that far in the course of the day without fitting in at least a 30-minute walk.

- **Buy Yourself a Pedometer** It's a small investment in your health. Nothing fancy is required. For $30 or less, you can get a dependable pedometer with a built-in clock so you don't lose track of time. All you have to do is measure your stride, enter it into the device's memory, press a button, and get going.

- **Start Out Sensibly** The folks at Shape Up America! suggest starting out by measuring your current fitness level. This means wearing your pedometer and going through your daily routine without changing a thing for a week or two. If you're like most people, you'll clock from around 900 to 3,000 steps in a day, but not much more. Your goal should be to add an extra 500 steps a day until you reach 10,000.

- **Step Up to the Challenge** Getting five miles in a day is quite a feat, but in the 10,000 Steps Club, every stride counts. Think of all the ways you can add a few active strides into your daily routines.

- **Invest in the Right Walking Shoes** You don't have to pay hundreds of dollars, but it is a good idea to exercise in solid, well-built walking shoes. Go to a store or website you trust to find running, walking, or all-purpose athletic shoes with a flexible cushioned sole. Wear socks that wick away rather than absorb moisture.

- **Keep an Account of Your Count** If you like to challenge yourself and watch yourself succeed, keep a walking diary. Competing with yourself is also a good way to fight boredom. Write down anything you want that will give you a sense of accomplishment—number of steps, distance covered, weather conditions, your weight. Keep a diary only if you enjoy this type of discipline. Otherwise, it will just become another excuse to quit.

- **Walk More at Work** Forget emails and interoffice phone calls. If you have a message to deliver, do it in person. Don't sit and think—pace and think. Keep your inbox in a place that requires you to get up and walk to it. Retire your outbox and make your own deliveries to the mailroom. Don't sit for more than an hour, even if you're at a meeting. Get up and move about. Eat lunch somewhere within walking distance, not driving distance.

- **At Home, Walk Around** Keep moving while talking on the phone. Do something active during commercial breaks when watching television. Walk the dog instead of letting him out to run in the yard. Retire the remote control to the television set, or at least keep it out of reach so you have to get out of your chair and walk to fetch it. Get rid of the lawn service and do the work yourself. Use a hand mower instead of a power mower.

- **Find a Way to Walk Wherever You Are** Park the farthest distance instead of trying to get the closest space in the parking lot. Use the stairs instead of the elevator. Walk the escalator at malls and the moving sidewalks in airports.

▶ | ACTIVE PLEASURES

The world's longevity superstars don't play competitive sports, run marathons, or swim a mile every day at the YMCA. Many of them have never even seen the inside of a gym. What they do, says Buettner, is engage in steady, consistent, low-intensity exercise. It's a part of their lifestyle. Their day-in, day-out routine involves keeping the body in motion. The key to keeping it up is this: They love what they're doing. Building entertaining activity into your lifestyle is the surest way to stick to your program.

---

good to know: ABOUT WALKING

- Walking 10,000 steps is the equivalent of burning 500 calories.
- If you ride an exercise bike with a calorie readout, you can figure burning 100 calories is equivalent to walking 2,000 steps.

Get Into the Act

- **Grow a Garden** There's nothing like gardening to challenge your physical stamina. Hoeing, planting, weeding, and harvesting all involve low-intensity, range-of-motion exercise on a regular basis. Okinawans—among the world's longest lived people—garden for hours every day during their long growing season, growing the food they put on their table, says Buettner.

- **Be More Like Ozzie and Harriet** Back in the good old days there were no remote control panels, power mowers, electric can openers, snow blowers, electric garage door openers, dishwashers, food processors, electric brooms, or vacuum cleaners that moved around the room on their own power. Ozzie used a shovel to remove snow and opened the garage door with his own muscle power. Harriet got down on her hands and knees to scrub the floor, and she washed and dried the dishes by hand. Putting a little inconvenience in your life is good for your body. You might be surprised to find out that it can also be quite satisfying.

- **Get Out and About With Others** Take walks in your community parks with friends, plan summer picnics and set up a badminton set, or start a neighborhood baseball or tennis league.

- **Take an Adventure Vacation** Instead of just going to the beach on your winter vacation south, sign up for scuba lessons. Instead of sitting in the spa, do laps in the pool. Take an adventure vacation that involves activities, such as hiking, horseback riding, or sailing.

- **Find a New Hobby** And choose something that gets you up and out! What about bird-watching? There are only so many species you can see out your living room window. See if a park or preserve near you offers weekly guided nature hikes. You're just not the outdoor type? Try antique refinishing. You stand, squat, lift, and move around as you do that. Low-impact sports like badminton, croquet, horseshoes, or even Ping-Pong can also add movement to your life, along with socializing and fun.

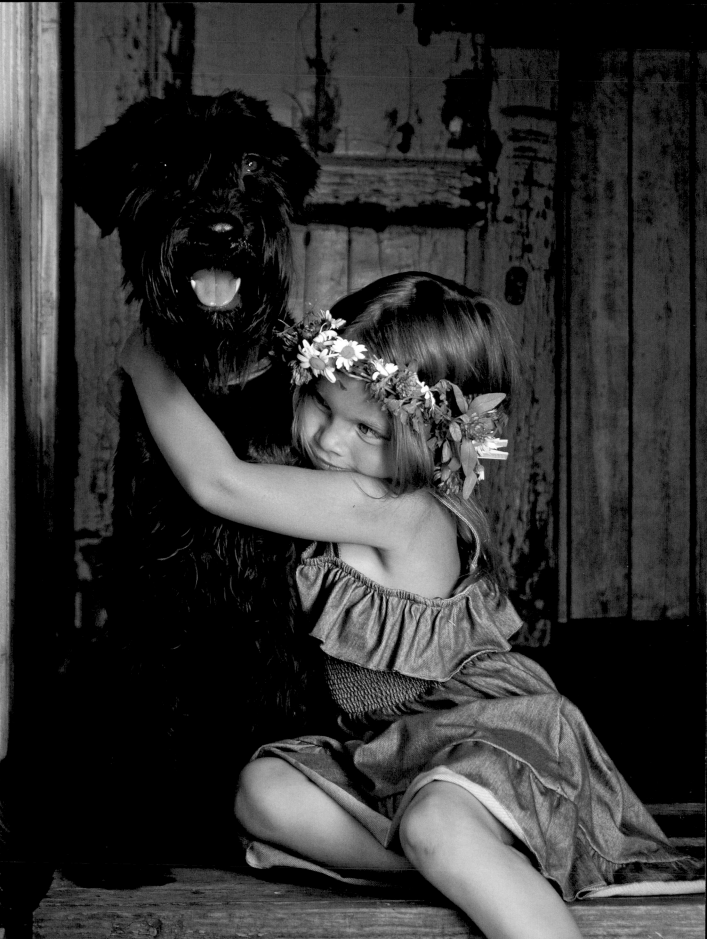

Get a Pet

13 WAYS TO FIND A FURRY FRIEND

More than half of all American households follow one of the best health practices known to medicine, and most probably don't even realize it. They own a pet. Pets have been found to offer enormous benefits to human health. Studies conducted during the last few decades found that having a pet in the household can help lower blood pressure, cholesterol, and triglycerides, which are all leading risk factors for heart disease. Pets can also help relieve stress and diminish feelings of loneliness. Studies show that, in general, pet owners are generally healthier and happier than people who don't have pets. One study found that just the presence of a pet, even more than a spouse or friend, has been found to be more effective at lowering stress levels.

▶ | BEST FRIENDS

Although any pet—be it dog, cat, bird, gerbil, or rabbit—has been shown to foster better health in humans, most of the credit for making us happier and healthier goes to man's best friend—a dog. In fact, the act of merely petting any dog, even a strange one, is enough to bring down blood pressure in even the most stressed individuals.

Dogs are trained for therapy to boost the happiness and health of people in hospitals and nursing homes. They are trained to be the eyes for the blind and the ears for the deaf. They have even proved useful for children having trouble learning to read—dogs listen very well!

Dogs are great for the health of their owners, too. Studies show that owning a dog increases physical activity because it gets you out and walking more often. One study suggests that kids are less likely to become obese in families that own a dog. In general, observational studies show that dog owners are healthier than people who don't have a dog.

Dogs reign in the pet kingdom for a lot of reasons. One is their domestication. You can't teach a gerbil to sit or a rabbit to roll over, but a dog can learn to do a lot of cute tricks to make the heart flutter and the owner proud. More than other pets, they offer us companionship and unconditional love. They offer us a means to take the focus off of our personal problems.

Canine Intervention

- **Be a Cool Cat and Get a Dog (or Cat)** If you have high blood pressure due to a stressful job or life situation, consider getting a dog. Researchers demonstrated this healthful tactic in an experiment with 48 people with high blood pressure in one of the standout stressful vocations: stockbroker. In the experiment, researchers intentionally reproduced two situations that mimicked the type of stress typical to a stockbroker. Each time, the brokers' blood pressure soared to dangerously high levels. All the brokers agreed to take medication, and half agreed to get a dog or cat. Six months later, the researchers called them back to repeat the experiment. However, the pet owners were asked to bring along and keep their furry friends by their sides. Sure enough, the experiments made blood pressure rocket, but the pet owners' pressure went up only half as much as their petless colleagues.

- **Find the Dog That's Right for You** It might seem to you that owning an Akita is the cat's meow, but if you're a 110-pound, 60-year-old woman who lives alone, getting a dog that weighs in the range of 75 to 100 pounds would literally be too much to handle. Downsize your desire. By the same token, if you have little kids who are going to be rolling around in the grass, sand, and mud with their four-legged friend, a breed with a coat like the corded mass of a komondor or a shaggy Old English sheepdog might fill you with regret and grooming debt.

▶ | THE RIGHT PET

Although there is no proof that owning a pet will make you live longer, there is substantial proof that it will enhance your quality of life. Americans love their pets, and the majority considers them just as important as any other member of the family.

Do Your Homework

- **Consider Purebred vs. Mutt** Both have their advantages and disadvantages. All pure-breds have basic traits that you can seek out to match your needs. Mutts are more of a crapshoot. By the same token, purebreds carry a higher risk of inherited disease and health issues. Many people prefer getting a dog from the pound because they feel good about giving it a home.
- **Go to the Rescue of a Dog in Need** If you're not dead set on having a pedigreed dog, con-sider getting a rescue dog that has been given up for adoption. Rescue facilities have trained personnel who can help match your lifestyle and needs with a pet. Almost all communities have an affiliate.
- **Find Your Hound at the Pound** Puppy love can last forever after a visit to an animal shelter. Pets need us even more than we need them. Consider finding your furry friends at your local animal shelter.
- **Be Weather Sensitive** It's okay to have an Alaskan malamute in California and a Mexican Chihuahua in Maine. Just keep in mind that all pets are more sensitive to weather than people. Heat prostration or heat

exhaustion is a common cause of illness in the summer. It can even kill. If your pet spends a lot of time outdoors in hot months, make sure it has a shelter from the sun and always has access to plenty of water. If Pepe shivers when you walk him in winter, get him a coat.

- **Recognize Your Life Patterns** In choosing a pet, take stock of how you live and how an animal fits into those habits. What is your schedule? How many hours per day and night can you give to your new animal? Pup-pies need round-the-clock attention at first. Choose the type and age of pet that suits the way you plan on living your life.
- **Consider the Menagerie** If you don't feel you're home enough to responsibly care for a dog, then consider a cat. They're more independent and can care for themselves for longer stretches of time. Even though dogs and cats interact more with people, even fish, parakeets, guinea pigs, or other less common pets can give daily doses of amusement and companionship.

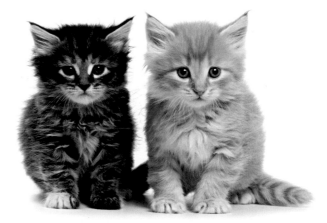

- **Get Your Pet Spayed or Neutered** In spite of all the love animals bring us, there isn't enough love to pay back. Pet overpopula-tion is a problem. An estimated four million homeless cats and dogs are put down every year. Many are the unwanted offspring of a family pet. If you have no intention of breed-ing responsibly, get your cat or dog spayed or neutered.

▶ | LOVE BOTH WAYS

Certainly one of the reasons that pets, and dogs in particular, have been found to contribute so greatly to healthy life and longevity is the love they express and evoke in those who care for them. You may be surprised to find that pets, especially dogs, can seem much like children. They may have their moods. And they may act like scamps. Or they can entertain you like skilled acrobats: Abyssinian cats—a particularly playful breed—can leap from the floor and alight atop a cabinet or open door as if stepping off an elevator. They are also quite bold. They might try to swipe something from your plate if you look away. Your dog will cock its head and listen for hours to anything you say as if comprehending every word. Getting a pet is a commitment to another living being as well as a promise of affection coming back to you.

Mutual Admiration Society

- *Be Ready to Take Responsibility* As an owner, you have an obligation to care for your pet. This means keeping it well nourished, exercised, properly groomed, and free of disease. It's also your responsibility to make sure it is trained to behave sociably at home, with strangers, and in public places.
- *Volunteer Your Love* Many people are unabashed dog lovers or cat lovers. If you're one of them, you can extend your love to a friend in need and fill yourself with joy at the same time by becoming a volunteer at a pet shelter.

▶ | FRIENDLY HELP

There are a number of resources for information that will help you and your pet enjoy your time together. The Humane Society of the United States offers all sorts of advice to help you address house training, barking, chewing or scratching, separation anxiety, and other behavioral issues involving your pet.

Info Central

- *Only the Best* What's in pet food? The website *www.dogfoodanalysis.com* carries standard test analyses for relative concentrations of ingredients and nutritional values of 1,500 brands of dog food. Also see *www.petfoodratings.com* for discussion of pet food ingredients, both for dogs and cats, and other nutrition- and health-oriented websites such as *wwww.catinfo.org* and *www.catster.com*.
- *Vet the Vet* Commit yourself and your pets to one veterinarian who can get to know you and them well. Some vets make home visits: Find out about those in your area who will come to you. And before you really need it, find out about emergency veterinary hospital and care centers available at night and on weekends in your area.

---

good to know: ABOUT GETTING A PET

- Many hospitals and nursing homes have pet visiting hours. Check the regulations at the medical facilities that you visit to find out if bringing your pet along is acceptable.
- If cost is a deterrent to having your pet spayed or neutered, consult your local humane society or rescue league. They often do it for free, though you may have to wait your turn.
- Household chemicals, certain foods, and garden plants can harm your pet. Be prepared: Check out poison control for pets at *www.animalpoisoncontrol.org* or *www.petpoisonhelpline.com*.
- Besides having a pet, there are lots of ways to get involved with the animals in your community. Begin by asking at your local humane society, or visit *www.aspca.org*.

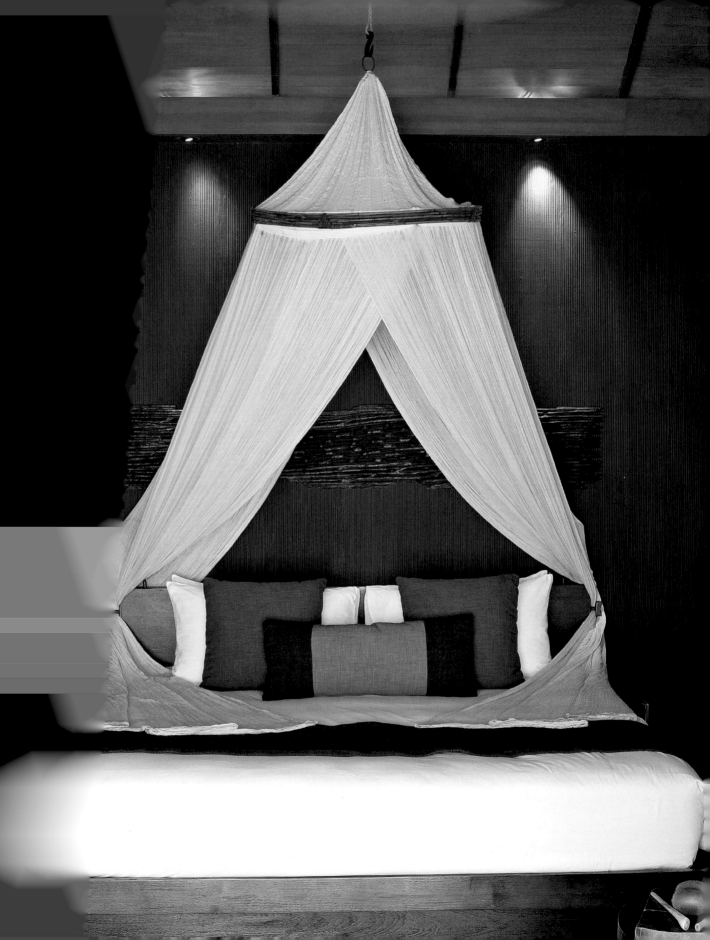

Get More & Better Sleep

15 SECRETS TO SUCCESSFUL SNOOZING

Sleep is like the dimmer switch to good health and longevity. While you sleep, heart rate slows and blood pressure relaxes to the lowest point of the day. A good night's sleep is essential to mental concentration, memory recall, and the repair of cell damage that took place during the day. Conversely, when you toss and turn in fits of interrupted sleep, your heart gets no downtime. Just one less hour of sleep at night can reduce daytime alertness by 35 percent. Continual lack of sleep is associated with a laundry list of health disorders including heart attack, obesity, diabetes, depression, and stroke.

Poor sleep quality can strain relationships and increase the risk of occupational and automobile accidents. It can also wreck your libido.

Although you may think that spending a third of your life sleeping is a waste of time, consider that it's the only way for you to truly enjoy your waking hours. So give sleep the respect it deserves. The following are things you can do to enhance the quality of your sleep so you will sleep like a baby through the night.

▶ | GOOD SLEEP

Sleep should not be considered a luxury. It is an important component of vital living. Though the number of hours required for a person to get restorative sleep differs from person to person, most sleep experts say we need a solid eight hours a night. Most Americans fall short of this by an hour or two. Kids aren't getting enough sleep either. Children between the ages of 7 and 12 should get 10 to 11 hours a night, and teens need 9 to 9½ hours.

Bad sleep—the inability to fall asleep at night or to sleep without interruption—takes a toll. It not only affects the ability to mentally respond; it taxes the heart. One study that followed more than 70,000 women between the ages of 45 and 65 found that those who routinely slept for eight hours or less had an increased risk of heart attack or heart-related death. At the greatest risk were those who slept five hours a night or less.

Tuck In Your Spirit

- **Lights Out** When it's time for bed, draw the blinds or drapes. Your body's built-in sleep cycle is largely controlled by the amount of light and darkness you are exposed to during the day. A darkened bedroom allows levels of the hormone melatonin to rise and facilitates sleep.
- **Skip the Stimulants in the P.M.** Avoid food, caffeine, and alcohol within a few hours of bedtime.
- **Exercise Early** One study found that people who exercise in the morning have less trouble getting to sleep at night. Don't engage in a vigorous workout just before you go to bed.
- **Get Into Position** The best sleeping positions are on your side or back, using a contoured pillow, which is thicker along the sides than in the center, to support your neck and keep your head and spine aligned. Avoid sleeping on your stomach,

which arches and strains the lower back and stretches the neck.

- **Don't Depend on Your Alarm Clock** You'll feel your best if you let your body wake you up naturally. That is what should happen when you get into the rhythm of your correct sleep cycle.

- **Cool Air Means Better Sleep** Keep the temperature in your bedroom low. Studies suggest that the best temperature for sleep is from 60°F to 68°F if you have blankets to snuggle or nestle under. Temperatures in this range help decrease core body temperature that, in turn, initiates sleepiness. But if you don't have blankets to keep you

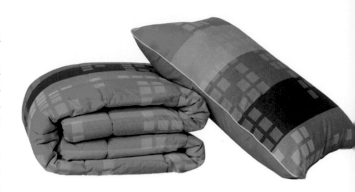

snug and comfortable in the cool air, then a slightly warmer temperature is better. You don't thermoregulate very well during sleep.

▶ | PAMPER YOURSELF

Don't short yourself when it comes to bedtime pampering. Set up a nighttime ritual that will ease you into relaxation. Take off your clothes and slip into a comfortable robe before heading for the bathroom to get ready for the night. Brush and floss. Wash and exfoliate. The following are some other ways to optimize the sleep experience.

Making Sleep the Place to Be

- **Take the Perfect Bath** An ideal way to unwind for sleep after a stressful day is with a desensitizing bath—in body temperature water (around 98°F) in complete darkness. You'll sense neither warmth nor cold, just sensory relief as your frayed nerves are soothed.

- **Optimize Your Bedroom for Sleep** The bedroom should be preserved as a place for sleeping and making love. This means it should be free of television sets, computers, sewing machines, gadgetry, bold blinking alarm clocks, and other distractions.

- **Wind Down** Give yourself some time in bed to do what you like to do—write in your journal, read magazines, even daydream. If you read before sleep, keep books or magazines

---

THE DANGERS OF SLEEP DEPRIVATION

Although most adults need an average of eight hours of sleep a night, surveys show that more than a third of Americans sleep fewer than seven hours a night. About 40 percent fail to get a good night's sleep on weekdays.

Like Scrooge tallying his shillings, your brain keeps track of your sleep and pressures you to pay back your debt. Let's say you shortchange your sleep an hour each night. By week's end, you're down nearly a full night's sleep. Daytime sleepiness mounts. Attention, concentration, alertness, and reaction times wane. Accidents happen. Mood sours.

Chronic sleep deprivation is serious. It depresses immune function and raises the risk of overweight, cardiovascular disease, and diabetes. Sadly, most people don't understand that their chronic malaise has a simple cure: more sleep. If you often have trouble sleeping, consult your health practitioner.

–Linda B. White, M.D.
Educator and author

---

good to know: ABOUT SLEEPLESSNESS

Lack of sleep can make you hungry. A study of 1,000 men and women found that those who slept poorly had increased levels of ghrelin, a hormone that increases feelings of hunger, and decreased levels of leptin, a hormone that helps suppress appetite. The researchers concluded that less than eight hours of sleep a night can contribute to a weight problem.

on your nightstand and a lamp close enough, so you only have to reach up to turn it off.

▶ | CAN'T SLEEP

It's one minute past midnight and your teenager has yet to "sneak" into the house. You lie awake and wait. The ten-hour flight from Cairo has left your body exhausted and your eyes wide open. Sleep is impossible. The crossword puzzle has your brain scrambling for a six-letter word for *altogether* that begins with an *i* and ends with an *o*. Sleep doesn't come until four hours later, after you get in toto.

Everyone experiences a sleepless night every now and then—and the dragged-out feeling the next day. When the sandman is eluding you, try these tactics.

WHEN TO CALL THE DR.: Chronic insomnia can have serious consequences, including psychological disturbances. If you have trouble falling asleep or can't sleep through the night for a month or so, it's time to discuss the problem with your doctor.

Eyes Wide Open

- *Sweeten Your Dreams With Lavender* The essential oil lavender is well known for its ability to bring sleep, and studies prove it. It can even help with insomnia (see pages 100–101).
- *Calm Your Mind* If worry or another emotion has you tossing and turning, calm yourself by focusing on counting slowly backward from 100.

- *Try a Glass of Warm Milk* This old wives' tale works for millions of fans, including many doctors (but avoid if you are lactose intolerant). Why it works is a matter of debate but the leading theory gives the credit to the sleep-inducing amino acid tryptophan, which is found in warm milk.

- *Snack on Nuts or Seeds* A number of seeds and nuts give you a boost of serotonin, a brain chemical that calms anxiety. Walnuts are perhaps the best nut to munch on for an added shot of serotonin. According to well-known medical botanist James Duke, many varieties of seeds and nuts contain tryptophan, an amino acid that the brain converts to serotonin. Other excellent sources of tryptophan include roasted pumpkin seeds and dry sunflower seeds. They provide a simple way to relieve mild insomnia.

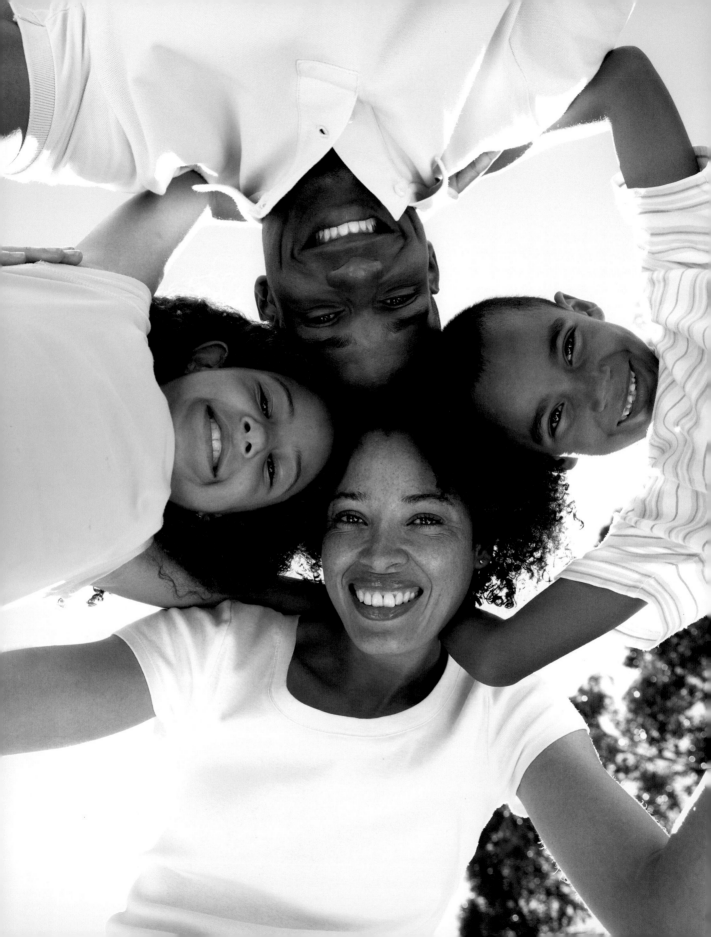

Have a Life Plan

16 STEPS TO SHARPENING YOUR FOCUS

When it comes to remembering the most satisfying moments of life, our memories tend to be unreliable. Research shows that we can recall the high points and low points, but not the minutiae in between. We tend to underrate some of the more subtle pleasures of life, like hanging out with friends, and overrate more fleeting moments, like buying a boat or some other materialistic pleasure. Then there's the distracting nature of modern living. Each day the average American is bombarded with 250 marketing messages encouraging us to eat the things that are bad for us and buy a lot of things we don't really need.

Studies show modern technology has us spending more time in front of a computer or television screen than interacting with people, and texting or sending emails rather than actually talking to one another. And to what end? The United States wasn't even on the list when it came to finding a country full of people who feel the most contented and fulfilled (though we do have pockets of happy places).

▶ | ART OF LIVING

When was the last time you assessed your life plan? Is your life's compass headed in the right direction? Are the things you have to show for your life what really matter to you? Do you even *have* a plan? To help you figure out the true art of living, let's take a look at the things happy people find to be most important in life.

Shaping a Life to Love

■ ***Create a Personal Mission Statement*** What's your reason for getting up in the morning? Richard Leider, author of the book *The Power of Purpose*, suggests taking a personal inventory by using the equation G+P+V=C. Are you using your Gifts—what

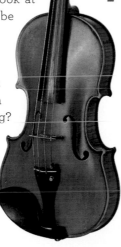

you have to offer the world—on something you feel Passionate about in an environment that Values you? If so, says Leider, you have your Calling.

■ ***Do the Kind of Work You Love*** A large part of our waking hours are spent on the job. The world's happiest people choose a profession steered by their passion, not by how much it pays or whom it will impress. The payoff is big in terms of personal satisfaction when you do work that you love.

■ ***Take an Interest in the Arts*** Researchers in Germany found a direct correlation between community funding of the arts and the well-being of its citizens. People who thrive have access to the arts—museums, theaters, orchestras, concert halls, and other cultural venues.

■ ***Write Your Story*** Taking some time to write down thoughts, memories, reflections can be an important step toward crafting your own life plan. It can take the form of a journal, in which you write every day—morning, afternoon, or night, reflecting on events of the day. Copy down quotations from books or articles you read that especially mean something to you. Keep your journal by your bed and write down your dreams when you wake up in the morning. Another way of writing your story is to take important events in your life, even your whole life story, and begin writing them down. Break the nervousness over writing by simply sitting down at the computer or with pen and notebook at a certain time every day and keep the words flowing. You don't even have to think about sharing what you write with anyone else—but maybe someday, you and they will both be glad you did.

▶ | START AT HOME

Do you lock your doors at night because you're afraid? People in the world who thrive the most are content with their surroundings. They know and trust their neighbors and community so much they don't feel a need to lock their doors at night. This doesn't mean you shouldn't lock *your* doors at night. Just consider if it's possible that you could leave them unlocked. The most valued secret to happiness isn't income; it is where you live.

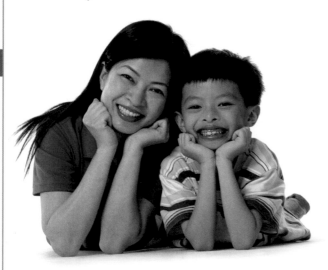

Valuing the Family

- **Rules to Live By** Sit down with your family and invite each member to write down what they consider to be their most important family values, suggests Dr. Robert Melillo in his book *Reconnected Kids*. Share and discuss them and jointly come up with the list by which your family can agree to live. Post them in a prominent place so everyone can be reminded of them daily.
- **Limit Your Work Week** Studies show that once a family income rises to $60,000, making more money does not necessarily bring more happiness. In fact, those who work long hours have less time for the family and social interactions, educational and cultural activities, sports, and volunteer work that make life worthwhile. Workaholics are also more likely to suffer chronic diseases. Don't make more work the goal of your new life plan.

▶ | INVEST IN HAPPY

Research shows we get greater happiness by giving to others to make them happy rather than spending on ourselves. To this end, economist Richard Thaler and former law professor Cass R. Sunstein, authors of the book *Nudge,* propose creating a "giving account"— say $1,000—at the beginning of each year and mentally commit to give it to a favorite charity at the end of the year. Should an emergency expense come up during the year, you have something to fall back on to soften the blow of an unplanned expense.

good to know: ABOUT WHERE YOU LIVE

— The book *Thrive* names Boulder, Colorado, as one of the happiest places in America to live. Much of the credit, according to the town fathers, goes to the preservation of open spaces for parks and recreational activities. Research shows that people are more active in cities that build sidewalks, add bike lanes, and create a feeling of safety.

— Studies show that people are adaptable to weather, but they don't adapt well to noise. In other words, neighborhoods near buzzing highways, airports, and noisy venues erode contentment.

— San Luis Obispo, California, banned drive-through restaurants in the 1980s. Why does that matter? Turns out the plan discouraged a car culture, encouraged walking and socializing, and also encouraged more healthy food choices.

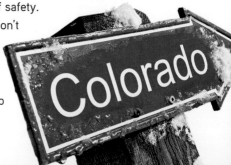

Money Can't Buy You Love

- *Give Back* Volunteer work benefits your community and society in general. It also gives you a sense of self-worth and satisfaction. It pays off in other ways as well. Research shows that people who donate time as a volunteer weigh less, feel healthier, have a lower risk of getting a heart attack, and score higher in every aspect that measures happiness.

- *Depend on One Credit Card* There is nothing that can trash your life's plan like a pile of debt. Limit yourself to one credit card and don't spend what you don't have, meaning you should be able to pay off the balance each month.

- *Invest Your Money in Experiences* Where does your disposable income go? Research shows that you'll get a longer-lasting sense of self-worth by spending it on experiences—ongoing education, taking the family to Disney World or Europe, learning how to play an instrument, taking up painting—than on material things, like a new car or a fur coat.

- *It Pays to Pay Off* Though your accountant may not agree, it feels a lot better knowing you have a house paid off than it does getting an interest deduction on your income taxes. The average American household has about $70,000 in mortgage debt. By making just one extra payment at the end of the year you can save thousands of dollars in interest and pay off your house around 10 years earlier on a typical 30-year mortgage, or around 5 years earlier on a 15-year mortgage.

▶ | THRIVE CENTERS

As Dan Buettner writes in *Thrive*, his research on the world's happiest people led him to recognize that even the environments they live in are constantly providing inducements to finding satisfaction in doing the right thing. Buettner identifies six life domains that you, too, can shape more deliberately in order to find your way to greater happiness. He calls these six domains "Thrive Centers." Here's a checklist of questions to ask yourself, spurring you on to shaping a healthy life plan.

Think Through Thrive Centers

- *Carve Out a Community* You may not be able to move, but you can help your community find ways to reshape itself. Support the arts. Encourage walking and bicycling. Use community spaces well.

- *Work on Work* Finding work that is important, fulfilling, and enjoyable is key—and, once you have, don't let it take over the rest of your life.

- *Sweeten Your Social Life* Okinawans, among the world's happiest people, create *moais*—groups of mutually committed friends—who enjoy activities together. Your moai might be a book group or a bird-watching club or a church choir. Belonging to a small group of people who know you through many ups and downs is key.

- *Discipline Dollars* Save mindlessly; spend thoughtfully—those are the rules by which the world's happiest people deal with their financial demands.

- *Happy Up Your Home* Find ways to enliven your home—a new pet, a new houseplant, or new flowers planted in your garden. The care and devotion required from you will give back many fold.

- *Find Your Passion* None of these pieces of advice is easy to follow. All amount to developing a personal sense of meaning and mission. Find that, focus on it, and don't forget it.

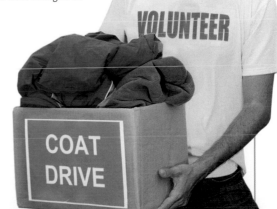

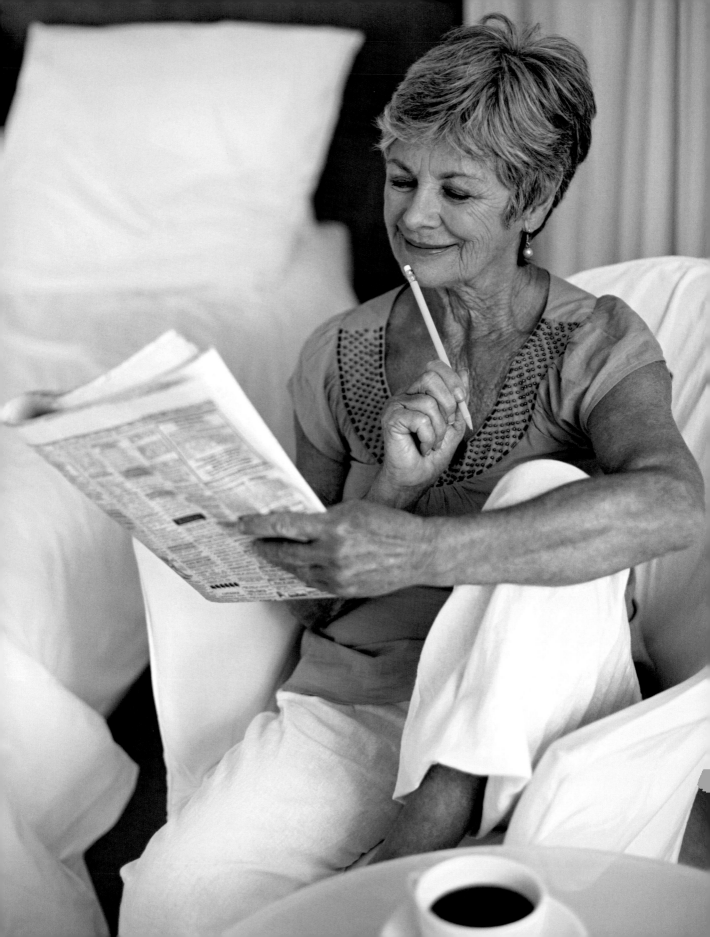

Improve Memory

14 WAYS TO JOG YOUR NOGGIN

Who were the Democratic and Republican candidates for U.S. president in 1984? If you can't remember in the time it would take to hit the buzzer in the TV quiz show *Jeopardy*, there's a good reason why. Your brain is getting old. In fact, it started aging around the time you cast your first presidential vote! By the time you reach your early 20s, the brain is already showing signs of change. These changes weaken memory, creating what some oldsters call "senior moments." You climb the stairs and before you get to the top, you already forgot what you went up there to get.

The word you want is on the tip of your tongue, but you just can't find it. You walk from room to room looking for your glasses that are sitting on top of your head. By age 50, nearly 50 percent of people complain about this type of age-related memory problem.

The brain is the organ of longevity, so you don't want to lose it. An agile body isn't going to do you much good if you don't have an agile mind to tell it what to do. But here's the good news: Studies show that about 65 percent of memory-zapping aging can be blamed on lifestyle, meaning you can do plenty of things to prevent it.

Before we tell what they are, you still might be stumped on the 1984 election question. The answer: Ronald Reagan and Walter Mondale. If you don't recall who won, you better keep on reading.

▶ | MEMORY AIDS

How much time do you think the average person spends over a lifetime looking for misplaced objects? By some estimates, a year—or more. Who needs that much aggravation in life! Try these memory-jogging tricks instead.

Cheat Sheet

- *Make Lists* Short-term memory is often fleeting because of limited brain capacity. It's amazing how much information you can sock away in your memory bank over the decades!

So, save some space and make lists. It'll free up your mind for remembering more important things.

- *Put Faces in Places* If you have difficulty remembering names, use your mind's eye to make an association between something physical about the person and his name. If you notice Chuck Kaminski laughs a lot, think *chuckles*. Or, if he has an upturned nose, think, *came in to ski*.

- *Click Your Parking Place* You're parked on level C, but you thought you parked on level B, where you're now roaming around looking for your vehicle—and you've found five that look like yours. Don't get yourself in such a pickle. When you get out of your car in a parking garage, get out your smart phone and click a photo that identifies your parking spot. Or write down the location on a piece of paper. Make it a habit.

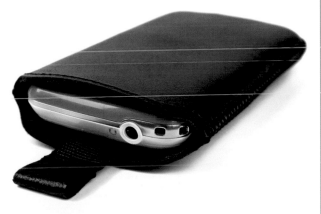

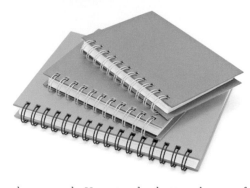

■ ***Chunk It*** Can't remember your bank account number or the router number on a missing package? That's understandable, because a series of numbers, say 2024561414, is hard to remember. Chunking them, like you do the many phone numbers you know off the top of your head, makes it possible, as in 202-456-1414. By the way, that's the telephone number for the White House.

▶ | TRAIN YOUR BRAIN

You don't have to be rounding the corner into your fifth, sixth, or seventh decade to need a little help remembering things sometimes. No matter what your age, you can pick up memory-enhancing habits that will help you into your later years.

Tricks of the Memory Trade

■ ***Make Up Your Own Acronym*** Okay, so you forgot the list. Now what? If you can't depend on yourself to remember your lists, there is a backup: acronyms. Let's say you have to go to the store to get milk, onions, nectarines, eggs, and yams. As an acronym, it's MONEY.

■ ***Repeat and Repeat*** Names are hard to remember, especially when you're meeting a lot of people at times when it's *really* important to remember, such as when you're at a meeting or moving into a new neighborhood. We're always told to repeat a person's name when introduced: Chuck says "Hi, I'm Chuck" and you say "Hi, Chuck, I'm Al." However, that doesn't always work. You stand a better chance of remembering by repeating the person's name in the initial course of conversation: "So, Chuck, what do you think of that merger?" And even again, "It was nice meeting you, Chuck." The more you can keep that name on the tip of the tongue, the more likely you'll be able to say, "Excuse me, Chuck," when you bump into him in the hallway.

▶ | MENTAL DECLINE

Dementia is a functional form of mental decline that is much more problematic than a really bad memory. People with dementia have impaired intellectual capacity, which makes it difficult for them to make decisions and think logically. People with dementia can seemingly go through a personality change. They also experience confusion and disorientation more and more frequently. Alzheimer's disease is the most common form of dementia, though there are several types.

No matter your age today, you can start right away with certain mental practices that will help you through to the end of your life by keeping your brain more nimble, sharp, and focused. All these practices have present-day rewards as well as the benefits they provide in longevity.

good to know: ABOUT MEMORY LAPSES

— Though vexing, memory glitches are natural, but the severe memory impairment known as dementia is not. Yet, one in seven Americans over the age of 70 suffers from a dementia severe enough to impact quality of life.

— Research in Portugal found that older people who drink several cups of coffee a day were less likely to experience lapses in memory than people who just drank one cup.

Forever Young

- **Practice Stress Reduction** Chronic stress releases hormones that can wear and tear on the brain. If you're under a lot of stress, practice the techniques recommended in this chapter on pages 317–318.

- **Do Puzzling Things** One well-known study, known as the Nun Study, found that those with the most education and language abilities were less likely to develop Alzheimer's disease. It's not schooling that counts the most, say the researchers, but how much time you actively spend challenging your brain. So put your brain through the hurdles with such things as trivia games, crossword puzzles, card games, and so on.

- **Take on a Challenge** You'll stimulate your mind as well as your personal satisfaction by continually challenging your abilities. For example, learn to play chess, take up playing an instrument, learn a new language, or take up sailing or ballroom dancing. If there's something you've always wanted to do, then do it. At first, these activities will feel novel and complex, just what your mind needs. When they start to feel as comfortable as an old pair of shoes, it's time to move on to a newer challenge.

▶ | BRAIN & BODY

Dementia is not reversible. If you have genes that put you at risk, you cannot entirely avoid it. But there are things you can do. Add a few practices to your life that represent exercise and valuable pampering to your brain cells. They'll thank you for it.

- **Sip a Cup of Cocoa** One small study found that sipping a cup of cocoa can help protect mental acuity by improving blood flow to the brain. In the study, 16 people drank a cup of the chocolate drink and then performed a mental task while researchers watched the activity in their brains on an MRI. The beverage caused a noticeable spike in blood flow in the brain. This is likely due to cocoa's rich content of antioxidant flavonols.

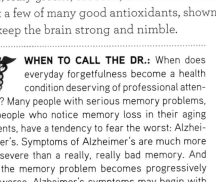

- **Consider a Supplement** Though research is inconsistent, Germany's Commission E, which tracks responsible research on herbs, stands behind ginkgo biloba as an effective remedy to slow the progression of dementia. Promising research also has begun to be published on the herb bacopa (*Bacopa monnieri*) as an aid to enhancing mental function and memory (see page 113).

- **Think B for the Brain** B vitamins—niacin, thiamin, B_6, and B_{12}—are important to the brain because they help repair brain tissue. Foods rich in these nutrients include bananas, chicken, nuts, turkey, wheat germ, and whole grains.

- **Watch Your Sugar** Simple carbohydrates, such as sugar and white flour, lead to diabetes, and diabetes slows circulation in the brain.

- **Eat Fruits and Vegetables** Apples and cherries, leafy greens, broccoli, and tomatoes are just a few of many good antioxidants, shown to keep the brain strong and nimble.

WHEN TO CALL THE DR.: When does everyday forgetfulness become a health condition deserving of professional attention? Many people with serious memory problems, or people who notice memory loss in their aging parents, have a tendency to fear the worst: Alzheimer's. Symptoms of Alzheimer's are much more severe than a really, really bad memory. And the memory problem becomes progressively worse. Alzheimer's symptoms may begin with not being able to find where the car is parked at the mall. But as the disease progresses, an Alzheimer's sufferer might forget that he drove and take the bus home, leaving the car at the mall. If you suspect a loved one is experiencing dementia—and especially if you fear that memory problems are causing safety concerns—set up a medical appointment for an evaluation.

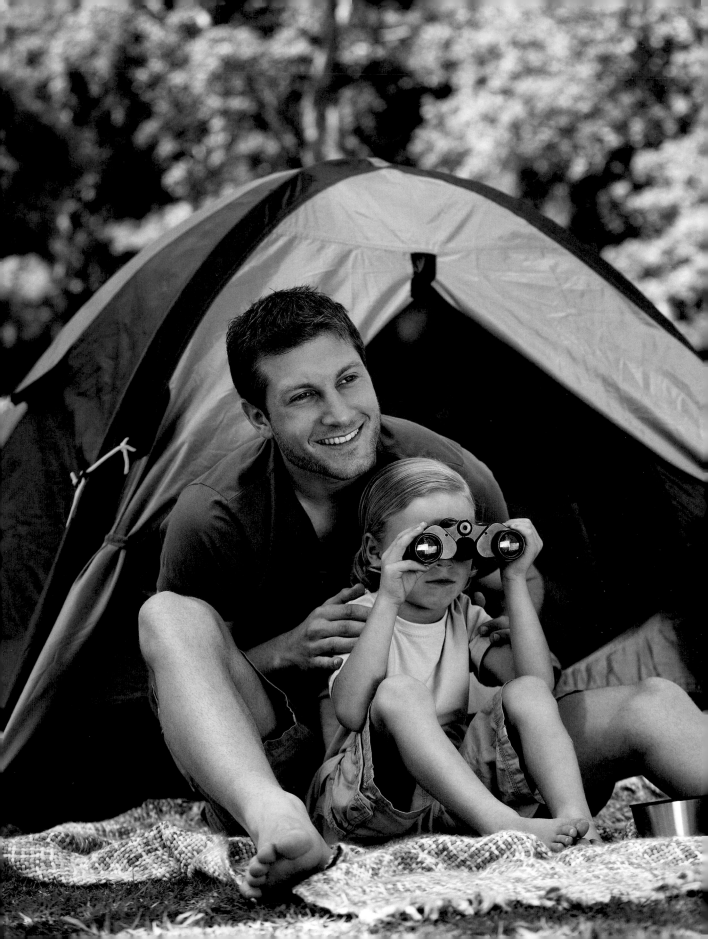

Learn New Skills

12 PLANS FOR NEWFOUND PLEASURES

At one time, scientists thought the prime time for learning something new was during childhood, when the brain is growing and forming. They thought the brain was like a hardwired machine, much like a computer, and that the brain we nourished from birth to early adulthood—primarily the years of formal education—formed our mental capacity for our lifetime. Scientists now know that this is not the case. The relatively new science of neuroplasticity shows that the brain is actually highly malleable. Though the brain maintains its basic conformation, nerves within the brain change, branch out, and make new connections (or disconnections). This new research is proof that learning something new is possible at any age.

▶ USE IT OR LOSE IT

When it comes to slowing down the aging process, studies show that staying mentally active is equally as important as physical fitness, a healthy diet, and stress reduction.

The Time Is Now

- **Stop Dreaming and Start Doing** Einstein didn't become a, well, Einstein until after he did poorly in college, failed to get into graduate school, and took a job as a clerk in a patent office. What he did was keep his mind stimulated. What others may have thought was eccentricity was actually the electricity of synaptic activity in the brain. At Einstein's death, an autopsy found that Einstein's brain was no bigger than average. It also had an average number of brain cells. However, his brain contained an enormous number of synapses.

- **Stay in Touch With Your Senses** Our senses are the primary driver of mental stimulation. Light, sound, touch, taste, smell, and also gravity send stimulation from the ends of sensory nerves in the skin, ears, eyes, and other organs, through the brain stem, and into the brain itself. People who say they feel more mentally vibrant after a beach vacation are not imagining it. Think of the powerful stimulation you can get just from a walk on the beach—the sound of crashing waves, the scent of sea air, the sensation of toes sinking in the sand, the warmth of the sun and touch of the sea breeze on your face. It's wonderful sensory overload.

- **Go on a Mental Adventure** Keep your mind stimulated by drawing on some of your dreams. If you've always dreamed of sailing around the world, take the initial steps and take sailing lessons. If you already know how to sail, then use your mental muscle to actually plan how such a trip would unfold. Do you wish you could dance as well as the professionals on *Dancing With the Stars*? Stop wishing and sign up for classes in ballroom dancing.

- **Learn a Little About a Lot** How often have you asked yourself, *I wonder why…?* or *I wonder how …?* A great way to exercise your brain is to exercise your curiosity. If you've always wondered what it's like to fly an airplane, find a place where you can have the experience through

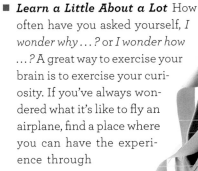

a flight simulator. Interested in the stars? Buy a telescope and take up amateur astronomy. If you enjoy feeding birds in your backyard bird feeder, take it one step further and join a bird-watching club.

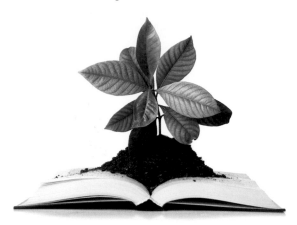

▶ BRAIN POWER

The brain continues to develop way beyond adolescence; it continues to have the ability to change and form new synapses throughout life. It's your challenge to keep it changing and growing as you age.

As one of many examples of the "use it or lose it" axiom, stimulation strengthens networks or nerves; disuse weakens them. In other words, your brain has a certain amount of plasticity. What's important is not so much how many cells you have in your noggin, but how well they're connected. Repeated stimulation causes brain cells to branch out and connect to their neighbors. It's why practice, practice, practice is the mantra of learning. World-famous cellist Yo-Yo Ma didn't play the Bach cello suites flawlessly his first time through.

A bit of struggle is good for your brain. At first, your new smart phone baffles you. Just when you're convinced the device is smarter than you, you're texting, emailing, and photographing like mad. You sweat for hours over a math problem. Then the ah-ha! moment arrives. Presto, you've made new neural connections. Learning is not just kids' stuff. It's never too late to develop new talents.

Forms of Engagement

- **_Limit TV Time in Your Household_** Too much TV is bad for the brain. Studies have found that activity in the brain slows down when watching TV. The American Academy of Pediatrics recommends that children under the age of two should not watch any TV at all. Studies show that every hour a day a preschooler spends watching television increases the child's risk of getting attention deficit/hyperactive disorder (ADHD) later in life by 10 percent.

- **_Get in the Flow_** Mastering a new challenge requires that you immerse fully in what you are doing, what experts call flow. Flow is concentration so strong that you can block out all sensory activity occurring around you. With flow, planes passing overhead, horns honking, or children screaming in play under your open window don't even exist. Your ability to achieve anything that requires a high degree of skill—playing an instrument, building a model plane, painting a landscape, or writing a book—is optimized when you can get into a state of flow.

- **_Take Up a Pursuit You Love_** We should all have a hobby that enhances our work. In Denmark, one of the happiest nations on Earth, 95 percent of its citizens belong to a club, be it for playing canasta, building model boats, or racing model airplanes. Some Danes are so invested in their hobbies, they'll even knock off work early in order not to miss out. Hobbies are important, says Buettner, because they offer another dimension in life that caters to our interests. It helps us get in a state of flow and heightens our happiness quotient.

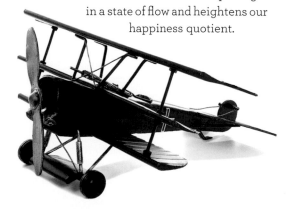

THE MODERN PORTAL TO ANCIENT KNOWLEDGE

Once relegated to special rooms of major libraries, rare books by the thousands are now accessible online. Google offers public domain herb, health, and medicine-related titles. Just go to the Books panel on Google, type in a title or author, and more often than not, there it is. If the book is in the public domain, you can download a pdf or e-pub format of the entire book or simply read it online. Hundreds of free e-book titles are also available from the Project Gutenberg (*www.gutenberg.org*). The Biodiversity Heritage Library (*www.biodiversitylibrary.org*) includes 50,000 titles. Many rare books, some centuries old, are now just a click away.

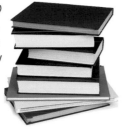

–Steven Foster
Herbalist and lecturer

▶ | HAVE FUN

Who says fun and games are just for kids? Interacting with others has big benefits— not just in building friendships, but also in building mental longevity. Studies show that socially active people are less likely to suffer from cognitive decline than people who prefer to be alone. Researchers believe this is likely due to the soothing effects of endorphins and serotonin, brain chemicals that are secreted when people are enjoying the company of others. This, in turn, reduces levels of the hormone cortisol, which has been linked to deterioration in the part of the brain that stores memory.

Never Too Young for Fun and Games

- **Work Out With Others** By that we mean share your brain workout with friends by finding games and puzzles you can enjoy together. Strategy games, such as chess, Scrabble, checkers, bridge, Monopoly, and any number of other board games, card games, and puzzles, will keep you both mentally and socially engaged.

- **Join a Game Online** If you're short on partners, there's a virtual world of competitors online. Researchers at the University of Michigan found that people who engaged in computer-based brain-training exercises for about 30 minutes daily increased their ability to reason and problem solve. Check out Luminosity.com, a research-based brain training site with exercises that are valuable—and fun,

- **Play "Neurobics"** Help your brain form new synapses with mind games that trick the brain. The basic idea is to take something you do every day without thinking— say brushing your teeth in front of the bathroom mirror— and do it in an unfamiliar way, say using the opposite hand and brush with your eyes closed. For example, if you drive the same route to the grocery store, go a new way. If you eat the same breakfast every day, challenge yourself to come up with something different every day for a week. Whatever new habits you form, disrupt the pattern to learn a new way of doing it.

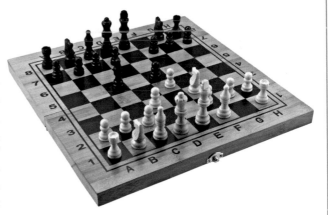

- **Shameless Crosswords** While once you may have considered crossword puzzles or Sudoku a waste of time, go ahead, indulge—these are the sorts of brain games that keep you thinking. If you have one type you've been doing for a while, try another. Most newspapers and many magazines include brain teasers or puzzles in every issue.

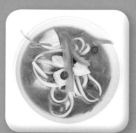
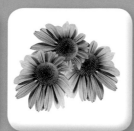
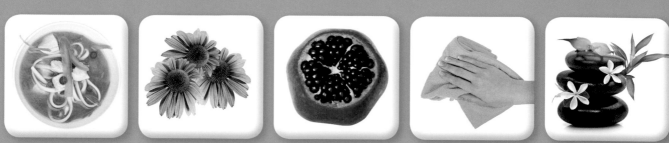
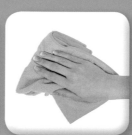
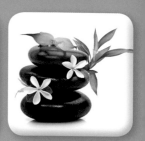

more on r

emedies

Further Reading

General

1,081 Home Remedies: Trustworthy Treatments for Everyday Health Problems. Editors of *Reader's Digest.* Reader's Digest Association, Inc., 2004.

Der Marderosian, Ara. *Folk Remedies, Healing Wisdom.* Publications International, Ltd., 1999.

The Doctors Book of Home Remedies: Quick Fixes, Clever Techniques, and Uncommon Cures To Get You Feeling Better Fast. Editors of *Prevention.* Rodale Books, 2010.

Evans, Mark. *Yoga, Tai Chi, Massage, Therapies & Healing Remedies: Natural Ways to Health, Relaxation, and Vitality: A Complete Practical Guide.* Hermes House, 2003.

Gaby, Alan R., ed. *The Natural Pharmacy Revised and Updated 3rd Edition: Complete A–Z Reference to Natural Treatments for Common Health Conditions.* Three Rivers Press, 2006.

Gottlieb, Bill. *Alternative Cures: The Most Effective Natural Remedies for 160 Health Problems.* Rodale, 2000.

Gottlieb, Bill, ed. *New Choices in Natural Healing: Over 1,800 of the Best Self-Help Remedies from the World of Alternative Medicine.* Rodale Press, 1995.

Hardy, Mary L., and Debra L. Gordon. *Reader's Digest Best Remedies: Breakthrough Prescriptions That Blend Conventional and Natural Medicine.* Reader's Digest Association, Inc., 2006.

Lad, Vasant. *The Complete Book of Ayurvedic Home Remedies.* Three Rivers Press, 1998.

Reader's Digest Food Cures: Fight Disease With Your Fork! Editors of *Reader's Digest.* Reader's Digest Association, Inc., 2007.

White, Linda B., and Steven Foster. *The Herbal Drugstore: The Best Natural Alternatives to Over-the-Counter and Prescription Medicines!* Rodale, 2000.

Worwood, Valerie Ann. *The Complete Book of Essential Oils and Aromatherapy: Over 600 Natural, Non-Toxic and Fragrant Recipes to Create Health, Beauty, a Safe Home Environment.* New World Library, 1991.

Yeager, Selene, and Editors of *Prevention. The Doctors Book of Food Remedies: The Latest Findings on the Power of Food to Treat and Prevent Health Problems—From Aging and Diabetes to Ulcers and Yeast Infections.* Rodale, 1998.

Chapter 1

Home Remedies on Hand

Dunne, Lavon J. *Nutrition Almanac.* 5th ed. McGraw-Hill, 2002.

Faelten, Sharon. *The Doctors Book of Home Remedies for Women: Women Doctors Reveal 2,000 Self-Help Tips on the Health Problems That Concern Women the Most.* Rodale Press, 1997.

Graedon, Joe, and Terry Graedon. *Favorite Home Remedies from The People's Pharmacy.* Graedon Enterprises, Inc., 2008.

Graedon, Joe, and Terry Graedon. *The People's Pharmacy Quick and Handy Home Remedies: Q&As for Your Common Ailments.* National Geographic, 2011.

Mars, Brigitte, and Chrystle Fiedler. *The Country Almanac of Home Remedies: Time-Tested & Almost Forgotten Wisdom for Treating Hundreds of Common Ailments, Aches & Pains Quickly and Naturally.* Fair Winds Press, 2011.

Mayo Clinic Home Remedies: 230 Treatments and Cures. Time Home Entertainment, 2010.

Murray, Michael, and Joseph Pizzorno. *Encyclopedia of Natural Medicine.* 2nd ed. Three Rivers Press, 1997.

Paragon staff. *The New Guide to Remedies.* Paragon Publishing, 2002.

White, Linda B., and Sunny Mavor, A.H.G. *Kids, Herbs, and Health.* Interweave Press, 1998.

Chapter 2

Herbs for Healing

Blumenthal, Mark. *The ABC Clinical Guide to Herbs.* American Botanical Council, 2003.

Chevallier, Andrew. *DK Natural Health Encyclopedia of Herbal Medicine: The Definitive*

Home Reference Guide to 550 Key Herbs With All Their Uses as Remedies for Common Ailments. 2nd ed. DK Adult, 2000.

Foster, Steven, and James A. Duke. Field Guide to Medicinal Plants: Eastern and Central North America. Houghton Mifflin, 2000.

Foster, Steven, and Rebecca L. Johnson. National Geographic Desk Reference to Nature's Medicine. National Geographic Society, 2006.

Foster, Steven, and Varro Tyler. Tyler's Honest Herbal. 4th ed. Haworth Press, 1999.

Gladstar, Rosemary. Rosemary Gladstar's Herbal Recipes for Vibrant Health: 175 Teas, Tonics, Oils, Salves, Tinctures, and Other Natural Remedies for the Entire Family. Storey Publishing, 2008.

Hobbs, Christopher, and Kathi Keville. Women's Herbs, Women's Health. Botanica Press, 2007.

Johnson, Rebecca L., Steven Foster, Tieraona Low Dog, and David Kiefer. National Geographic Guide to Medicinal Herbs: The World's Most Effective Healing Plants. National Geographic Society, 2010.

Richardson-Gerson, Rosamond. The Little Herb Book. Piatkus Books, 1988.

Chapter 3
Foods for Health

Berthold-Bond, Annie. Better Basics for the Home: Simple Solutions for Less Toxic Living. Three Rivers Press, 1999.

Bond, Annie B., Melissa Breyer, and Wendy Gordon. True Food: Eight Simple Steps to a Healthier You. National Geographic Society, 2009.

Edible: An Illustrated Guide to the World's Food Plants. National Geographic Society, 2008.

Graedon, Joe, and Terry Graedon. Favorite Foods from The People's Pharmacy: Mother Nature's Medicine. Graedon Enterprises, Inc., 2009.

Jaret, Peter. Heart Healthy for Life: The Ultimate Guide To Preventing and Reversing Heart Disease. Reader's Digest Association, Inc., 2002.

Seaver, Barton. For Cod and Country: Simple, Delicious, Sustainable Cooking. Sterling Epicure, 2011.

Chapter 4
Clean, Safe, & Beautiful

Bond, Annie, B. Home Enlightenment: Create a Nurturing, Healthy, and Toxin-Free Home. Rodale, 2005.

Burnes, Deborah. Look Great, Live Green: Choosing Bodycare Products That Are Safe for You, Safe for the Planet. Hunter House, 2009.

Gabriel, Julie. Green Beauty Recipes: Easy Homemade Recipes To Make Your Own Organic and Natural Skincare, Hair Care and Body Care Products. Petite Marie Ltd., 2010.

Green Guide: The Complete Reference for Consuming Wisely. Editors of Green Guide Magazine. National Geographic Society, 2008.

Green Living: The E Magazine Handbook for Living Lightly on the Earth. Editors of E/The Environmental Magazine. Plume, 2005.

Hunter, Linda Mason, and Mikki Halpin. Green Clean: The Environmentally Sound Guide to Cleaning Your Home. Melcher Media, 2005.

Jeffery, Yvonne, Liz Barclay, Michael Grosvenor, Elizabeth B. Goldsmith, Betsy Sheldon, Eric Corey Freed, Rik DeGunther, Ann Whitman, Owen E. Dell, and The National Gardening Association. Green Your Home All in One for Dummies. For Dummies, 2009.

Khechara, Star. The Holistic Beauty Book: Over 100 Natural Recipes for Gorgeous Healthy Skin. Green Books, 2008.

Nikogosian, Narine. Return to Beauty: Old-World Recipes for Great Radiant Skin. Atria Books, 2009.

Chapter 5
Healing Traditions

Anderson, John W., ed., Larry Trivieri, ed., and Burton Goldberg. Alternative Medicine: The Definitive Guide. 2nd ed. Celestial Arts, 2002.

Calvert, Robert Noah. The History of Massage: An Illustrated Survey From Around the World. Healing Arts Press, 2002.

Damian, Peter, and Kate Damian. Aromatherapy: Scent and Psyche: Using Essential Oils for Physical and Emotional Well-Being. Healing Arts Press, 1995.

Dubitsky, Carl. *Bodywork Shiatsu: Bringing the Art of Finger Pressure to the Massage Table.* Healing Arts Press, 1997.

Keville, Kathi, and Mindy Green. *Aromatherapy: A Complete Guide to the Healing Art.* Crossing Press, 2009.

Leddy, Susan Kun. *Integrative Health Promotion: Conceptual Bases for Nursing Practice.* 2nd ed. Jones & Bartlett Publishers, 2006.

Maizes, Victoria, and Tieraona Low Dog, eds. *Integrative Women's Health.* Oxford University Press, 2010.

Wooten, Heather Green. *The Polio Years in Texas: Battling a Terrifying Unknown.* Texas A&M University Press, 2009.

Chapter 6

A Healthy Lifestyle

Aggarwal, Bharat, with Debora Yost. *Healing Spices: How To Use 50 Everyday and Exotic Spices To Boost Health and Beat Disease.* Sterling, 2011.

Anderson, Douglas M., et al. *Mosby's Medical, Nursing & Allied Health Dictionary.* 6th ed. Mosby, 2002.

Bertin, Mark, M.D. *The Family ADHD Solution: A Scientific Approach To Maximizing Your Child's Attention and Minimizing Parental Stress.* Palgrave MacMillan, 2011.

Bottom Line's Health Breakthroughs 2009. Bottom Line, 2009.

Bottom Line Yearbook 2009. Editors of *Bottom Line Personal.* Boardroom, 2010.

Buettner, Dan. *The Blue Zones: Lessons for Living Longer from the People Who've Lived the Longest.* National Geographic Society, 2008.

Buettner, Dan. *Thrive: Finding Happiness the Blue Zones Way.* National Geographic Society, 2010.

Cooksley, Valerie Gennari, RN. *Aromatherapy: Soothing Remedies to Restore, Rejuvenate and Heal.* Prentice Hall Press, 2002.

De la Cerda, P., et al. "Effect of an Aerobic Training Program as Complementary Therapy in Patients with Moderate Depression." *Perceptual and Motor Skills* (June 2011): 761–69.

Diener, Ed, and Robert Biswas-Diener. *Happiness: Unlocking the Mysteries of Psychological Wealth.* Wiley-Blackwell, 2008.

Doherty, Bridget, Julia VanTine, and *Prevention Health Books for Women. Growing Younger: Breakthrough Age-Defying Secrets.* Rodale Press, 1999.

Fogle, Bruce. *The New Encyclopedia of the Dog.* DK Adult, 2000.

Gottlieb, Bill. *Bottom Line's Breakthroughs in Drug-Free Healing.* Boardroom, 2008.

Growing Younger: Breakthrough Age-Defying Secrets. Women's Edge series. Rodale, 1999.

Heart Disease and Stroke Statistics 2011 Update. American Heart Association, 2011.

Melillo, Robert, Dr. *Disconnected Kids: The Groundbreaking Brain Balance Program for Children With Autism, ADHD, Dyslexia, and Other Neurological Disorders.* Perigee Trade, 2009.

Melillo, Robert, Dr. *Reconnected Kids: Help Your Child Achieve Physical, Mental, and Emotional Balance.* Perigee Trade, 2001.

Trechsel, Jane Goad. *A Morning Cup of Yoga: One 15-Minute Routine for a Lifetime of Health and Wellness.* Sweetwater Press, 2002.

Westgarth, C., et al. "Family Pet Ownership During Childhood." *International Journal of Environmental Research in Public Health* 7(10) (2010): 3704–29.

Yost, Debora. *The Anti-Cancer Food and Supplement Guide: How To Protect Yourself and Enhance Your Health.* St. Martin's Press, 2010.

Yost, Debora. *Heal Your Heart With Wine and Chocolate.* Stuart, Tabori and Chang, 2006.

Index

Illustrations Credits

All images used under license from Shutterstock.com except for the following: 7, Quentin Bacon; 17, Charles B. White; 54, Jose Luis Pelaez Inc/Getty Images; 77, © Steven Foster, Steven Foster Group, Inc.; 82, Mike Kiev/iStockphoto.com; 90, Rice/Buckland/Getty Images; 106, lenka/Bigstock.com; 110, Image Source/Corbis; 118, © Steven Foster, Steven Foster Group, Inc.; 120 (UP), Neil Fletcher and Matthew Ward/Getty Images; 120 (LO), Organics Image Library/Alamy; 121 (UP), Siri Stafford/Getty Images; 126, f.Olby/Getty Images; 129, Photolibrary/Getty Images; 137, Katie Stoops; 189 (UP), Ju-Lee/iStockphoto.com; 197, Teresa Lee; 253, Reed Rhan; 254, George Doyle/Getty Images; 255, amriphoto/iStockphoto.com; 256, Doable/amanaimagesRF/Getty Images; 257 (UP), Courtesy Helmut Breitinger, Travelband International; 262, Dragan Trifunovic/iStockphoto.com; 266, ersler/Bigstock.com; 273 (UP), WPCasey/Bigstock.com; 282, Sharon Smith; 284, Sharon Smith; 285, Qiao Qiming/Xinhua Press/Corbis; 288 (LO), lilly3/iStockphoto.com; 290, Aifos/iStockphoto.com; 292 (LO), Gary Conner/Phototake; 299, josh webb/iStockphoto.com; 307, David McLain; 312, RonTech2000/iStockphoto.com; 325, Daniela Jovanovska-Hristovska/iStockphoto.com; 330 (UP), Lauri Patterson/iStockphoto.com; 348, 4FR/iStockphoto.com.

IMPORTANT NOTE TO READERS:

This book is meant to increase your knowledge about home remedies and recent developments in possible ways to care for your health at home, and to the best of our knowledge the information provided is accurate at the time of its publication. It is not intended as a medical manual, and neither the authors nor the publisher is engaged in rendering medical or other professional advice to the individual reader. The illustrations in this book are for general informational purposes, and they are not intended to be used as guides to identification or instruction. You should not use the information contained in this book as a substitute for the advice of a licensed health care professional. Because everyone is different, we urge you to see a licensed health care professional to diagnose problems and supervise the use of any of these home remedies to treat individual conditions.

The authors, advisers, and publisher disclaim any liability whatsoever with respect to any loss, injury, or damage arising directly or indirectly from the use of this book.

NATIONAL GEOGRAPHIC

COMPLETE GUIDE TO
natural home remedies

Prepared by the Book Division

Hector Sierra, *Senior Vice President and General Manager*
Anne Alexander, *Senior Vice President and Editorial Director*
Jonathan Halling, *Design Director, Books and Children's Publishing*
Marianne R. Koszorus, *Design Director, Books*
Susan Tyler Hitchcock, *Senior Editor*
R. Gary Colbert, *Production Director*
Jennifer A. Thornton, *Director of Managing Editorial*
Susan Blair, *Director of Photography*
Meredith C. Wilcox, *Administrative Director, Illustrations*

Staff for This Book

Barbara H. Seeber, *Text Editor*
Melissa Farris, *Art Director*
Linda Makarov, *Illustrations Editor, Designer*
Rebecca L. Johnson, *Contributing Writer*
Deborah Yost, *Contributing Writer*
Linda B. White, M.D., *Medical Consultant*
Andrew Knauss, *Researcher*
Judith Klein, *Production Editor*
Lisa A. Walker, *Production Manager*
Marshall Kiker, *Illustrations Specialist*

Manufacturing and Quality Management

Christopher A. Liedel, *Chief Financial Officer*
Phillip L. Schlosser, *Senior Vice President*
Chris Brown, *Vice President*
Nicole Elliott, *Manager*
Rachel Faulise, *Manager*
Robert L. Barr, *Manager*

Since 1888, the National Geographic Society has funded more than 13,000 research, exploration, and preservation projects around the world. National Geographic Partners distributes a portion of the funds it receives from your purchase to National Geographic Society to support programs including the conservation of animals and their habitats.

National Geographic Partners
1145 17th Street NW
Washington, DC 20036-4688 USA

Get closer to National Geographic explorers and photographers, and connect with our global community. Join us today at nationalgeographic.com/join

For information about special discounts for bulk purchases, please contact National Geographic Books Special Sales: specialsales@natgeo.com

For rights or permissions inquiries, please contact National Geographic Books Subsidiary Rights: bookrights@natgeo.com

ISBN: 978-1-4262-1260-4 (paperback)
ISBN: 978-1-4262-0943-7 (regular)
ISBN: 978-1-4262-0944-4 (deluxe)
ISBN: 978-1-4262-1867-5 (special sales paperback)
ISBN: 978-1-4262-1869-9 (Canadian special sales edition)
ISBN: 978-1-4262-2110-1 (special sales hardcover)

Printed in China

19/RRDH/1